LLOFACIAL SURGERY SECRETS

A. Omar Abubaker, DMD, PhD

Associate Professor
Department of Oral and Maxillofacial Surgery
School of Dentistry
Division of Oral and Maxillofacial Surgery
Department of Surgery
School of Medicine
Medical College of Virginia
Virginia Commonwealth University
Richmond, Virginia

Kenneth J. Benson, DDS

Private Practice, Oral and Maxillofacial Surgery
Raleigh, North Carolina

HANLEY & BELFUS, INC./Philadelphia

Publisher: HANLEY & BELFUS, INC.
Medical Publishers
210 South 13th Street
Philadelphia, PA 19107
(215) 546-7293; 800-962-1892
FAX (215) 790-9330
Web site: http://www.hanleyandbelfus.com

Note to the reader: Although the information in this book has been carefully reviewed for correctness of dosage and indications, neither the authors nor the editors nor the publisher can accept any legal responsibility for any errors or omissions that may be made. Neither the publisher nor the editors make any warranty, expressed or implied, with respect to the material contained herein. Before prescribing any drug, the reader must review the manufacturer's current product information (package inserts) for accepted indications, absolute dosage recommendations, and other information pertinent to the safe and effective use of the product described. This is especially important when drugs are given in combination or as an adjunct to other forms of therapy.

Library of Congress Cataloging-in-Publication Data

Oral and maxillofacial surgery secrets / edited by A. Omar Abubaker, Kenneth J. Benson.
       p. ; cm.—(The Secrets Series®)
    Includes index.
    ISBN 1-56053-401-X (alk. paper)
     1. Mouth—Surgery—Examinations, questions, etc. 2. Maxilla—Surgery—
Examinations, questions, etc. 3. Face—Surgery—Examinations, questions, etc.
I. Abubaker, A. Omar. II. Benson, Kenneth J, 1966– III. Series.
    [DNLM: 1. Surgery, Oral—Examination Questions. 2. Oral Surgical
Procedures—Examination Questions. WU 18.2 O63 2000]
RK529.O675 2000
617.5'2'0076—dc 21

                                                                00-040900

ORAL AND MAXILLOFACIAL SURGERY SECRETS   ISBN 1-56053-401-X

Last digit is the print number: 9   8   7   6   5   4   3   2   1

DEDICATION

To all my teachers, especially those in the early years of my education, for planting the seeds of scientific curiosity and thirst for knowledge.

To my mentors, who recognized and nourished the potential in me to learn and teach.

To my students and residents, who taught me by asking me questions.

To my family, who supported me throughout all this.

AOA

CONTENTS

VI. MANAGEMENT OF THE ORAL AND MAXILLOFACIAL SURGERY PATIENT

CONTRIBUTORS

A. Omar Abubaker, D.M.D., Ph.D.
Associate Professor, Department of Oral and Maxillofacial Surgery, School of Dentistry; Division of Oral and Maxillofacial Surgery, School of Medicine, Medical College of Virginia, Virginia Commonwealth University, Richmond, Virginia

Kathy A. Banks, D.M.D.
Department of Oral and Maxillofacial Surgery, University of Medicine and Dentistry of New Jersey, Newark, New Jersey

Timothy S. Bartholomew, D.D.S.
Department of Oral and Maxillofacial Surgery, Medical College of Virginia, Virginia Commonwealth University, Richmond, Virginia

Kenneth J. Benson, D.D.S.
Oral and Maxillofacial Surgeon in Private Practice, Raleigh, North Carolina

Paul W. Brinser III, M.D., D.D.S.
Department of Oral and Maxillofacial Surgery, Medical College of Virginia, Virginia Commonwealth University; Medical College of Virginia Hospitals, Richmond, Virginia

William A. Carvajal, D.D.S., M.D.
Department of Oral and Maxillofacial Surgery, Medical College of Virginia, Virginia Commonwealth University, Richmond, Virginia

Matthew R. Cooke, D.D.S.
Pediatric Dentist and Dental Anesthesiologist, Department of Dentistry, Medical College of Virginia, Virginia Commonwealth University; Medical College of Virginia Hospitals; Richmond Eye and Ear Hospital, Richmond, Virginia

Robert E. Doriot, D.D.S.
Department of Oral and Maxillofacial Surgery, Medical College of Virginia, Virginia Commonwealth University; Medical College of Virginia Hospitals, Richmond, Virginia

Sonia E. Francioni, D.M.D.
Department of Oral and Maxillofacial Surgery, University of Medicine and Dentistry of New Jersey, Newark, New Jersey

James A. Giglio, D.D.S., M.Ed.
Professor, Department of Oral and Maxillofacial Surgery, Medical College of Virginia, Virginia Commonwealth University; Medical College of Virginia Hospitals, Richmond, Virginia

Steven G. Gollehon, D.D.S., M.D.
Department of Oral and Maxillofacial Surgery, Louisiana State University Medical Center; Charity Hospital; University Hospital, New Orleans, Louisiana; Earl K. Long Hospital, Baton Rouge, Louisiana

Bradley A. Gregory, D.M.D.
Department of Oral and Maxillofacial Surgery, Medical College of Virginia, Virginia Commonwealth University, Richmond, Virginia

Hamid Hajarian, M.S., D.D.S., M.D.
Lecturer, Department of Oral and Maxillofacial Surgery, University of California, Los Angeles, UCLA School of Medicine, Los Angeles, California

Lubor Hlousek, D.M.D., M.D.
Oral and Maxillofacial Surgeon in Private Practice, Annapolis, Maryland

Frank P. Iuorno, Jr., D.D.S.
Oral and Maxillofacial Surgeon in Private Practice, Richmond, Virginia

Maria J. Iuorno, M.D.
Assistant Professor of Medicine, Division of Endocrinology and Metabolism, Medical College of Virginia, Virginia Commonwealth University; Medical College of Virginia Hospitals, Richmond, Virginia

Jeffrey S. Jelic, D.M.D., M.D.
Department of Oral and Maxillofacial Surgery, University of North Carolina Dental School, Chapel Hill, North Carolina

John N. Kent, D.D.S.
Boyc Professor and Head, Department of Oral and Maxillofacial Surgery, Louisiana State University Health Sciences Center; Chief, Oral and Maxillofacial Surgery, Medical Center of Louisiana at New Orleans; Active Staff, Doctor's Hospital of Jefferson; Active Staff, East Jefferson General Hospital, New Orleans, Louisiana

Jennifer Lamphier, D.M.D.
Department of Oral and Maxillofacial Surgery, University of Medicine and Dentistry of New Jersey, Newark, New Jersey

Lt. Richard G. Long, D.D.S.
United States Navy, Naval Dental Center, Camp Lejeune, North Carolina

Christopher L. Maestrello, D.D.S.
Assistant Professor of Pediatric Dentistry and Dental Anesthesiology, Department of Dentistry, Medical College of Virginia, Virginia Commonwealth University; Medical College of Virginia Hospitals; Richmond Eye and Ear Hospital, Richmond, Virginia

Renato Mazzonetto, D.D.S., Ph.D.
Assistant Professor, Department of Oral and Maxillofacial Surgery, Piracicaba Dental School, University of Campinas, Piracicaba, Sao Paulo, Brazil

Ian McDonald, M.D., D.M.D.
Oral and Maxillofacial Surgeon in Private Practice, Escondido, California

Mark A. Oghalai, D.D.S.
Department of Oral and Maxillofacial Surgery, Medical College of Virginia, Virginia Commonwealth University, Richmond, Virginia

Vincent J. Perciaccante, D.D.S.
Oral and Maxillofacial Surgeon in Private Practice, Tucker, Georgia

Noah Sandler, D.M.D., M.D.
Department of Oral and Maxillofacial Surgery, Medical College of Virginia, Virginia Commonwealth University, Richmond, Virginia

Chris A. Skouteris, D.M.D., DRDENT(Path)
Associate Professor, Department of Oral and Maxillofacial Surgery, University of Athens School of Dentistry; Evangelismos General Hospital, Athens, Greece

Daniel B. Spagnoli, D.D.S., Ph.D.
Clinical Assistant Professor, Department of Oral and Maxillofacial Surgery, Louisiana State University University Health Scinece Center, New Orleans, Louisiana

Robert A. Strauss, D.D.S.
Associate Professor and Director, Residency Program, Department of Oral and Maxillofacial Surgery, Medical College of Virginia, Virginia Commonwealth University; Medical College of Virginia Hospitals, Richmond, Virginia

Vincent B. Ziccardi, M.D., D.D.S.
Assistant Professor and Residency Program Director, Department of Oral and Maxillofacial Surgery, University of Medicine and Dentistry of New Jersey; University Hospital, Newark, New Jersey

FOREWORD

Students, residents, and practitioners are constantly bombarded by questions from patients, colleagues, and teachers. When they do not know the answer, they usually turn to their textbooks for the information. However, there are times when textbooks do not provide the appropriate information, the available information is not specific enough, or the correct answer is difficult to find among all of the details that are provided. Thus, the need became apparent for another source of concise information on a variety of topics that are specific to a particular area of specialization. Until now, this source has not existed in oral and maxillofacial surgery. Drs. Abubaker and Benson are to be congratulated on filling this niche with *Oral and Maxillofacial Surgery Secrets*.

Following the format used in the other books in this series, *Oral and Maxillofacial Surgery Secrets* covers the broad scope of the specialty, providing precise answers to the most common questions that arise during clinical practice. Therefore, it contains information under one cover that ordinarily could be found only by referring to multiple textbooks. In this way, the book makes an important contribution to the field of oral and maxillofacial surgery. Readers will find it valuable as a handy, quick way to obtain answers and also as an excellent review of what is current in the field.

Daniel M. Laskin, D.D.S., M.S.
Professor and Chairman
Department of Oral and Maxillofacial Surgery
Schools of Dentistry and Medicine
Virginia Commonwealth University

PREFACE

With the expanding scope of oral and maxillofacial surgery, the breadth of information to be acquired both by the neophyte to the field and by the practicing clinician is increasing daily. Although conventional textbooks contain a great deal of valuable information, it is often difficult, especially for residents and students, to identify and remember the most relevant information. According to the Socratic method, the best way to teach is to question, and this book uses this effective teaching approach to help guide students, residents, and clinicians to acquire and retain the significant knowledge in the field.

Oral and Maxillofacial Surgery Secrets is intended not only to answer questions, but also to provide the additional information an oral and maxillofacial surgeon must have to provide the best care to a patient with a particular problem. With the generous help of the contributors, we have covered the topics that are important for building an adequate knowledge base necessary for supplying appropriate patient care. Of course, no one book can be the source of all the information that a good practitioner needs to know. However, for a quick, concise, and to-the-point way to find the answers to most clinical questions and issues that residents and clinicians face on a daily basis, this part of the Secrets Series® is a valuable first step.

A. Omar Abubaker, D.M.D., Ph.D.
Kenneth J. Benson, D.D.S.

I. Patient Evaluation

1. HISTORY AND PHYSICAL EXAMINATION

James A. Giglio, D.D.S., M.Ed.

1. Which portion of a complete medical history is recorded in the patient's own words?
The chief complaint.

2. Describe the review of systems.
This is an outline for review of the patient's medical history that inquires about specific symptoms associated with each organ system of the body.

3. What is the difference between a physical sign and a symptom?
In general, a symptom is an abnormal sensation felt by the patient, whereas a sign can be seen, felt, or heard by the examiner.

4. Name the four vital signs.
Pulse
Blood pressure
Temperature
Respiration rate

5. What are the four methods employed in a physical examination?
Inspection
Palpation
Percussion
Auscultation

6. What is the difference between a remittent fever and an intermittent fever?
A remittent fever has a diurnal variation of more than 2°F but has no normal readings. Intermittent fever refers to episodes of fever separated by days of normal temperature.

7. What is quotidian fever?
A daily recurring fever often associated with hepatic abscess or acute cholangitis.

8. What fever pattern is associated with Hodgkin's disease?
Pel-Ebstein fever. This pattern describes several days of continuous remittent fever followed by remissions for an irregular number of days.

9. Define macule, papule, and nodule.
Macules are localized changes in skin color that occur in various shapes, sizes, and colors and are not palpable. Papules are solid and elevated, with a diameter of less than 5 mm. Nodules are also solid and elevated but extend deeper into the skin than papules and usually have diameters greater than 5 mm.

10. What is PERRLA?

PERRLA refers to the eye examination findings of *p*upils *e*qual, *r*ound, and *r*eactive to *l*ight and *a*ccommodation.

11. What is a pterygium?

A raised, yellow plaque termed the pinguecula is normal and found on a horizontal plane between the canthus and limbus of the eye. In response to chronic irritation, the pinguecula will grow to extend a vascular membrane, termed *pterygium*, over the limbus toward the center of the cornea. Vision may become obstructed.

12. When examining the ear, where is the light reflex normally located and what conditions will alter its location or appearance?

The light reflex is normally noted at about the five o'clock position. Conditions that can alter its appearance include retracted drumhead, serous otitis, bulging drumhead, air bubbles in serous otitis, and a perforated drumhead.

13. What is Darwin's tubercle?

Darwin's tubercle is a fusiform swelling that occasionally develops on the surface of the pinna above the midpoint of the helix on the ear.

14. What is the difference between bone conduction and air conduction when applied to tuning fork tests of hearing?

Air conduction implies sound transmission through the ear canal, tympanic membrane, and ossicle, to the cochlea, and finally to the eighth or auditory nerve. Bone conduction relies on the transmission of sound through the skull to the cochlea and to the auditory nerve.

15. Describe the difference between the Rinne and Weber tests of auditory function.

The Rinne test makes use of air conduction and bone conduction whereas the Weber test makes use of bone conduction. A Rinne test is considered normal or positive when sound is heard better by air conduction rather than bone conduction. In a Weber test of hearing, a conductive deafness will cause sound to be referred to the side of the deaf ear. The Weber test checks lateralization.

16. What chain of lymph nodes is palpable along the anterior border of the sternocleidomastoid muscle?

The superior cervical chain, which drains lymph from the skin and neck.

17. Where is Erb's point?

On the side of the neck where applied pressure on the roots of the fifth and sixth cervical nerves causes paralysis of the brachial muscles. Muscles involved are of the upper arm (e.g., deltoid, biceps, brachialis anterior).

18. Which ribs are referred to as "floating" ribs?

The 11th and 12th ribs.

19. Where is the angle of Louis?

It is located at the junction between the manubrium and the body of the sternum; it marks the articulation of the second rib on the sternum. It is also known as the angle of Ludwig.

20. What structure lies under the clavicle?

The 1st rib.

21. What is Kussmaul breathing?

This is an increase in both rate and depth of respiration and is synonymous with hyperventilation.

22. What is the difference between hyperventilation and hyperpnea?
Hyperventilation is an increase in both rate and depth of respiration whereas hyperpnea is an increase in depth only.

23. What is Cheyne-Stokes breathing?
Alternating hyperpnea, shallow respiration, and apnea.

24. What is stridor?
A high-pitched respiratory sound such as the inspiratory sound heard often in acute laryngeal obstruction.

25. Where is the intercostal angle?
The inferior margins of the 7th, 8th, and 9th costocartilages meet in the midline (at the infrasternal notch) to form the intercostal angle. It normally measures less than 90° and is increased in obstructive lung disease.

26. At what level of reduced hemoglobin does a patient become cyanotic?
5 gm/dl.

27. What is the diaphragmatic effect on the heart?
During inspiration, the diaphragm descends, stretching the heart from its anchorage in the fascia surrounding the aorta and pulmonary artery. The vertical cardiac axis becomes elongated, the transverse direction narrowed, and filling of the right ventricle is delayed.

28. When does blood from the coronary arteries perfuse the heart muscle?
During diastole.

29. What is the PMI?
The *p*oint of *m*aximum *i*mpulse of the heart. At the beginning of systole the heart is rotated forward toward the chest wall where the impulse can be felt. The PMI is normally felt at the 5th interspace between the ribs, 1–2 cm medial to the left midclavicular line.

30. What causes the heart sounds?
At the beginning of systole, the ventricles contract, increasing the ventricular pressure and causing the mitral and tricuspid valves to close. Blood rebounds in the ventricles, transmitting vibrations to the chest wall which can be heard with the stethoscope as S_1. Blood then courses silently through the aorta and pulmonary arteries. The second sound occurs when the ventricles relax in diastole, ventricular pressure decreases, and the aortic and pulmonary valves close. The backflow of blood against these valves sets up another series of vibrations audible as the second heart sound S_2.

31. What is the difference between a physiologic and an organic heart murmur?
Heart murmurs are caused by disruption of the normal laminar flow of blood. Causes include regurgitation of blood, blood flow through narrowed or stenotic valves or vessels, shunting of blood, increased rate of blood flow, and decreased blood viscosity. An organic murmur is pathologic and caused by some intrinsic cardiac disease or defect such as deformed or stenotic heart valves, ventricular septal defects, or a patent ductus arteriosus. Physiologic murmurs are not pathologic and usually result from an altered metabolic state such as in pregnancy or early childhood.

32. What is a flow murmur?
A flow murmur is induced when the velocity of normal blood is increased as it courses through a normal heart.

33. What are the grades of intensity of heart murmurs?

Intensity of heart murmur is graded on a scale of 1 to 6. The subjectivity of this scale is minimized by the following guidelines:

Grade 1: very faint and heard only when paying close attention
Grade 2: faint, but unmistakably present
Grade 3: clearly louder than faint, but not associated with a thrill
Grade 4: loud and associated with a thrill
Grade 5: very loud but requiring a stethoscope partly on the chest to be heard
Grade 6: able to be heard with stethoscope off the chest

34. What are Korotkoff sounds?

These are the sounds produced by the turbulence created when the inflated blood pressure cuff disrupts normal arterial laminar blood flow.

35. How high should the cuff be inflated when measuring blood pressure?

The cuff should be placed over the antecubital fossa and the brachial artery palpated at the lower edge of the cuff. The radial pulse should be palpated while the cuff is being inflated. Inflation should continue to 30 mm of pressure above where the radial pulse is last palpated. This technique is recommended to compensate for the possible presence of an auscultatory gap. This is a period of silence that can occur during the systolic measurement and primarily in hypertensive patients. Arbitrary inflation of the cuff may cause the initial systolic reading to fall somewhere in this gap, or silent period resulting in an inaccurately (too low) measured systolic pressure.

36. What is the result of using a blood pressure cuff that is too large or too small for the diameter of the patient's arm?

Too large a cuff will result in an erroneously low pressure recording whereas too small a cuff will result in an erroneously high measurement.

37. When does one use the bell and when does one use the diaphragm of the stethoscope?

A stethoscope is equipped with bell and diaphragm components on the chest piece. The diaphragm of the stethoscope is best for picking up relatively high-pitched (high-frequency) sounds such as S_1 and S_2, the murmurs of aortic and mitral regurgitation, and pericardia friction rub. The bell is best for hearing low-pitched (low-frequency) sounds such as S_3, S_4, and the diastolic murmur of mitral stenosis.

38. What maneuvers or special positions are used to accentuate abnormalities of heart sounds?

For accentuation of aortic regurgitation, ask the patient to sit up, lean forward and exhale completely, and hold breath in expiration. For bringing out mitral murmurs or S_3, ask the patient to roll onto his or her left side, then listen at the apical area.

39. Define pulse pressure.

The pulse pressure is the numeric difference between the systolic and diastolic blood pressures. The normal pulse pressure is in the range of 30–40 mmHg. Causes of an increased or widening pulse pressure include hyperkinetic states (anxiety, fever, exercise, hyperthyroidism), aortic regurgitation, and increased aortic rigidity (aging, atherosclerosis). A decrease or narrowing of the pulse pressure can be caused by obstructed ventricular output as in aortic stenosis or decreased stroke volume from shock or heart failure.

40. If clinical measurement of the blood pressure is not possible in either arm, where are alternative sites to measure blood pressure?

Blood pressure can be auscultated over the dorsal pedis artery with the cuff placed on the lower leg above the malleolus. Pressure measured here is comparable to pressure recorded over the brachial artery. Blood pressure can also be measured over the popliteal artery with a wide (thigh) cuff placed over the femoral artery. Here the blood pressure is higher (10 ± 5 mmHg) than in the brachial artery.

41. Where in the abdomen is the appendix located?
Lower right quadrant.

42. Where on the abdomen is the liver percussed?
Upper right quadrant. A liver span of 6–12 mm in the midclavicular line is considered normal.

43. What is the significance of rebound tenderness in the abdomen?
Peritoneal inflammation.

44. What is the Hering-Breuer reflex?
When the lungs become overly inflated, stretch receptors activate an appropriate feedback response to limit further inspiration. These stretch receptors are located in the walls of the bronchi and bronchioles throughout the lungs that, when overstretched, transmit inhibitory signals through the vagus nerve in the inhibitory center. It seems to be a protective mechanism to prevent overinflation rather than normal control of ventilation.

45. How are deep tendon reflexes graded?
0 = no response   3+ = more brisk than average
1+ = diminished; low normal   4+ = hyperactive
2+ = normal

46. How is the Babinski sign elicited?
It is done by lightly stroking the lateral aspect of the sole of the foot vertically from the heal to the base of the toes. The course of stimulation is changed as you approach the toes by medially directing the path of stimulation along the base of the toes toward the great toe. Normal response is plantar flexion while abnormal response is dorsiflexion of the toe, fanning of the other toes, and dorsiflexion of the ankles.

47. What is anisocoria?
Anisocoria refers to inequality of the pupils. It is a common normal variation of pupil size.

48. What is the Glasgow Coma Scale?
Glasgow Coma Scale (GCS) is a quantitative measure of the patient's level of consciousness. The GCS is the sum of scores for three areas of assessment: (1) eye opening, (2) verbal response, and (3) best motor response. The minimum GSC score that can be obtained is 3, and the maximum is 15.

AREA OF ASSESSMENT	PATIENT RESPONSE	SCORE
Eye opening	Spontaneous	4
	Responds to verbal command	3
	Responds to pain	2
	No response	1
Motor response	To verbal command	6
	Localizes pain (e.g., moves hand to push yours away)	5
	Withdraws	4
	Flexor response	3
	Extensor response	2
	No response	1

(*Table continued on next page.*)

AREA OF ASSESSMENT	PATIENT RESPONSE	SCORE
Verbal response	Oriented	5
	Confused conversation	4
	Inappropriate words	3
	Incomprehensible sounds	2
	No response	1

49. What is Homans' sign?

Pain in the calf when the toe is dorsiflexed. This is an early sign of deep venous thrombosis.

50. What are the components of the corneal reflex?

Sensory limb: fifth cranial nerve (V3)

Motor response: seventh cranial nerve—look for eye blinking

51. What is the oculocardiac reflex?

The trigeminal-vagal reflex. Pressure applied to the globe or stretching of the extraocular muscles results in 10–15% reduction in heart rate. It also can cause junctional rhythm and possible premature ventricular contractions (PVCs). Atropine is not useful in treating this situation.

52. What is the direct light reflex?

When a light is shone into the eye to the retina, the pupil constricts (retina–optic nerve–optic tract).

53. What is the consensual light reflex?

When a light is shone into the eye to the retina, the pupil of the opposite eye constricts. There are many forms of strabismus depending on the direction of the strabismus, whether the condition is affecting one eye or both, and what is the cause of the condition.

54. What is nystagmus?

Nystagmus is an involuntary, rapid, rhythmic movement of the eyeball, which may be horizontal, vertical, rotatory, or mixed. There are various forms of nystagmus, some of which may be indicative of certain disease of the vestibular system.

55. What is strabismus?

Strabismus is a deviation of the eye that the patient cannot overcome. The visual axis deviates from that required by the physiologic conditions.

BIBLIOGRAPHY

1. Bates B, Bickley L, Hoekelman R: A Guide to Physical Examination and History Taking, 6th ed. Philadelphia, J. B. Lippincott, 1995.
2. DeGowin E, DeGowin R: Bedside Diagnostic Examination, 2nd ed. London, Macmillan, 1965.
3. Handler B: History and physical examination. In Kwon PH, Laskin DM (eds): Clinician's Manual of Oral and Maxillofacial Surgery, 2nd ed. Carol Stream, IL, Quintessence, 1997, pp 1–12.
4. Seidel HM, Ball JW, Dains JE, Benedict GW: Mosby's Guide to Physical Examination. St. Louis, Mosby, 1987.

2. ECG INTERPRETATION

Frank P. Iuorno, D.D.S.

1. Describe the PQRS complex as it relates to the physiology of the myocardium.

The **P wave** represents atrial depolarization and contraction. It originates in the sinoatrial (SA) node. Usually, depolarization is noted on an ECG with repolarization usually too small or obscured by other waves. Normal < 0.12 sec. The **PR interval** represents conduction of an impulse through the atrioventricular (AV) node. Normal < 0.2 sec. The **QRS complex** represents the electrical activity of ventricular depolarization and contraction. Normal < 0.12 sec. The **ST segment** represents the maintenance depolarization of the ventricles. The **T wave** represents electrical repolarization of the ventricles and is not associated with any physical event.

2. What do the various types of PR interval indicate?

The *normal* PR interval (< 0.2 seconds) represents the lag in electrical conduction through the AV node. It allows time for ventricular filling. A *narrow* PR interval (< 0.12 sec) may reveal accelerated AV conduction (as in Wolfe-Parkinson-White syndrome) or premature junctional complexes. *Wide* PR intervals (> 0.2 sec) indicate first-degree AV block. *Progressively lengthening* PR intervals indicate second-degree AV block or multifocal atrial tachycardia.

3. What are the intrinsic automatic firing rates of the sinus node, the AV node, and the ventricles?

The sinus node fires at an intrinsic rate of 60–100 beats/min. The AV node and the ventricles fire intrinsically at about 60 and 30–40 beats/min, respectively.

4. What is the normal route of conduction?

Via sinus node → AV node → HIS-Purkinje fibers

5. Describe the markings of an ECG.

1 small square (light lines) = 1 mm = 1 mV = 0.04 sec
1 large square (dark lines) = 5 mm = 5 mV = 0.2 sec
Normal paper speed = 25 mm/sec

6. How do I determine the heart rate from an ECG?

Atrial rate (**P to P interval**) may be different from ventricular rate (**R to R interval**), if atria and ventricles are not conducting impulses in a 1:1 fashion. Ventricular rate governs cardiac output, and is most critical. Count P-P or R-R along 5 mm large squares:

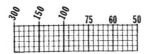

Alternatively, you can multiply the number of beats in 6 seconds (two 3-second marks) by 10.

7. How are leads placed to determine the direction of the cardiac impulse in the frontal plane?

An ECG measures the electrical impulse between two leads. By measuring these impulses using several leads at different angles, the axis (or overall vector) of the impulse can be derived. The limb leads are used to determine the impulse direction in the frontal plane. Leads are placed on the right arm, left arm, and left leg. Impulses that travel toward the positive lead have a positive deflection on the ECG. Using a common ground, two leads may be averaged to yield three more vectors named **aVR**, **aVL**, and **aVF**.

8. How are leads placed to determine the axis of the cardiac impulse in the axial or horizontal plane?

Chest leads V1–V6 are used to determine the direction of an impulse in the axial plane. They are placed sequentially: V1 (right of sternum in 4th intercostal space), V2 (left of sternum), V3 (midway between V2 and V4), V4 (midclavicular line in 5th intercostal space), V5 (midway between V4 and V6), and V6 (lateral chest in 5th intercostal space).

9. When analyzing ECGs what are the five factors to consider?

Rate, rhythm, axis, hypertrophy, and infarction.

10. Define tachycardia and bradycardia.

Sinus tachycardia indicates a rate > 100 bpm and bradycardia a rate < 60 bpm.

11. How do I determine the axis of the heart's electrical impulse?

Consider leads I and aVF. Remember that the more positive the deflection in each lead indicates the axis following in the same direction. Lead I flows from right to left, and lead aVF flows from superior to inferior. A normal axis shows positive deflections in both I and aVF. Left axis deviation shows positive in lead I and negative in aVF, and the patient may have left ventricular hypertrophy or bundle branch block. Right axis deviation shows negative in lead I and positive in aVF, and the patient may have right ventricular hypertrophy or bundle branch block. Extreme right axis deviation is negative in both leads I and aVF and rare.

12. How do potassium and calcium affect the ECG?

Hypokalemia causes U waves (small, positive deflections following T waves). Hypokalemia may also be seen as ST depression and flat T waves. Hyperkalemia causes tall, narrow, peaked T waves, QRS widening, and P wave flattening, and can progress to ventricular fibrillation. Hypocalcemia causes prolonged QT intervals. Finally, hypercalcemia causes shortened QT intervals.

13. Identify the following rhythm.

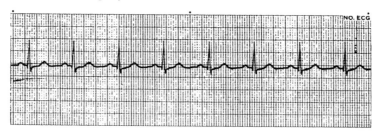

Sinus rhythm. The rate is normally 60–100 bpm. The PR interval is 0.12–0.2 seconds. The QRS complex is 0.04–0.12 seconds. The rhythm is regular.

14. Identify the following rhythm.

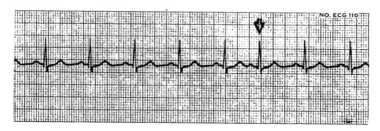

Premature atrial contractions. Here the rate varies depending on the number of these contractions. A different P wave (originating from an ectopic focus in the atrium) and a shortened PR interval are evident. The QRS complex is normal, however, and the rhythm is basically normal with the exception of occasional prematurities (*arrow* indicates premature wave).

15. Identify the following rhythm.

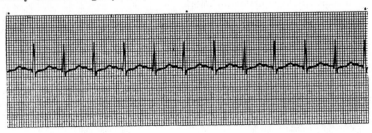

Sinus tachycardia. By definition, the rate at rest is greater than 100 bpm. The P waves, PR intervals, and QRS complexes are normal. The rhythm is regular.

16. Identify the following rhythm.

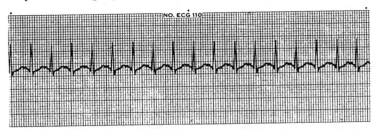

Supraventricular tachycardia. Generally, the rate is 150–250 bpm. The P waves differ from normal and may be coincident with the previous T waves, with a noticeable lack of PR interval. The QRS complexes are again normal.

17. Identify the following rhythm.

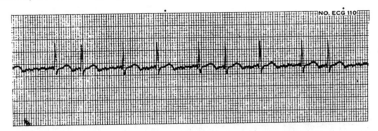

Atrial fibrillation. Commonly remembered as an irregularly irregular rhythm. The rate is usually 300–500 bpm, with a ventricular capture rate of 150–180 bpm. P waves are not usually discrete, and PR intervals are virtually impossible to distinguish. The QRS complexes are normal.

18. Identify the following rhythm.

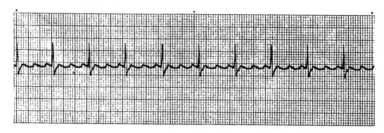

Atrial flutter. The "sawtooth" rhythm. The atrial rate averages 220–350 bpm; the ventricular rate is also variable at 100–220 bpm. P waves give the characteristic sawtooth appearance to this rhythm (flutter or "F" waves). PR intervals are usually regular, and the QRS complexes are normal.

19. Identify the following rhythm.

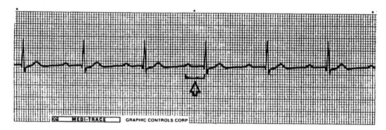

First-degree AV block. The only unusual finding on this ECG is a prolonged PR interval (> 0.2 seconds; see *arrow*).

20. Identify the following rhythm.

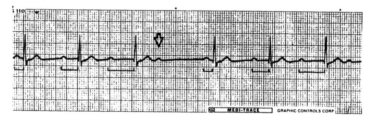

Second-degree AV block, Mobitz type I (Wenckebach). The atrial rate is usually fixed, but the ventricular rate is slower. Here the P waves are normal, but the PR intervals lengthen until eventually a QRS complex is dropped. The QRS complexes are normal. *Brackets* indicate increasing PR intervals; *arrow* indicates P wave that is not conducted to ventricles ("dropped beat").

21. Identify the following rhythm.

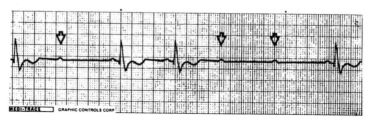

Second-degree AV block, Mobitz type II. The rate is usually normal in the atrium, but the ventricular rate is slower by a factor of two (2:1) or three (3:1). Here the P waves are normal, and when conducted the PR interval is usually normal. There are simply missed QRS complexes for P waves. *Arrows* indicate intermittent nonconducting P waves.

22. Identify the following rhythm.

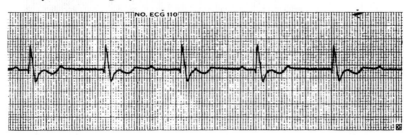

Third-degree AV block. There is total dissociation of the atrium and the ventricles. Thus, the P waves and QRS complexes are regular, but do not coincide, leaving a rate of 20–60 bpm. The QRS complexes may be normal to wide.

23. Identify the following rhythm.

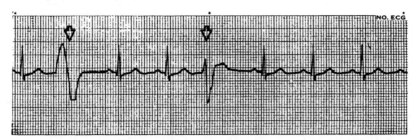

Premature ventricular contractions. The overall rate is normal, but the P waves are usually indistinguishable from the QRS complex. The PR interval is not measurable, and the QRS complex is prolonged (> 0.12 seconds). *Arrows* indicate premature complexes.

24. Identify the following rhythm.

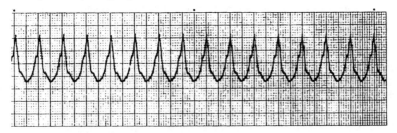

Ventricular tachycardia. P waves and PR intervals are not seen. The rate is usually > 100 bpm and the QRS complexes are wide (> 0.12 seconds).

25. Identify the following rhythm.

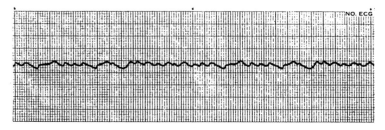

Ventricular fibrillation. The rate is not calculable because there are no actual QRS complexes. There are no P waves or PR intervals to speak of. The patient is usually without a pulse.

26. Identify the following rhythm.

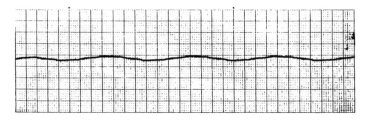

Asystole.

27. What are typical ECG signs of ischemia, injury, and infarction?

Ischemia shows inverted T waves in the leads nearest the part of the affected myocardium most easily identified in the chest leads. ST depression may also be seen. *Injury* to heart muscle is indicated by ST elevation and tall, positive T waves. *Infarction* shows Q waves that are 0.04 seconds or longer, or greater than one-third the size of the entire QRS complex. Location can be determined from the lead. Anterior leads show Q waves in V1 and V2; inferior leads in II, III, and aVF; and lateral leads in I, aVL, V5, and V6.

28. What is Wolff-Parkinson-White (WPW) syndrome?

WPW syndrome is a pre-excitation syndrome caused by conduction from the SA node to the ventricle through an accessory pathway that bypasses the AV node. Early depolarization of the ventricles produces a short PR interval and a delta wave (a delay in initial deflection of the QRS complex) on ECG just before normal ventricular depolarization is initiated. Clinically, this syndrome is manifested as tachyarrhythmias

29. How is digitalis toxicity seen on ECG?

Digitalis toxicity has several ECG manifestations, including SA and AV node blocks, tachycardia, premature ventricular contractions, ventricular tachycardia, atrial fibrillation, and possible sloping of the ST segment.

30. What is the ECG manifestation of hypothermia?

Hypothermia is seen on ECG as sinus bradycardia, AV junctional rhythm, or ventricular fibrillation. Typically there is an elevated J-point, and there may be an intraventricular conduction delay and prolonged QT interval.

BIBLIOGRAPHY

1. Dubin D: Rapid Interpretation of EKG, 5th ed. Tampa, Cover Publishing Company, 1997, pp 61–190.
2. Gomella LG: Basic ECG Reading. In Clinician Pocket Reference, 7th ed. Norwalk, CT, Appleton & Lange, 1993, pp 325–347.
3. Steeling C: Simplified EKG Analysis. Philadelphia, Hanley &-Belfus, 1992, pp 3–45.
4. Strauss R: ECG Interpretation. In Kwon PH, Laskin DM (eds): Clinician Manual of Oral and Maxillofacial Surgery, 2nd ed. Chicago, Quintessence Books, 1996, pp 55–74.

3. LABORATORY TESTS

Paul W. Brinser III, M.D., D.D.S.

1. What is included in a complete blood count (CBC) and how are the results charted?
The CBC or heme 8 typically includes:

Complete Blood Cell Count

	DEFINITION	NORMAL RANGE
White blood cell (WBC) count		$4–11 \times 10^3$ cells/mm^3
Red blood cell (RBC) count		$4.5–6 \times 10^6$ cells/mm^3
Hemoglobin (Hgb)		Men: 14–18 gm/dl Women: 12–16 gm/dl
Hematocrit (Hct)	Percentage of RBC mass in blood volume	Men: 40–54% Women: 37–47%
Platelets (Plt)		$150–400 \times 10^3$/mm^3
Red blood cell indices:		
Mean corpuscular volume (MCV)	Average RBC volume in femtoliters (fl)	80–100 fl
Mean corpuscular hemoglobin (MCH)	Estimates weight of Hgb in average RBC	27–31 pg
Mean corpuscular hemoglobin concentration (MCHC)	Estimates average concentration of Hgb in average RBC	32–36%

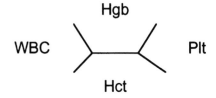

2. What information does a white blood cell differential provide?
The total WBC count is made up of neutrophils (50–70%), lymphocytes (20–40%), monocytes (0–7%), basophils (0–1%), and eosinophils (0–5%). Most laboratories also provide the absolute number of each cell type as well as percentage. Differentials for alterations in the WBC fractions are:

Polymorphonuclear neutrophils (PMNs)

Increased:
Bacterial infection
Tissue damage (myocardial infection, burn, or crush injury)
Leukemia
Uremia
Diabetic ketoacidosis (DKA)
Acute gout
Eclampsia
Physiologic:
  Severe exercise

Decreased:
Aplastic anemia
Viral infection
Drugs
Radiation
Kidney dialysis

Late pregnancy
Labor
Surgery
Newborn

Lymphocytes (lymphs)

Increased (lymphocytosis):
Viral infections
Acute or chronic lymphocytic leukemia
Tuberculosis (TB)
Mononucleosis

Decreased:
Uremia
Stress
Burns
Trauma
Steroids
Normal in 20% of population

Monocytes

Increased (monocytosis):
Subacute bacterial endocarditis
TB
Protozoal infection
Leukemia
Collagen disease

Decreased:
Aplasia of bone marrow

Basophils

Increased (basophilia):
Chronic myeloid leukemia
Polycythemia
After recovery of infection or hypothyroidism
    (rarely)

Decreased:
Acute rheumatic fever
Lobar pneumonia
Steroid treatment
Stress
Thyrotoxicosis

Eosinophils

Increased (eosinophilia):
Allergy
Parasite

Malignancy
Drugs
Asthma
Addison's disease
Collagen vascular diseases

Decreased:
Steroids
Stress (infection, trauma, and burn)
Increased adrenocorticotropic
    hormone (ACTH)
Cushing's syndrome

3. What is a "left shift" and how is it significant?

PMNs are subdivided morphologically on the blood smear into segmented neutrophils ("segs" or "polys") and band forms ("bands") based on the nuclear lobes and their chromatin connections. The segs are more mature neutrophils, having 2–5 nuclear lobes and thin strands of chromatin and comprising 50–70% of total PMNs. The bands are immature neutrophils, make up 0–5% of total PMNs, and have a thick band of chromatin connecting 1–2 nuclear lobes. On the early manual neutrophil counting machines, the keys that represented the bands were on the left side and the keys representing segs were on the right. If the bands increased to > 20% of the WBC total, or the PMNs were > 80% of the WBC total, the result was said to have a "left shift." This shift increases the likelihood of bacterial infection, sepsis, or hemorrhage as the etiology of an elevated WBC count.

4. How are the RBC indices used clinically?

The indices are used to diagnose and classify anemia, which is defined as a decreased RBC mass or Hgb content below physiologic needs. The MCV and MCHC are the most useful in determining the etiology of the anemia.

- $MCV = (Hct \times$ unit constant$)/RBC$

  Macrocytic (> 100 fl): megaloblastic anemia (B_{12} or folate deficiency), chronic liver disease, alcoholism, reticulocytosis, physiologic for newborn.

  Microcytic (< 80 fl): iron deficiency, thalassemia, chronic disease (cancer, renal, infection), or lead toxicity.

- $MCH = Hgb/RBC$

  MCH helps to diagnose chromaticity of cells because increased Hgb content cells will have more pigment (hyperchromic) and will be hypochromic in the reverse situation. This tends to parallel changes in MCV in that macrocytic cells are usually hyperchromic and microcytic or hypochromic cells have low MCH.

- $MCHC = Hgb/Hct$

  This is increased with prolonged, severe dehydration, heavy smoking, intravascular hemolysis, and spherocytosis. The MCHC will be decreased in overhydration, iron deficiency anemia, thalassemia, and sideroblastic anemia.

5. What does the reticulocyte count mean?

Reticulocytes are immature RBCs. These cells are larger, continue hemoglobin synthesis, and are bluer in color on smears than mature erythrocytes. The normal count is 1% of total RBCs but will increase if the need for erythrocytes has risen. A "corrected count" is made by multiplying the reticulocyte count by the measured Hct divided by 45; the result should be $<$ 1.5%. If the count is increased, then erythropoiesis is usually due to bleeding, hemolysis, and correction of iron, folate, or B12 deficiencies. Decreased reticulocyte counts are often due to transfusions or aplastic anemia.

6. What information is obtained from the hemoglobin and hematocrit values?

The Hgb concentration is an indicator of oxygen-carrying capacity of blood. It is dependent primarily on the number of RBCs and much less significantly (or treatable) on the amount of hemoglobin per cell. Additionally, Hgb is known to vary by as much as 1 gm/dl diurnally, with peaks in the morning. Studies have also shown a 1-gm/dl variation between Hgb values drawn on admission and those taken following one night of bed rest. The relation between Hgb and Hct is given by:

$Hgb \times 3* = Hct$ (*Note: this varies between 2.7 and 3.2 based on the MCHC)
RBC (millions) $\times 3 = Hgb$
RBC $\times 9 = Hct$

Increased Hgb and Hct values may result from polycythemia, dehydration, heart disease, increased altitude, heavy smoking, or birth physiology. **Decreased** levels may indicate anemia, hemorrhage, dilution, alcohol, drugs, or pregnancy.

7. Are hemoglobin and hematocrit primary indicators of blood loss and the need for transfusion?

No! These are poor early measures of bleeding because one loses plasma and RBC in equal measures. It takes 2–3 hours or following fluid resuscitation before the Hgb/Hct will reflect blood loss. Previously, surgical transfusion guidelines were 10 gm/dl or 33% Hct, then 9 gm/dl or 25–30%. Today most patients are transfused for Hgb < 7 gm/dl but the best guidelines are the vital signs and symptoms such as shortness of breath and exercise tolerance. Initially low Hct values suggest chronic blood loss, which should be supported by low MCV and a high reticulocyte count.

8. Name some common terms and significant morphologic changes on smears.

Poikilocytosis—irregularly shaped RBCs
Anisocytosis—irregular RBC size
Sickled cells—crescent or sickle-shaped RBCs seen with decreased oxygen (O_2) tension
Howell-Jolly bodies—large RBC basophilic inclusions (megaloblastic anemia, splenectomy, hemolysis)

Basophilic stippling—small RBC blue inclusions (lead poison, thalassemia, heavy metals)

Spherocytes—spherical RBC (autoimmune hemolytic anemia, hereditary)

Burr cells—spiny RBC (liver disease, anorexia, ↑ bile acids)

Schistocyte—helmet RBCs (severe anemia, hemolytic transfusion reaction)

Döhle's inclusion bodies—PMNs (burns, infection)

Toxic granulation—PMNs (burns, sepsis, fever)

Auer bodies—acute myelogenous leukemia

Hypersegmentation—PMNs with 6–7 lobes (megaloblastic anemia, liver disease)

9. What is clinically useful about the platelet count?

Thrombocytopenia (low platelet count) that is less than $50,000/mm^3$ is an absolute contraindication to elective surgical procedures because of the possibility of significant bleeding. Patients with less than 10,000–20,000 platelets have been known to bleed spontaneously. Platelet counts between 50,000 and 100,000 have not been associated with significant bleeding provided platelet function is normal. Possible etiologies for low platelet counts are idiopathic thrombocytopenic purpura (ITP), disseminated intravascular coagulation (DIC), marrow invasion or aplasia, hypersplenism, drugs, cirrhosis transfusions, and viral infections (mononucleosis).

10. How is platelet function assessed and what drug most commonly affects the test?

Bleeding time is a screening test that assesses platelet number and function. The test is performed by inflating a blood pressure cuff to 40 mmHg, making a standard incision in the patient's forearm, and recording the time until the bleeding stops (Ivy method). It has been recommended that this test be used to diagnose specific hemorrhagic diseases and to monitor therapy of these diseases, but not to screen preoperative patients who have no history of bleeding or abnormal coagulation studies. The bleeding time is increased by platelet counts < 100,000 and by presence of aspirin, antibiotics (synthetic penicillins), uremia, alcoholism, chronic liver disease, vasculitis, Ehlers-Danlos syndrome, and von Willebrand's disease. There is an undefined risk of bleeding with elevated test times until about double the control time. Aspirin irreversibly blocks cyclooxygenase function, inhibiting platelet aggregation for their 7–10-day life span. Because approximately 10% of platelets are replaced each day, it takes an average of 2–3 days for bleeding time to normalize, but most experts recommend allowing 7 days without aspirin prior to surgery. Other nonsteroidal anti-inflammatory drugs (NSAIDs) will alter platelet function only temporarily, usually < 24 hours. Capillary fragility is also assessed in bleeding time values.

11. What tests monitor the extrinsic clotting system?

Prothrombin time (PT) is normally 11.5–13.5 seconds but requires separate control per reagent. The PT measures the function of clotting factors V, VII, X, II (prothrombin), and I (fibrinogen). It will be increased by warfarin, vitamin K deficiency, fat malabsorption, liver disease, DIC, and, artificially, increased tourniquet time. Warfarin blocks vitamin K use, while broad-spectrum antibiotics elevate PT by killing normal bowel flora, which decreases vitamin K absorption. Heparin in high doses also will increase PT by altering factor X. In dental extractions, few bleeding effects are seen with PT ≤ 2.5 control. Fresh frozen plasma (FFP) will reverse warfarin effects immediately, while vitamin K requires 12–24 hours to begin decreasing the PT.

International normalized ratio (INR, normal ≤ 1.0) was developed to allow comparison between tests and test centers of PT values though different reagents are used. This test should not be used for routine coagulation evaluation but only to follow chronic warfarin therapy.

$$INR = [PT (sample)/PT (mid\ lab\ range)]^x$$

where x = thromboplastin reagent of lab compared with international sensitivity index: human brain = 1.0, > 1 less sensitivity, < 1 greater sensitivity.

12. How is the intrinsic clotting system examined?

Normal activated partial thromboplastin time (APTT) is 27–38 seconds. This test monitors the function of factors V, VIII, IX, X, XI, XII, II, and I. APTT is increased by heparin, clotting factor deficiency, hemophilia A (VIII), hemophilia B (IX), increased tourniquet time, and, partially, warfarin. Heparin's primary effect is to activate antithrombin III, which blocks coagulation by inhibiting mostly IX and X factors. Antithrombin III amounts are significantly decreased in severe malignancy, severe liver disease, nephrotic syndrome, deep venous thrombosis (DVT), septicemia, major surgery, malnutrition, and DIC. Low–molecular-weight heparin (Enoxaparin) also works on antithrombin III. Heparin's peak effect is at 30 minutes to 1 hour after intravenous use and 3–4 hours after subcutaneous dose. Its duration of effect is approximately 3–4 hours when given intravenously and 6 hours subcutaneously.

13. Why are fibrin degradation products (FDPs) and fibrin "split" products (FSPs) important?

The result of the clotting cascade is insoluble polymeric fibrin meshwork. Naturally occurring fibrinolysin (plasmin) attacks and breaks down fibrinogen and fibrin leaving split products behind. Physiologically, this occurs after trauma or surgery and is quickly regulated. Pathologically, plasmin may be activated in DIC, DVT, malignancy, emboli, infections (especially gram-negative sepsis), necrosis, or infarctions. This will result in an elevated fibrin split product assay. Fibrinogen assays will be decreased (< 150 mg/dl) in DIC, burns, surgery, neoplasia, severe acute bleeding, snakebites, and some hematologic diseases. Protamine sulfate and d-dimer (a specific FSP) are other tests that look for abnormal clotting activity. Though not very specific, the d-dimer assay is used to screen for DVT in the emergency department because a normal value virtually excludes the possibility of this clotting problem.

14. What is measured in a blood chemistry test (also called basic metabolic, chem 7, or SMA 7)?

The basic electrolytes, renal function evaluation, and blood glucose are tested.

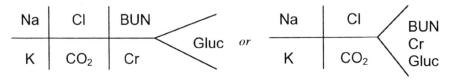

	Normal Ranges
1. Sodium (Na)	136–145 mEq/L
2. Potassium (K)	3.5–5.2 mEq/L
3. Chloride (Cl)	95–108 mEq/L
4. Carbon dioxide (CO_2)	24–30 mEq/L
5. Blood urea nitrogen (BUN)	6–20 mg/dl
6. Creatinine	0.7–1.4 mg/dl
7. Glucose	65–110 mg/dl (fasting)

15. What are common causes of basic electrolyte disturbances?

	INCREASE	DECREASE
Sodium (Na)	Dehydration	Diuretics
	Glycosuria	CHF
	Diabetes insipidus	Renal failure
	Cushing's syndrome	Vomiting
	Excessive sweating	Diarrhea

(Table continued on next page.)

	INCREASE	DECREASE
Sodium (Na) (*cont.*)		Liver failure
		Nephrotic syndrome
		SIADH
		Hypothyroidism
		Pancreatitis
		Hyperlipidemia
		Multiple myeloma
		Hyperglycemia—corrected Na = 1.6
		$\times$ 1/100 gm glucose over 100 gm/dl
Potassium (K)	Factitious (sample hemolysis, probably most common cause)	Diuretics
		Nasogastric suctioning
	Dehydration	Vomiting
	Renal failure	Alkalosis
	Acidosis	Mineral corticoid excess
	Addison's disease	Zollinger-Ellison syndrome
	Iatrogenic	
Chloride (Cl)	Dehydration	Vomiting
	Metabolic acidosis (nonanion gap)	Excessive sweating
		CHF
	Diarrhea	Chronic renal failure
	Diabetes insipidus	Diuretics
	Medications	DKA
	Aldosterone deficiency	SIADH
		Aldosterone excess
Carbon dioxide (CO_2)	Dehydration	Metabolic acidosis
	Respiratory acidosis	Respiratory alkalosis
	Vomiting	Renal failure
	Emphysema	Diarrhea
	Metabolic alkalosis	Starvation

CHF = congestive heart failure; SIADH = syndrome of inappropriate secretion of diuretic hormone; DKA = diabetic ketoacidosis

16. What tests are used as markers for liver function or disease?

Serum albumin, total protein, bilirubin, aspartate aminotransferase (AST = SGOT), alanine aminotransferase (ALT = SGPT), alkaline phosphatase (ALP), gamma-glutamyl transferase (GGT), lactate dehydrogenase (LDH), PT, bile acids, and blood ammonia.

17. How is the synthetic function of the liver evaluated?

Serum levels of albumin, total protein, PT, bile acids, conjugated bilirubin, BUN, and ammonia are used to examine liver function. Although not widely used, the most sensitive test for liver or bile tract abnormality is for bile acids. These are water soluble compounds produced from cholesterol metabolism in the liver. This test is best done 2 hours after eating and will show abnormailites in inactive cirrhosis and resolving hepatitis where other tests are normal. More commonly used is albumin level, which is decreased with liver damage as well as starvation, inflammatory bowel disease, nephrotic syndrome, leukemia, and hemorrhage or burns. Albumin is produced almost exclusively by the liver and makes up almost 75% of the total protein in serum so these tests usually parallel each other. Prothrombin is synthesized by the liver using vitamin K and will be abnormal in severe, most often end-stage, chronic liver disease. The absence of conjugated bilirubin in the blood with severely elevated unconjugated bilirubin could indicate severely decreased liver function. The ammonia level is used to diagnose and follow hepatic encephalopathy when failure of the liver is already known.

18. What is the clinical significance of liver enzymes?

Any increase of "hepatic" enzymes indicates cellular damage. AST is made in the liver, heart, skeletal muscle, and red blood cells so elevations may be due to liver disease, acute myocardial infarction (AMI), pancreatitis, muscle trauma, hemolysis, congestive heart failure (CHF), surgery, burns, or renal infarction. Increased specificity for liver damage occurs with elevation of ALT, GGT, or 5'nucleotidase. ALP is found in liver cells, bile duct epithelium, and osteoblasts. Therefore, elevations of ALP should be confirmed to involve the liver or bile ducts by checking a liver specific fraction (GGT, ALT, or 5'nucleotidase level). These tests will help rule out bone diseases, bone growth, healing of fractures, pregnancy, or childhood physiology as the cause of ALP elevation. Lastly, LDH also is increased in liver cell damage with the LDH_5 subfraction showing about the same sensitivity and somewhat greater specificity as AST.

19. What are the causes of bilirubin abnormalities?

Bilirubin is produced by the breakdown of hemoglobin in the reticuloendothelial system. This newly formed bilirubin (indirect or unconjugated) circulates through the bloodstream bound to albumin. Liver cells extract the bilirubin and conjugate it to a water-soluble pigment (direct or conjugated bilirubin) that is excreted in bile. Elevations of total bilirubin in the blood cause jaundice (yellowing of skin and sclera, and pruritis) and may be due to bile obstruction or excessive hemolysis. Elevation of indirect bilirubin occurs with obstruction and hepatocellular disease, and hemolytic anemia and physiologically in newborns. The direct bilirubin increases primarily with obstruction to bile flow and should be associated with an increase in ALP.

20. What are common laboratory trends in liver disorders?

	AST	ALT	ALP	BILI-RUBIN TOTAL	CONJU-GATED	UNCON-JUGATED	GGT	BILE ACID
Acute viral hepatitis	↑↑↑↑	↑↑↑↑	↑	↑ varies	↑↑	↑	↑–↑	↑↑↑
Chronic-resolving hepatitis	N–↑	N–↑	N–↑	N	—	—	N–↑	↑↑
Cirrhosis (active)	↑↑↑	↑↑	↑	N–↑	—	—	↑↑	↑↑↑
Cirrhosis (inactive)	N–↑	N–↑	N–↑	N–↑	—	—	N–↑	↑↑↑
ETOH hepatitis	↑↑↑	↑–↑↑	↑	N–↑	—	—	↑↑↑	↑↑
Obstruction (intrahepatic)	↑↑	N–↑↑	↑↑–↑↑↑	↑↑	↑↑	↑↑	↑↑↑	↑↑↑
Obstruction (extrahepatic)	N–↑	N–↑	↑↑↑	↑↑↑	↑↑↑	N–↑	↑↑↑	↑↑
Metastatic disease	N	N	↑↑	+/- ↑	—	—	↑↑	↑↑

21. What tests monitor calcium (Ca) in the body?

Ca is the fourth most common extracellular cation and plays a vital role in membrane permeability. The metabolically active Ca in the body is the ionized Ca^{2+} portion, which represents approximately 50% of total serum Ca. The range that is considered normal covers only 0.44 mg/dl, an indication of its physiologic importance. The other half of serum Ca is bound by albumin (45%) and complexed with anions. So the total Ca level will be lowered by decreases in albumin such that for each 1mg/dl drop of albumin, Ca will decrease by 0.8 mg/dl. That is, "corrected" total Ca = 0.8 × (normal albumin − measured albumin) + measured Ca. Possible causes of hypercalcemia include hyperparathyroidism, Paget's disease, metastatic bone tumor, hyperthyroidism, hypervitaminosis D, multiple myeloma, osteoporosis, immbolization, thiazide drugs, and parathyroid secreting tumors (lung, breast). Causes of hypocalcemia include hypoparathyroidism (commonly after thyroid surgery), insufficient vitamin D, chronic renal failure, hypomagnesemia, seizures, acute pancreatitis, and factious due to hypoalbuminemia.

22. What two body elements are commonly linked to Ca metabolism?

Magnesium (Mg) and phosphorous (Ph) play important nutritional roles in the body and are associated with Ca metabolism. Mg is the second most abundant intracellular cation and is found mostly in muscle, soft tissues, and bones (50%). Less than 5% of magnesium circulates in the blood, and 30% of this is bound to albumin. Ph is used interchangeably with phosphate because much of the body's store is as the anion compound. About 80–85% of Ph is found in bones and 10% in muscle, and it is the most common intracellular anion.

Common Causes of Calcium Metabolism Abnormalities

	INCREASED LEVELS	DECREASED LEVELS
Magnesium (Mg)	Renal failure Mg antacid overdose Specimen hemolysis DKA Lithium intoxication Hypothyroidism	Alcoholism Malnutrition Severe diarrhea Hypercalcemia Hemodialysis Loop/thiazide diuretics Hypoalbuminemia Nasogastric suction Pancreatitis Acidosis compensation
Phosphorous (Ph)	Hypoparathyroidism Chronic renal failure Bone diseases Healing fracture Childhood Hemolysis	Hyperparathyroidism Alcoholism Vitamin D deficiency Glucose or insulin administration Hypomagnesemia Diuretics Antacids Nasogastric suction Alkalosis Hypokalemia Gram-negative sepsis

23. What blood tests are used to follow renal function?

BUN (normal: 6–20 mg/dl) and creatinine (normal: 0.7–1.4 mg/dl) blood levels are the products of protein and muscle metabolism, respectively, that are excreted by the kidneys. Decreased levels of creatinine are rarely significant whereas drops in BUN may be due to liver failure (site of urea production), starvation, protein deficiency, overhydration, nephrotic syndrome, or late pregnancy. Elevations of these compounds indicate severely decreased glomerular or tubular function. This can be due to reduced blood volume to kidneys (dehydration, shock, pump failure), increased protein intake, or catabolism. It can also be due to direct parenchymal damage (glomerulonephritis, chronic pyelonephritis, acute tubular necrosis, acute glomerular damage) or obstruction of urine flow (stones, strictures, tumor). These etiologies are often grouped as "prerenal," "renal," and "postrenal," respectively, and may be responsible, separately or in combination, for elevations of the BUN or creatinine.

24. Are there more sensitive indicators of kidney dysfunction?

Yes. Urine clearance of creatinine, specific gravity, osmolality, electrolyte excretion, and free water clearance are tests used to evaluate kidney function. Clearance studies are most sensitive at defining mild-to-moderate, diffuse glomeruler disease by providing an estimate of glomerular filtration rate (GFR). Creatinine is most often used because it estimates GFR with approximately 90% accuracy while urea only approximates to 60%. These studies are very difficult to perform because they require a 24-hour collection and all urine needs to be obtained accurately. In addition, the creatinine clearance must be corrected for variation in muscle mass, age, and sex. Urine specific gravity and osmolality tests measure the renal tubules' ability to concetrate urine and also involve protracted preparation and collection times. All of the above tests give more sensitive information regarding both glomerular and tubular function than BUN or creatinine; however, all are more expensive and difficult to obtain.

25. What information is obtained from a urinalysis?
- **pH** (4.5–8.0). Provides little useful information.
- **Specific gravity** (1.001–1.035). Provides spot view of kidney tubule concentrating ability.
- **Osmolality** (500–1200 mOsm/L). Provides similar information as specific gravity.
- **Blood or hemoglobin**. Results may indicate stone, trauma, tumor, infection, or menstruation.
- **Glucose/acetone**. Negative results may indicate diabetes mellitus, pancreatitis, tubular disease, or shock.
- **Bilirubin**. Negative results may indicate hepatitis or obstructive jaundice.
- **Protein**. Negative results might indicate fever, hypertension, glomerulonephritis, nephrotic syndrome, myeloma, or heavy exercise.
- **Nitrite**. Negative results indicate infection.
- **Leukocyte esterase**. Negative results indicate infection.
- **Ketones**. Negative results may indicate starvation, DKA, vomiting, diarrhea, or pregnancy.
- **Microscopic:**
  Squamous epithelial cells. None may indicate contamination.
  RBC. None may indicate tumor, stone, or pyelonephritis.
  WBC. Count < 5/hpf indicates infection.
  Casts indicate tubular kidney disease or crystals/stones.

26. What laboratory studies are used to evaluate the pancreas?

Because the pancreas is vital for digestion and maintenance of homeostasis, the effects of pancreatic disease are seen in many tests. However, serum levels of amylase (starch-digestion), lipase (fat digestion), and trypsin (protein digestion) allow a direct indication of pancreatic cell damage. Amylase levels peak about 29 hours after the onset of acute pancreatitis as does lipase; however, once active cell damage has stopped, the amylase returns to normal within 72 hours while lipase does not normalize for 7–10 days. Amylase levels may also be elevated because of common bile duct lithiasis, cholecystitis, tumor, peritonitis, peptic ulcer, intra-abdominal hemorrhage, intestinal obstruction or infarction, acute salivary gland disease, DKA, pregnancy, burns, and renal failure. Lipase shows an increased specificity to the pancreas because lipase levels are elevated in pancreatitis, pancreatic duct obstruction, renal failure, and, much less significantly, intestinal obstruction or infarction and cholangitis. Trypsin is the most pancreatic specific exocrine enzyme but this assay is not widely available. Lastly, Ca levels also are followed in acute pancreatitis because it decreases with lipase's digestion of peritoneal fat (fat necrosis) and provides prognostic information.

27. How is blood glucose regulation monitored by the laboratory?

Glucose is regulated primarily by the liver in response to hormones released from structures such as the pancreas (insulin, glucagon), adrenal medulla (epinephrine), and adrenal cortex (cortisol/cortisone). Blood glucose is used most commonly to diagnose diabetes mellitus and to explain altered mental status. A fasting level above 140 mg/dl or nonfasting glucose greater than 200 mg/dl is indicative of diabetes. A glucose tolerance test provides a more accurate assessment of the patient's ability to process glucose but may be inaccurate in cases of fever, stress, afternoon testing, inactivity, advancing age, trauma, or MI. Glycosylated hemoglobin or HgbA1c (normally 6–7% of total Hgb) is used to monitor patient compliance and treatment effectiveness. The amount of Hgb glycosylated is a function of degree and duration of RBC exposure to glucose and illustrates average blood glucose over a 2–4-month period.

An **increase** in glucose levels may indicate diabetes mellitus (type I or II), acute pancreatitis, hyperthyroidism, Cushing's syndrome, acromegaly, epinephrine (e.g., exogenous, pheochromocytoma, stress, burn), advancing age, or sample drawn above intravenous access.

A **decrease** in glucose levels may indicate oral hypoglycemics or exogenous insulin, pancreatitis, starvation, liver disease, sepsis, hypothyroidism, or postprandial "reactive" hypoglycemia (after gastric surgery).

28. What is measured by a "blood gas"?

This test is drawn from an artery (usually radial or femoral) and is sent to the laboratory in ice with the patient's temperature and current oxygen supplementation recorded.

Blood Gas Measurements

	DEFINITION	NORMAL RANGE
pH	Negative logarithm of hydrogen ion concentration	7.35–7.45
pCO_2	Partial pressure of CO_2 gas in blood that is proportional to the amount of dissolved CO_2	34–45 mmHg
HCO_3^-	Concentration of bicarbonate in serum	20–28 mEq/L
Base difference or excess/deficit	The "normal" base amount is calculated using measured Hgb and normal values for pH and HCO_3^- then this is compared to measured amount of blood base	$^+2–^-2$
pO_2	Blood oxygen tension or dissolved O_2 content of plasma	80–95 mmHg. If > 60 years old, the lower limit is dropped 1 mmHg/year until 60 is reached
% SaO_2	Amount of Hgb bound with O_2 compared to the amount of Hgb available	Should be > 90%

29. What components of the blood gas are used in determining acid-base status?

The essential test values are the pH, pCO_2, HCO_3^-, base difference, and anion gap (AG) from the basic metabolic formula:

$$AG = [Na^+] - ([Cl^-] + [HCO_3^-]$$

with a normal value of 8–12 mEq/L. The major buffering system of the blood is bicarbonate-carbonic acid:

$$CO_2 + H_2O \leftrightarrows H_2CO_3 \rightleftarrows H^+ + HCO_3^-$$

where H_2CO_3 = carbonic anhydrase, which is found in RBC and kidney tubule epithelium. pH is determined as follows:

$$pH = pKa + log (base/acid) = pKa + log ([HCO_3^-]/0.03 \times pCO_2)$$

The normal $HCO_3^-/CO_2 = 20/1$.

The lung is the major regulator of pCO_2 with an increase of 10 mmHg in hypoventilation corresponding to a pH drop of 0.08 units. The kidney regulates $[HCO_3^-]$ with response to acid-base abnormalities, taking 1–2 days for correction. Hemoglobin accounts for 75% of nonbicarbonate-based buffering of blood, while phosphate and other extracellular proteins account for the rest.

30. How are acid-base abnormalities determined and classified?

The first step is to evaluate pH. If pH < 7.35, then the finding is **acidosis**. A pH > 7.45 indicates **alkalosis**. The next step uses pCO_2 and HCO_3^- to classify the primary abnormality as **respiratory** or **metabolic**, respectively. Metabolic acidosis is then further classified as an anion gap or nonanion gap problem. There will be a response to the primary disturbance by the opposite component in an attempt to compensate or normalize the pH. Any pH changes beyond 6.8–7.8 are incompatible with life. If the blood gas does not match the calculated compensation then a **mixed acid-base disorder** should be suspected—that is, a respiratory acidosis and metabolic acidosis occurring simultaneously.

31. What are the common causes and compensations in the primary acid-base disorders?

- **Respiratory acidosis** (hypoventilation). pCO_2 > 45 mmHg; HCO_3 increase = change $pCO_2/10$ (acute) or $4 \times \Delta pCO_2/10$ (chronic 2–5 days). Possible etiology: chronic obstructive pulmonary disease (COPD), asthma, cardiac arrest, severe pulmonary edema or pneumonia, injury to airway or chest wall, cerebrovascular accident (CVA), drugs (narcotics, sedatives), foreign body, muscular dystrophy, or myasthenia gravis.
- **Respiratory alkalosis** (hyperventilation). pCO_2 < 35 mmHg; HCO_3 decrease = $2 \times \Delta pCO_2/10$ (acute), $5 \times \Delta pCO_2/10$ (chronic). Possible etiology: anxiety, pain, fever, pulmonary embolus, mechanical overventilation, head injury, hypoxia, increased altitude, interstitial lung disease, pregnancy, hyperthyroidism, hepatic insufficiency, aspirin overdose, or early sepsis.
- **Metabolic acidosis**. HCO_3^- < 20 mEq/L; pCO_2 decrease = $8 + (1.5 \times HCO_3)$. Possible etiology:
  1. Anion gap normal: diarrhea, fistula, renal tubular acidosis
  2. Anion gap increased = extra acid:
     Exogenous: aspirin, methanol, ethylene glycol, ETOH ketoacidosis, hyperalimentation
     Endogenous: lactic acidosis, diabetic or starvation ketoacidosis, uremia, severe dehydration
- **Metabolic alkalosis**. HCO_3^- > 28 mEq/L; CO_2 increase = $0.6 \times \Delta [HCO_3^-]$. Possible etiology: nasogastric suction, vomiting, diuretics, cystic fibrosis, post hypercapnia, Cushing's syndrome, hyperaldosteronism, exogenous steroids, or hypoparathyroidism.

32. What components of the blood gas evaluate oxygenation?

The pO_2 and % SaO_2 are used to monitor oxygenation. The pO_2 gives an estimate of the alveolar gas exchange with inspired air, so that the patient likely has normal ventilation if the pO_2 is normal. The amount of oxygen available to cells is given by the percent oxygen saturation that may also be obtained using pulse oximetry. The "pulse ox" has been shown to measure Hgb O_2 saturation accurately between 70% and 100% or pO_2 > 35–40 mmHg. The oxygen saturation is influenced by temperature, pH, level of 2,3-diphosphoglycerate (DPG), and pO_2 as seen on the sigmoid-shaped O_2 dissociation curve. Hgb's affinity for O_2 is decreased by acidosis, fever, elevated 2,3-DPG, and hypoxia, which causes a shift of the curve to the right, and is increased with alkalosis, hypothermia, decreased 2,3-DPG, and banked blood, which causes a shift to the left.

33. How is an acute myocardial infarction ruled in or ruled out by the lab?

Much like the liver and pancreas, the heart has enzymes and proteins that are released from its cells in damage or death. A single measure of these substances is not adequate to rule out an AMI alone, and they should be checked at least twice in a 12-hour time frame.

1. **AST (SGOT)** is found to increase in 90–95% of AMIs, begins elevation in 8–12 hours, peaks at 1–2 days, and is normal in 3–8 days. There is a rough correlation between degree of elevation and extent of damage to the heart but low specificity for heart muscle.

2. **LDH** levels are elevated in 92–95% of AMIs with slightly increased sensitivity over AST. LDH begins to rise at 24–48 hours, peaks at 2–3 days, and is normal at 5–10 days. Fractionating of isoenzymes shows improved specificity. $LDH_1/LDH_2 > 1$ is seen in 80–85% of AMIs. LDH_1 is found in RBCs, heart, and kidney, and normal values at 24 and 48 hours effectively rule out AMI.

3. **Creatine kinase** (CK) is increased in 90–93% of AMIs. Levels begin to rise in 3–6 hours, peak in 12–24 hours, and are normal in 1–2 days. Fractionated isozymes are MM (skeletal muscle, 94–100% of total), BB (brain and lung, usually 0% of total), and MB (heart fraction usually less than 6% of total) and allow greater test specificity. There is a rough correlation with size of increase and amount of heart infarcted. Levels are usually checked at 0, 12, and 24 hours or 0, 8, 16, and 24 hours.

4. **Troponin-T** is an antibody that detects the cardiac-specific regulatory proteins. It has approximately the same specificity and sensitivity as CK-MB but rises in 4–6 hours, peaks at 11 hours, and is normal in 4 days.

5. **Troponin-I** is the same as above, but its timing is different; it begins to rise after 4–6 hours, peaks 10–24 hours, and is normal after 10 days or more.

34. What tests are used to evaluate possible collagen vascular diseases?

Several nonspecific laboratory tests are used to help diagnose these enigmatic diseases:

- **Rheumatoid factor**—Positive in collagen vascular diseases, rheumatoid arthritis (RA), systemic lupus erythematosus (SLE), scleroderma, polyarteritis nodosa, infections, CHF, inflammation, subacute bacterial endocarditis, MI, and lung disease
- **Lupus erythematosus (LE) preparation**—No cells = normal; positive in SLE, RA, scleroderma, and drug-induced lupus
- **Antinuclear antibody (ANA)**—Negative result = normal; positive in SLE, scleroderma, drug-induced lupus, mixed connective tissue disease, RA, polymyositis, and juvenile RA
- **Antimicrosomal**—Detects Hashimoto's thyroiditis
- **Anticentromere**—Tests for scleroderma, Raynaud's disease, CREST syndrome
- **Anti–SCL 70**—Detects scleroderma
- **Anti-DNA**—Detects SLE, mononucleosis, chronic active hepatitis

35. What are C-reactive protein (C-RP) and erythrocyte sedimentation rate (ESR) tests used to evaluate?

The C-RP and ESR are nonspecific but very sensitive markers for infections and inflammatory diseases. The ESR measure changes in plasma proteins (mainly fibrinogen) and is evaluated using several scales (zeta sedimentation ratio, Wintrobe method, Westergren method). The ESR is increased by any infection, inflammation, rheumatic fever, endocarditis, neoplasm, or AMI. The C-RP is a glycoprotein produced by acute inflammation and tissue destruction. Its levels are noted to begin elevating 4–6 hours after onset of inflammation and should be normal 5–7 days postoperatively or at least decreasing by day 3 after surgery, otherwise an infection is likely. Other than inflammation or infection, the C-RP is also increased by pregnancy, oral contraceptives, and malignancies.

36. What tests are used to screen for thyroid disease?

The most sensitive screening test for thyroid disease is the thyroid stimulating hormone (TSH) level. It is elevated in hypothyroidism and low in hyperthyroidism. The thyroxine total (T_4 Tot) screens for hyperthyroidism with 95% sensitivity but is less accurate for hypothyroidism. Triiodothyronine (T_3) resin uptake (RU) is an indirect measurement of T_4. By measuring the protein thyroid binding sites that are unbound, the test is elevated in hyperthyroidism, as a result of low thyroid binding globulin (TBG), or if the patient is taking medications that bind TBG (e.g., phenytoin, aspirin, steroids, heparin). The T_3 RU is 80% sensitive for hyperthyroidism but only 40% for hypothyroidism. The free thyroxine index (FTI) is determined by multiplying the T_4 Tot by the T_3 RU and has a 95% sensitivity for hyperthyroidism and 90–95% sensitivity for hypothyroidism. The FTI attempts to balance the TBG effects on T_4 measurement. TBG is elevated in pregnancy, estrogen use, liver disease, and hypothyroidism. Total serum T_3 (T_3-RIA) is also measured in some labs and is equivalent to T_4 Tot measurements.

37. What tests can be used to evaluate possible bone disease?

The Ca and phosphorous levels (discussed previously). Alkaline phosphatase can also be used and is elevated in hyperparathyroidism, Paget's disease, osteoblastic bone tumors, osteo-malacia, rickets, pregnancy, childhood, healing fractures, hyperthyroidism, and liver disease. The liver disorders may be ruled out using fractionated enzyme levels or checking GGT or 5'-nucleotidase.

38. What procedures are done to evaluate body fluids and pathology specimens for organisms?

The most definitive test to isolate infectious agents is culturing but this requires 24 hours at minimum. Staining allows for rapid screening identification to assist in selecting empiric antibiotics. The most common stains are:

- **Gram:** "Positive" organisms turn violet color because the microorganisms' thick cell walls of peptidoglycan and teichoic acid resist decolorization. "Negative" organisms have a thin cell wall and outer lipoprotein or lipopolysaccharide coat that decolorize in alcohol and pick up the counterstain (red).
- **Acid-fast:** These organisms do not decolorize in strong acid and are usually mycobac-terium species.
- **Potassium hydroxide** (KOH): 10% KOH dissolves most cellular elements except for fungus species.
- **Wayson** is used for general bacteria screening.
- **India ink** identifies mostly fungus in cerebrospinal fluid (CSF).
- **Giemsa** stains intracellular organisms (chlamydia, malaria) and viral inclusion bodies.

Newer technology with DNA/PCR probes and enzyme-linked immunosorbent assay (ELISA) tests allow rapid detection of organisms (e.g., *Gonozyme*, *Streptozyme*) or monospot tests.

39. What tests are used to evaluate viral hepatitis?

Hepatitis A. Oral/fecal hepatitis is usually self-limited. Acute infection tests positive IgM plus or minus IgG. Old infection or convalescence tests negative IgM but positive IgG. The antigen may be detected in stool but usually is gone prior to symptoms.

Hepatitis B. Blood-borne disease with 1% acute fatality, 5–15% develop chronic disease, 3% develop hepatoma:

- HBsAg—surface antigen from viral outer envelope indicates current or active HBV in-fection; DNA PCR Probe is most accurate indicator of activity, infectivity, and progres-sion to chronicity.
- Anti-HBs—indicates immunity and end of acute HBV.
- Anti-HBcAg (presence of antibody to core viral protein)—indicates a recent or acute infection and is present during "core window" while HBsAg and anti-HBs are negative; drops out after 3–6 months.
- Anti-HBc Tot—stays positive for life, shows old infection if HBsAg and HBc-IgM are negative.
- HBeAg/Anti-HBe—indicate infectivity, because as anti-HBe increases, the infectivity decreases.

• Chronic hepatitis B states:
 Carrier—positive HBsAg but negative biopsy and liver function tests (LFTs).
 Persistent hepatitis B—as above with negative biopsy and abnormal LFTs.
 Active hepatitis B—as above with positive biopsy and abnormal LFTs.
  Hepatitis C. Post-transfusion transmission; low severity acutely but 60% for chronic disease. HCV nucleic probe shows current infection but this is still investigational, and anti-HC indicates current, convalescing, or old HCV infection.
  Hepatitis D. Requires HBV infection to be present, parenteral transmission, 5% acute fatality, 5% chronic. HDAg indicates infection; may follow with antibody levels.

40. What tests are used to detect and monitor HIV infection?

HIV antigen detection is used by blood banks because they may detect viral presence as early as 1–2 weeks. Antibodies are used to detect core proteins p24 or p55 and envelope glycoproteins gp41, 120, or 160. They are about 80–90% sensitive if patients have symptoms but 60–65% without. Nucleic acid probe with PCR amplification is also being used with 98% sensitivity at 3 months but 40–60% at 1–2 weeks. More commonly, patients are screened for the presence of antibodies in their serum, which take an average of 6–10 weeks to develop or "seroconvert." The ELISA screens the patients' blood for antibodies. A positive ELISA is confirmed by Western blot, which looks for the most specific antibodies to gp41 and p24 or group-specific antigen (gag) core protein. Once HIV infection is determined, the CD4 T-cell count, viral load, and beta$_2$-microglobulin levels are followed for infection severity, prognosis, and activity and to direct therapy. The CD4 count (normal 600–1600 cells/mm^3) is a useful indicator of immune system damage and ability to respond effectively to pathogens. Immune suppression occurs with counts below 500 cells/mm^3 denoting an advanced risk of opportunistic infections and need for prophylactic antibiotics. Viral load assays appear to be the best prognostic marker for a patient's long-term clinical outcome and are used in conjunction with CD4 counts to direct antiviral therapy. Beta$_2$-microglobulin is a soluble marker for immune system activation and can be used to evaluate disease progression or exacerbation.

41. What tests screen or assist diagnosis of cancer?

  Alphafetoprotein (AFP). Elevated in hepatoma, testicular tumors, occasionally benign hepatic disease (hepatitis, alcoholic cirrhosis), and in pregnancy, neural tube defects, multiple gestation, or fetal death.
  Cancer antigen 19-9 (CA 19-9). Elevated in 80–85% pancreatic adenocarcinoma, 40–50% gastric adenocarcinoma, 30–40% colorectal cancer, 50% hepatoma, 16–20% lung cancer, and 14–27% of breast cancer.
  CA 125. Increased in ovarian, endometrial, colon cancers also endometriosis, inflammatory bowel disease, pelvic inflammatory disease, pregnancy, breast lesion, and teratomas.
  Carcinoembryonic antigen (CEA). Not used to screen but is a good monitor of recurrence and response to treatment (if checked before started). Elevated in colon, pancreas, lung, and stomach cancers as well as in smokers and those with Crohn's disease, liver disease, and ulcerative colitis.
  Prostate specific antigen (PSA). Good for screening and monitoring after treatment. Levels above 10 mg/dl are associated with cancer > 90%. Also, a "velocity" of 0.75 mg/ml/year indicates high suspicion for cancer. Differential for elevation includes prostate cancer, acute prostatitis, benign prostate hypertrophy, prostate surgery, and vigorous prostate massage. Normal rectal has no influence.

42. What basic tests are used to evaluate cerebrospinal fluid?

  Opening pressure. Normal is 100–200 mmHg; most significantly elevated in bacterial infections (meningitis) and subarachnoid hemorrhage (SAH).
  Color or appearance. Normal is clear and colorless, but is bloody or xanthochromic (yellow from Hgb breakdown) after 2–8 hours in SAH and is white or cloudy in bacterial infections.

Glucose. Normal is $\frac{1}{2}$ serum glucose (45–80 mg/dl), but will be < 20 mg/dl in meningitis and between 20 and 40 mg/dl in granulomatous infection (TB or fungal).

Protein. Normal range is 15–45 mg/dl but the upper limit is debated. Levels will be 50–1500 mg/dl in meningitis and will be increased but < 500 mg/dl in granulomatous disease.

Cell count. Normal is up to 5/mm^3 with all being lymphocytes; any condition that affects the meninges will cause CSF leukocytosis, the degree being determined by type, duration, and severity of irritation. The highest counts are seen in meningitis with PMNs dominating, while viral and granulomatous disease cause elevations to 10–500 cells, with lymphocytes predominant. SAH and traumatic taps will have increased cell counts made up of RBCs and WBCs in a ratio about equal to blood (1 WBC per 500–1000 RBCs). However, no good formulas exist to confirm that the WBC elevation is an artifact from a traumatic tap versus infective or inflammatory increase. Gram stain and culture are performed in all suspected infective taps.

43. What tests can be done to verify or exclude a cerebrospinal fluid leak in craniofacial trauma?

Confirmation of CSF oto- or rhinorrhea in trauma can be challenging. Typically, one looks for a colorless fluid, glucose about 45 mg/dl (nasal secretions < 30 mg/dl and blood > 80 usually), and low protein and potassium compared to nasal secretions or serum. Trauma patients, however, often exhibit a complex mixture of these body fluids blocking chemical analysis. The most sensitive and specific test requires about 2–10 µl of fluid, protein electrophoresis, and about 3 hours to complete in a modern laboratory. The beta$_2$-transferrin isozyme will be isolated correctly in the presence of any mixture of fluid, and a beta$_1$ subset allows reduction of cirrhotic false-positive results. This test helps prevent the need for more invasive radiologic studies to rule out CSF leak.

BIBLIOGRAPHY

1. Aziz N, Detels R, Fahey JL, et al: Prognostic significance of plasma markers of immune activation, HIV viral load and CD4 T-cell measurements. AIDS 12:1581–1590, 1998.
2. Burns ER, Lawrence C: Bleeding time. A guide to its diagnostic and clinical utility. Arch Pathol Lab Med 113:1219–1224, 1989.
3. Fauci A (ed): Harrison's Principles of Internal Medicine, 14th ed. New York, McGraw-Hill, 1997.
4. Gomella LG (ed): Clinician's Pocket Reference, 8th ed. Stamford, CT, Appleton & Lange, 1997.
5. Jacobs DS, et al: Laboratory Test Handbook, 4th ed. Hudson, OH, Lexi-Corp, 1996.
6. Kaiser R, Kupfer B, Rockstroh JK, et al: Role of HIV-1 phenotype in viral pathogenesis and its relation to viral load and CD4+ T-cell count. J Med Virol 56:259–263, 1998.
7. Keane CB, Miller BF: Encyclopedia and Dictionary of Medicine, Nursing, and Allied Health, 6th ed. Philadelphia, W.B. Saunders, 1997.
8. Kwon P, Laskin D (eds): Clinical Manual of Oral and Maxillofacial Surgery, 2nd ed. Chicago, Quintessence, 1997.
9. Little JW, Falace DA, Miller CS, Rhodus NL (eds): Dental Management of the Medically Compromised Patient, 5th ed. St. Louis, Mosby, 1997.
10. Malley W: Clinical Blood Gases: Application and Noninvasive Alternatives. Philadelphia, W.B. Saunders, 1990.
11. Patton LL, Shugars DC: Immunologic and viral markers of HIV-1 disease progression: Implications for dentistry. J Am Dent Assoc 130:1313–1322, 1999.
12. Peacock MK, Ryall RG, Simpson DA: Usefulness of beta$_2$-transferrin assay in the detection of cerebrospinal fluid leaks following head injury. J Neurosurg 77:737–739, 1992.
13. Ravel R: Clinical Laboratory Medicine, 6th ed. St. Louis, Mosby, 1995.
14. Schwarz SI, Shires GT, Spencer FC (eds): Principles of Surgery, 7th ed. New York, McGraw-Hill, 1998.
15. Tietz N: Clinical Guide to Laboratory Tests, 3rd ed. Philadelphia, W.B. Saunders, 1995.
16. Zaret DL, Morrison N, Gulbranson R, Keren DF: Immunofixation to quantify beta2-transferrin in cerebrospinal fluid to detect leakage of cerebrospinal fluid from skull injury. Clin Chem 38:1908–1912, 1992.

4. DIAGNOSTIC IMAGING FOR THE ORAL AND MAXILLOFACIAL REGIONS

A. Omar Abubaker, D.M.D., Ph.D., Robert E. Doriot, D.D.S., and James A. Giglio, D.D.S., M.Ed.

1. Describe the radiographic patterns of disease on an x-ray examination of the chest.

The patterns of disease on a chest radiograph are limited. The three most common patterns are:

1. **Alveolar.** Pulmonary alveolar disease is the most common pattern and appears as a localized, homogeneous, fluffy density. It can represent water, blood, pus, or tumor within the alveoli.

2. **Interstitial.** The interstitial pattern may be reticular (linear), nodular, or a combination of the two (reticulonodular). The reticular pattern usually is bilateral and diffuse.

3. **Nodular.** The nodular pattern of disease appears as discrete, well-circumscribed, radiopaque masses in the lung field.

2. What is the diagnostic value of posteroanterior (PA) chest films?

A PA chest film is taken by directing an x-ray beam from posterior to anterior on the chest. This radiograph is useful to evaluate the soft tissue and bony tissues of the chest, the diaphragm, the heart and mediastinum, the hila of the lungs, and the entire PA view of the lung fields.

3. What are the main uses of a lateral chest film?

• Localizing lesions to a specific area of the lungs or mediastinum
• Diagnosing small pleural effusions (blunting of the posterior costophrenic angles)
• Diagnosing vertebral and sternal abnormalities

4. Describe the chest x-ray appearance of a pneumothorax.

Pneumothorax is usually represented by a thin, linear density that parallels the chest wall. No long markings should be seen peripheral to this line. In tension pneumothorax, a shift in the mediastinum is seen, especially with a large tension pneumothorax.

5. What radiographic changes are associated with chronic obstructive pulmonary disease (COPD)?

Hyperexpanded lung fields
Flattening of the diaphragm
A large, radiolucent zone behind the sternum
Elongated heart

6. How do lung masses show up on chest film?

Lung masses usually follow the nodular pattern of disease. Masses within the lung fields can be divided into **cavitary** and **noncavitary lesions** and represent either tumor or infection. Other causes of masses include vascular malformations, but these are far less common than tumor and infection.

7. What is a lordotic chest radiograph used for?

A lordotic chest radiograph permits better visualization of the apices of the lung. This view should be obtained when a questionable lesion is seen in these areas on a standard chest radiograph.

8. Describe the common radiographic finding of chest radiographs in AIDS patients.

Infectious pulmonary disease. *Pneumocystis carinii* pneumonia, the most common infection, usually has the pattern of a fine, diffuse reticular process.

9. Which views are included in an acute abdominal series? When are they used?

1. Supine and upright abdominal films (to view the kidneys, ureter, and bladder)
2. Chest radiograph

These views are used for the initial evaluation of acute abdominal pain or trauma.

10. What is a KUB?

KUB is a radiographic view to evaluate the *k*idneys, *u*reters, and *b*ladder. The series, which is also known as a **supine abdominal radiograph**, is useful in the initial work-up of abdominal pain, distention of the bowel, and change of bowel habits. It is also used for evaluation of urinary tract problems. Renal stones and 10–20% of gallstones are visualized by a KUB. Evaluation of the KUB views involves examining the bowel gas pattern and looking for calcifications and radiopaque foreign bodies. The psoas; renal, liver, and splenic shadows; flank stripes; vertebral bodies; and pelvic bones are also examined.

11. What is a barium swallow (esophagram)?

An esophagram, usually performed with barium, a water-soluble contrast agent, is used to evaluate the swallowing mechanism and to look for esophageal lesions or abnormal peristalsis. No preparation is required for this study.

12. What is the upper gastrointestinal series (UGI)?

UGI, which includes an esophagram, is used to study the stomach and duodenum. This double-contrast study uses barium and air and is useful for detection of gastritis, ulcers, masses, hiatal hernias, and gastrointestinal reflux. It is also an important part of the work-up of heme-positive stools and upper abdominal pain.

13. Define intravenous pyelogram (IVP).

This imaging technique uses intravenous contrast to evaluate the kidneys, ureters, and bladder. This test is indicated for patients with hematuria, kidney stones, urinary tract infection, and suspected malignancy of the kidney or bladder and is used for the work-up of patients with flank pain.

14. Describe the different nuclear scans and their uses.

In nuclear scans, or nuclear medicine studies, radionuclides are injected intravenously, and results are based on detection of the tissue uptake of these radionuclides, specifically the degree of uptake, the time intervals between the study, and the injection of the radionuclides.

1. **Bone scan** is a nuclear scan study used in metastatic work-ups, especially in patients with cancer that has a predilection to metastasize to bone (e.g., breast, prostate, kidney, lung, thyroid). It is also used as a screening test for primary tumors, osteomyelitis, avascular necrosis, and stress fractures.

2. **Gallium scan** is used to locate abscesses that are over 5–10 days old. When used in combination with a bone scan, the gallium scan is very specific for osteomyelitis. **Indium 111 white blood cell scans** can be substituted for gallium scanning to detect osteomyelitis.

3. **Cardiac scan** has become increasingly popular in recent years and is used for many purposes, including detection of myocardial infarction and ischemia, stress testing, and evaluation of ejection fractions, cardiac output, and ventricular aneurysms.

4. **Liver-spleen scan** is used to estimate parenchymal disease, abscess, tumors, and cysts in these organs. The current preference for computed tomography (CT) scanning has significantly decreased the use of the liver-spleen scan.

5. **Ventilation-perfusion lung scan** is used principally for the evaluation of pulmonary emboli. Although not as sensitive or specific as a pulmonary angiogram, the ventilation-perfusion scan is less invasive and often is obtained following a chest radiograph when the diagnosis of pulmonary embolus is suspected.

15. What views are included in a facial series?

Facial series usually include Caldwell's view, Waters' view, lateral skull view, and submentovertex view (view of the zygomatic arches). These studies are used for the initial work-up of facial trauma.

16. What is the purpose of a mandibular series?

Mandibular series includes a Towne's view, a PA skull view, both oblique views of the mandible, and a panoramic view. This series is used mainly for evaluation of the mandible following facial trauma.

17. What views are included in a nasal bone series?

Nasal bone series includes an anteroposterior (AP) skull view and both lateral views of the nasal bones. This series is used for evaluation of trauma to the nose.

18. Describe the sinus series.

A sinus series is used for evaluating the paranasal sinuses, including the frontal, ethmoid, maxillary, and sphenoid sinuses. The views taken usually include a Caldwell's, Waters', lateral, and submentovertex. This series is used for the initial evaluation of sinusitis or sinus masses.

19. What views are included in the cervical spine series?

The cervical spine series usually includes PA and lateral views, both oblique views, and odontoid views of the cervical spine. This series is useful for evaluating traumatic injury, neck pain, and neurologic symptoms referable to the upper extremities. All seven cervical vertebrae must be seen for the examination to be considered acceptable.

20. What views are included in airway films?

Airway films include AP and lateral views of the neck to provide good visualization of the airways and adjacent soft tissues. It is used as the initial step in the work-up of masses, foreign bodies, and infections of the airway.

21. Explain the uses and advantages of plain film tomography.

With the advent of CT, plain film tomography now has only limited utility in the evaluation of problems within the head and neck. Its principal advantage is that it does not show the metallic artifact that often obscures the CT evaluation of postoperative patients. It also has the advantage of allowing three-plane evaluation of bony structures, which can only be accomplished with CT scans by reconstruction of axial views. In evaluating temporomandibular joints (TMJs), sagittal tomography frequently provides more information about the bony architecture of this joint than axial CT scans do.

22. Define sialography.

Sialography is an imaging study used for the radiographic demonstration of the salivary gland ductal system. It is accomplished by cannulating the ducts of the submandibular and parotid glands and injecting a radiopaque contrast medium.

23. When is sialography indicated?

- To detect or confirm small radiopaque or radiolucent sialoliths or foreign bodies
- To evaluate damage secondary to recurrent inflammation

- To provide a more detailed evaluation of suspected neoplasms such as size, location, and extension into adjacent tissues
- To evaluate fistulas, strictures, and diverticula of the ductal system, especially in post-traumatic cases
- To detect chronic sialadenitis and chronic stricture (rarely used)

24. When is sialography contraindicated?
- In patients with known sensitivity to iodine compounds
- In acute salivary inflammation

25. What does the obstructive form of salivary gland disease look like on a sialogram?
In the acute form of obstructive salivary gland disease and acute sialadenitis, sialography is rarely performed and mostly contraindicated. However, a sialogram performed during a clinically quiescent period of the disease in a patient with the obstructive form of the disease usually shows a focal narrowing (stricture) of the main duct and a central dilatation (sialecta-sia) with these ducts tapering dramatically to normal peripheral ducts. If the acini are compressed and destroyed by the cellular infiltrate, the peripheral ducts and acini are not visualized, even on a technically good sialogram.

26. What is the appearance of Sjögren's syndrome on a sialogram?
Sjögren's syndrome initially involves only the peripheral intraglandular ducts and acini. Accordingly, the early stages of the disease are manifested on a sialogram as normal central duct system and numerous, uniform, peripheral punctate collections of contrast material throughout the gland. These changes are the earliest sialographic features and are diagnostic of the disease. As the disease progresses, the sialogram is said to resemble a leafless fruit-laden tree or a mulberry tree. The advanced form of the disease is seen on a sialogram as di-latation of the central ducts and, eventually, a large peripheral collection of the contrast material and the associated changes of sialadenitis superimposed on the punctate and globular findings of Sjögren's syndrome.

27. How are disc perforations of the TMJ diagnosed?
Although magnetic resonance imaging (MRI) is usually the first choice for soft tissue imaging of the TMJ in most clinical situations, the best imaging modality available to diagnose disc perforations is arthrography. Because of the recent decrease in use of arthrography, diagnosis of disc perforation currently is based on clinical examination.

28. What are the main disadvantages to arthrography?
TMJ arthrography is an invasive imaging modality that requires a skilled, well-trained, and knowledgeable radiologist. It also can be associated with some degree of pain and discomfort.

29. List the advantages and disadvantages of MRI for the diagnosis of TMJ pathology.
Advantages
Provides an image of both hard and soft tissue structures of the TMJ in multiple planes
Does not use radiation
Is not technically demanding
Disadvantages
Is expensive for patients
Is not well tolerated by patients suffering from claustrophobia

30. When is MRI contraindicated?
MRI is absolutely contraindicated in patients with cerebral aneurysm clips and cardiac pacemakers. However, it should be noted that titanium in bone plates and dental implants do not affect the MRI examination.

31. How can CT assist in dental implant treatment planning?

Historically, implant patients were evaluated with panoramic, intraoral, and cephalometric films to determine the location of the inferior alveolar nerve, sinus location, and ridge height. However, exact measurements are not possible, and these films do not allow assessment of the average width of the ridge. Hence, a CT program was developed (DentaScan) that provides direct axial images of the mandible and maxilla to permit accurate measurements for implant length and width and visualization of internal anatomy.

32. How is diagnostic and interventional angiography used by the oral and maxillofacial surgeon?

Diagnostic and interventional angiography assists the oral and maxillofacial surgeon in the diagnosis and delineation of uncontrollable hemorrhage and vascular tumors in the maxillofacial region. When coupled with CT and MRI examinations, the surgical approach and definitive treatment can be planned. The use of interventional angiography for embolization of vascular tumors prior to or instead of surgical resection has become a popular modality in the management of these tumors.

33. What is the role of radionuclide scintigraphy in oral and maxillofacial surgery?

Oral and maxillofacial surgeons use radionuclide scintigraphy to evaluate bone and joint diseases because it provides more sensitive bone imaging than conventional radiologic techniques. Specifically, scintigraphy or bone scanning can assist in the evaluation of arthritic changes to the TMJ, condylar hyperplasia, idiopathic condylar resorption (active and inactive), metabolic disorders, viability of bone grafts, trauma, dental disorders, osteomyelitis, and malignancies. However, it should be noted that scintigraphy has a low specificity for abnormal findings, and 20–50% of patients referred for routine bone scan may have abnormal activity in the mandible or face.

34. What diagnostic imaging modalities are useful for the diagnosis of cysts and benign odontogenic tumors of the jaw?

Most pathologies in the oral and maxillofacial region can be demonstrated through conventional radiographs. The panoramic radiograph is still the primary screening film for the oral and maxillofacial surgeon, but CT and MRI have proven to be useful adjuncts, especially when planning surgical intervention. CT is extremely helpful for illustrating cysts and tumors of the mandible and maxilla especially if the lesion extends beyond the bony cortex with encroachment on the adjacent soft tissue structures. MRI is useful in differentiating cysts from solid tumors and differentiating fluid within the cystic lumen from other cystic components such as keratin and blood degradation products.

35. What diagnostic imaging modalities are used for evaluation of malignant diseases of the jaws?

CT

MRI

Panoramic radiography

Polycycloidal tomography

Radionuclide scanning techniques

Radiologic evaluation of jaw lesions requires an image that accurately differentiates bone and soft tissue. CT permits the accurate assessment of tumor size, location, and extent of spread and detects subtle bony involvement and calcifications. However, MRI provides high-resolution, thin tomographic images with superior soft tissue contrast. In addition, MRI allows visualization of blood vessels without intravenous contrast agents and some information regarding tissue composition.

36. What are the uses of the different imaging techniques for mandibular fractures?

Plain films are the most cost-effective and adequate means to image mandibular injuries. The panoramic radiograph is still the primary imaging modality used by the oral and maxillofacial surgeon to evaluate mandibular fractures. AP, lateral skull, Waters', and Towne's views also can be helpful. Additionally, CT examination in the axial and coronal planes can assist in the diagnosis of mandibular fractures, especially in the condylar-subcondylar region.

37. Which imaging modalities are used to diagnose midfacial fractures?

The initial radiographic survey of patients with midface trauma should include Waters', Towne's, AP, lateral skull, and submentovertex views. However, because the facial bone diverges in a posterior-to-anterior direction, AP views distort bone anatomy and produce magnified and overlapping structural images. Hence, CT is the definitive means of imaging midfacial trauma. Generally, axial views are easily obtained and quite useful, but they should be supplemented with views in the coronal plane. Direct coronal views are obtained to appreciate the orbital roof, floor, palate, and maxillary alveolar processes. However, direct coronal views are attainable only after the patient's cervical spine is clear because the patient must assume a position with the neck in hypertension. If direct coronals are not possible, reconstruction data from axial images may be used to obtain coronal images. These reconstructed images are usually somewhat deformed and misleading because the pixel edges of each slice give a serrated appearance to bone surfaces; they will, however, demonstrate gross discrepancies in position or size of structures.

38. What imaging techniques are used for evaluation of maxillary sinus pathology?

Radiographic examination of the maxillary sinus is routinely conducted as a standard sinus series in three imaging planes with the patient in the upright position, allowing fluid and air to be separated horizontally. The standard sinus series generally includes Waters', Caldwell, lateral skull, and submentovertex views, but it can be supplemented with panoramic radiography. If indicated by the plain film examination, a CT can be performed to allow visualization of both bony and soft tissues. In addition, CT allows visualization of the extent of bone destruction and soft tissue reactions to disease including infiltrations. Recently, MR tomography has proven to be a useful imaging modality for the sinuses owing to its superior soft tissue imaging and ability to demonstrate edematous and inflammatory changes with great clarity. Furthermore, MRI is not affected by the beam-hardening artifacts from dental amalgam or dense cortical bone.

39. What imaging modalities are used for diagnosis of inflammatory disorders of the jaw?

Most inflammatory disorders of the jaw can be evaluated by plain radiographs, but plain films may require supplementation by CT, MRI, or radionuclide scanning techniques. MRI and CT are helpful in determining the extent of the pathology and any localized destruction and invasion, especially in cases of osteomyelitis. Scintigraphy or radionuclide imaging is the most definitive way of demonstrating bone changes and clinical activity caused by inflammation or suspected osteomyelitis.

40. Which imaging techniques will reveal soft tissue infection in the head and neck regions?

The primary imaging modalities to evaluate infection in the head and neck are CT and MRI. CT and MRI both differentiate abscess from cellulitis, indicate the presence of venous thrombosis and airway compromise, and show the exact location and extent of the infectious process. CT is better than MRI in evaluating the integrity of cortical bone, and CT takes less time, costs less, and is more readily available than MRI. MRI, on the other hand, allows imaging in the sagittal, coronal, and axial planes with the patient supine, does not use radiation, and is not affected or degraded by artifacts from dental amalgam.

BIBLIOGRAPHY

1. Abrams JJ: CT assessment of dental implant planning. Oral Maxillofac Surg Clin North Am 4:1–18, 1992.
2. Barsotti JB, Westesson PL, Ketonen LM: Diagnostic and interventional angiographic procedures in the maxillofacial region. Oral Maxillofac Surg Clin North Am 4:35–50, 1992.

 3. Conway WF: Diagnostic imaging. In Kwon PH, Laskin DM (eds): Clinical Manual of Oral and Maxillofacial Surgery, 2nd ed. Chicago, Quintessence Books, 1996, pp 41–54.
 4. Dolan KD, Ruprecht A: Imaging of mandibular and temporomandibular joint fractures. Oral Maxillofac Surg Clin North Am 4:113–124, 1992.
 5. Dolan KD, Ruprecht A: Imaging of midface fractures. Oral Maxillofac Surg Clin North Am 4:125–152, 1992.
 6. Holliday RA, Prendergast NC: Imaging inflammatory processes of the oral cavity and suprahyoid neck. Oral Maxillofac Surg Clin North Am 4:215–240, 1992.
 7. Miles DA: Imaging inflammatory disorders of the jaw: simple osteitis to generalized osteomyelitis. Oral Maxillofac Surg Clin North Am 4:207–214, 1992.
 8. O'Mara RE: Scintigraphy of the Facial Skeleton. Oral Maxillofacial Surg Clin North Am 4:51–60, 1992.
 9. Som PM, Brandweir M: Salivary glands. In Som PM, Curtin HD (eds): Head and Neck Imaging, Vol 2. St. Louis, Mosby, 1996, pp 823–914.
10. Sune, Ericson: Conventional and oral computerized imaging of maxillary sinus pathology related to dental problems. Oral Maxillofac Surg Clin North Am 4:153–182, 1992.
11. van Rensburg LJ, Nortje CJ: Magnetic resonance imaging and computed tomography of malignant disease of the jaws. Oral Maxillofac Surg Clin North Am 4:75–112, 1992.
12. Wandtke JC: Chest imaging for the oral and maxillofacial surgeon. Oral Maxillofac Surg Clin North Am 4:241–252, 1992.
13. Weber AL: Imaging of cysts and benign odontogenic tumors of the jaw. Oral Maxillofac Surg Clin North Am 4:61–74, 1992.
14. Westesson P: Magnetic resonance imaging of the temporomandibular joint. Oral Maxillofac Surg Clin North Am 4:183–206, 1992.
15. White SC: Computer-assisted radiographic differential diagnosis of jaw lesions. Oral Maxillofac Surg Clin North Am 4:261–272, 1992.

II. Anesthesia

5. LOCAL ANESTHETICS

Christopher L. Maestrello, D.D.S.

1. What is the maximum amount of 2% lidocaine with 1:100,000 epinephrine (in milligrams) that can be administered to a healthy 150-pound man?

477 mg. The maximum dose of 2% lidocaine with 1:100,000 epinephrine for the adult patient is 7 mg/kg. Convert pounds to milligrams by dividing by 2.2.

$$150 \text{ lb} \div 2.2 \text{ lb/kg} = 68 \text{ kg}$$

$$68 \text{ kg} \times 7 \text{ mg/kg} = 477 \text{ mg}$$

Adult Dosages for Commonly Used Local Anesthetics in Dentistry*

AGENT	MG/CARTRIDGE	MAXIMUM DOSE MG/KG	MAXIMUM DOSE MG/LB	MAXIMUM DOSE
2% lidocaine	36	4.5	2	300
2% lidocaine with 1:100,000 epinephrine	36	7	3.3	500
3% mepivacaine	54	5.5	2.6	400
2% mepivacaine with 1:20,000 levonordefrin	36	5.5	2.6	400
4% prilocaine	72	8	4	600
4% prilocaine with 1:200,000 epinephrine	72	8	4	600
0.5% bupivacaine with 1:200,000 epinephrine	9	1.3	0.6	90
1.5% etidocaine with 1:200,000 epinephrine	27	5.5	2.6	400
4% articaine† with 1:100,000 epinephrine	68	7	3.2	500

* Maximum dosages are based on an adult weight of 150 lb or 70 kg and taken from the following manufacturers: Astra (Xylocaine, prilocaine, Citanest, Duranest), Cook-Waite (Marcaine), and Septodont (Septocaine)
† Articaine (Septocaine) dosages are based on a 1.7-cc cartridge.

2. In the above scenario, how many dental cartridges does this equal?

Thirteen cartridges. One dental cartridge of 2% lidocaine with 1:100,000 epinephrine contains 20 mg/cc of lidocaine. A 1.8-cc cartridge contains 36 mg of lidocaine.

$$477 \text{ mg} \div 36 \text{ mg/cartridge} = 13.25 \text{ cartridges.}$$

Outside the United States, anesthetic manufactures also provide 2.2-cc dental cartridges of 2% lidocaine with 1:100,000 epinephrine, with the total amount of comparable local anesthetic being 44 mg. *Note:* Articaine is packaged as a 1.7-cc cartridge in the United States.

3. How many dental cartridges of lidocaine or mepivacaine can be administered to a 30-pound child? What should be considered when selecting a local anesthetic for children?

The pharmaceutical industry generally is not required to perform drug testing on the pediatric population; therefore definitive maximum drug dosages are often unknown. In addition, pharmaceutical manufacturers are reluctant to recommend maximum pediatric dosages of a drug because of variations in age and weight. Two standard formulas can be used to calculate pediatric drug dosages: Young's rule, which is based on the child's age, and Clark's rule, which is based on the child's weight. Clark's rule, the preferred formula, is as follows:

Maximum pediatric dose = (weight child in lb. ÷ 150) × (maximum adult dose in mg)

The maximum number of cartridges has been calculated for the following local anesthetics:

2% lidocaine with 1:100,000 epinephrine	2.7 cartridges
2% lidocaine	1.6 cartridges
2% mepivacaine with 1:20,000 levonordefrin	2.2 cartridges
3% mepivacaine	1.5 cartridges

It is easy to exceed the maximum dose of local anesthetics with the pediatric patient. The practitioner needs to be especially careful if, for example, a child requires extraction of four abscessed teeth that are located in different quadrants. If all four teeth are to be extracted in one appointment, the practitioner has to be very careful with the amount of local anesthetic administered in each quadrant. Vasoconstrictors are another consideration. They limit the uptake of local anesthetic by the vasculature and thereby decrease systemic effects, allowing for an increase in dosage. Therefore, the solution concentration and the use of a vasoconstrictor will change the maximum dose of local anesthetic that can be administered.

The safest local anesthetic to use in the pediatric patient is 2% lidocaine with 1:100,000 epinephrine. A simple method for remembering the pediatric dose of 2% lidocaine with or without vasoconstrictor is to use one cartridge for every 20 pounds.

4. What effect does narcotic sedation have on the maximum pediatric dose of local anesthetic?

Amide local anesthetics and narcotics have an additive effect thereby increasing the chance of a toxic reaction. Lowering the calculated pediatric maximum dose (e.g., 4.4 mg/kg of 2% lidocaine with 1:100,000 epinephrine) is recommended to prevent possible respiratory depression or acidosis that may decrease the seizure threshold. Opioids (fentanyl, meperidine, and morphine) may cause this amide local anesthetic additive effect because of their similar chemical structures (both are basic lipophilic amines) and a first-pass pulmonary effect. The lungs may serve as a reservoir for these drugs with a subsequent release back into the system.

5. How are local anesthetics classified?

All local anesthetics contain an aromatic ring linked to amide groups. The link is either an amide or an ester and thus determines the classification.

AROMATIC GROUP — INTERMEDIATE CHAIN — N $< \begin{array}{c} C_nH_n \\ C_nH_n \end{array}$ — AMINE GROUP

An easy way to identify amide local anesthetics is to remember that the drug name contains an *i* plus *-caine* (lidocaine, mepivacaine, and bupivacaine). Esters such as Novocain, procaine, benzocaine, and tetracaine contain no *i*.

A new local anesthetic, articaine, was approved for use in the United States in April of 2000, though it has been used in other countries for some time. This local anesthetic contains both an amide and an ester link, though it is classified as an amide.

6. How are local anesthetics metabolized?

Amide local anesthetics are metabolized mainly by the liver (microsomal enzymes) while the ester types are metabolized by the plasma (pseudocholinesterase). An easy way to remember how the most commonly used local anesthetic is metabolized is *l*idocaine and *l*iver.

7. Describe the mechanism of action of local anesthetics.

Once injected into the tissue, local anesthetics exist in both an ionized and a nonionized form. The nonionized base is able to penetrate many layers of tissue. The base, guided by its lipophilic aromatic ring, passes through the lipid nerve sheath and membrane. Reequilibration between the ionized and nonionized forms occurs once passage is completed. While in the nerve axon, the ionized form is able to block sodium (Na⁺) channels, prevent the inflow of Na⁺, slow the rate of depolarization, and thus prevent an action potential from occurring (see Figure).

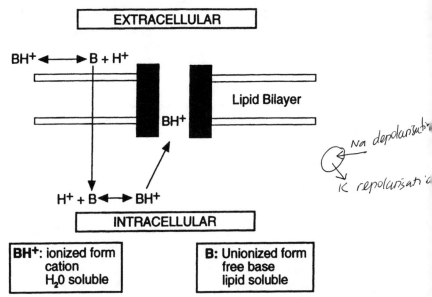

From Fitzpatrick K: Local anesthetics. In Duke J (ed): Anesthesia Secrets, 2nd ed. Philadelphia, Hanley & Belfus, 2000, pp 63–68, with permission.

8. Describe how a nerve impulse is transmitted on the cellular and microanatomic level.

A nerve impulse is generated when an electrical gradient occurs across the nerve membrane. An initial stimulus with sufficient intensity (–90 mV to –60 mV) must occur to allow depolarization of the nerve, propagation of the impulse, and restoration of the Na⁺-K⁺ pump to equilibrium. During depolarization, Na⁺ flows from the extracellular to the intracellular space. Repolarization occurs when K⁺ flows from the intracellular to the extracellular space (see Figure, next page).

The electrical gradient generated across the nerve membrane is initiated at the outer most surface of the nerve (mantle) and continues toward the center of the nerve (core). The outer surface is responsible for innervating the proximal structures while the core is responsible for innervating distal structures. Proximal structures are innervated more rapidly than distal structures. Following a mandibular inferior alveolar injection, one notices an almost immediate local anesthetic effect at the site of injection, while a delayed effect is noticed at the peripheral tissues (tongue then lip).

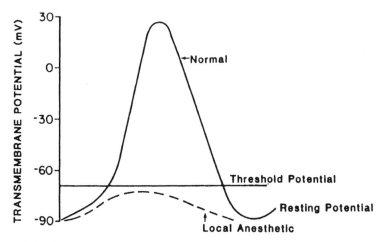

Local anesthetics slow the rate of depolarization of the nerve action potential such that the threshold potential is not reached. (From Stoelting RK, Miller RD: Local anesthetics. In Stoelting RK, Miller RD (eds): Basics of Anesthesia, 3rd ed. New York, Churchill Livingstone, 1994, pp 73–82, with permission.)

9. Following a local anesthetic injection, anesthetic effects will disappear and reappear in a definite order. List the sensations in increasing order of resistance to conduction.
  1. Pain
  2. Cold
  3. Warm
  4. Touch
  5. Deep pressure
  6. Motor

10. What are the causes and clinical manifestations of local anesthetic toxicity?
  Local anesthetic toxicity is due to elevated plasma levels of the anesthetic. This may be caused by an inadvertent vascular injection or by iatrogenically violating the maximum milligram per kilogram dose. A classic sign of systemic local anesthetic toxicity is circumoral numbness. However, if circumoral numbness is the desired effect of a nerve blockade, additional signs need to be recognized. Toxicity involves the cardiovascular and central nervous systems. Initial signs include tachycardia, hypertension, drowsiness, confusion, tinnitus, and a metallic taste. Progressive signs include tremors, hallucinations, hypotension, bradycardia, and decreased cardiac output. Late signs include unconsciousness, seizures, ventricular dysrhythmias, and respiratory and circulatory arrest.

11. Who is at greatest risk for local anesthetic toxicity?
  The potential for local anesthetic toxicity is greatest in the geriatric and pediatric patients. Older individuals generally metabolize drugs at a slower rate. A geriatric patient who takes multiple medications may experience adverse drug reactions when lidocaine is administered. Cimetidine (Tagamet), a histamine H_2-receptor antagonist, inhibits the hepatic oxidative enzymes needed for metabolism, thereby allowing lidocaine to accumulate in the circulating blood. This adverse reaction is seen only with cimetidine and not with other H_2-receptor antagonists. Propranolol (Inderal), a beta-adrenergic blocker, can reduce hepatic blood flow and reduce lidocaine clearance. Therefore, a local anesthetic toxic reaction would not be expected with a routine injection of lidocaine in a patient who takes cimetidine or propranolol, but may result if high doses of lidocaine are given.
  In addition, a possible additive adverse drug reaction exists with the administration of local anesthetics and opioids in the geriatric and pediatric populations.

12. What is methemoglobinemia, what are its causes and clinical manifestations, and how can it be treated?

A hemoglobin deficiency occurring when hemoglobin has been oxidized to methemoglobin. Oxidized hemoglobin cannot bind or carry oxygen. Excessive doses of prilocaine (above 600 mg) or articaine (above 500 mg) may result in the accumulation of an oxidized metabolite, ortho-toluidine, that is capable of allowing this conversion. Clinical manifestations include a decreased pulse oximeter reading, cyanosis, and chocolate-colored blood in the surgical field. This condition can be reversed with intravenous administration of 1–2 mg/kg of methylene blue over a 5-minute period.

Benzocaine also has the potential to cause methemoglobinemia. Benzocaine can be found in certain topical liquids, gels, ointments, and sprays (e.g., Hurricaine, Cetacaine). Methemoglobinemia formation can occur with benzocaine doses of 15–20 mg/kg. Benzocaine gels typically contain 18–20% benzocaine. Sprays containing 14–20% benzocaine can deliver 45–60 mg of benzocaine in 1 second.

Prilocaine is marketed as a 4% solution. A 4% solution contains 72 mg of prilocaine, with eight cartridges needed to obtain 600 mg. The use of a benzocaine topical along with prilocaine will reduce the maximum amount of injectable local anesthetic that can be used. In some countries other than the United States and Canada, prilocaine is marketed as a 3% solution. A 3% solution is less likely to cause an excessive delivery of this local anesthetic.

EMLA (eutectic mixture of local anesthetic) cream, used preoperatively prior to venous access, contains both lidocaine and prilocaine. EMLA cream should be used with caution in children, and it is not recommended for use in children younger than 12 months of age because of potential methemoglobinemia development.

13. Why are epinephrine and levonordefrin added to local anesthetics?

These substances are added to local anesthetics because of their vasoconstrictive properties. Vasoconstriction at the site of injection is beneficial because it limits the uptake the anesthetic by the vasculature, thereby increasing the duration of the anesthetic and diminishing systemic effects.

14. What is the maximum amount of epinephrine or levonordefrin that can be administered to a 70-kg patient with a history of coronary artery disease?

An average adult patient with a history of coronary artery disease should receive no more than 0.04 mg (40 µg) of epinephrine or 0.20 mg (200 µg) of levonordefrin. Each dental cartridge of 1:100,000 epinephrine contains 0.01 mg/ml of epinephrine; therefore no more than two cartridges (3.6 ml) should be administered. Each dental cartridge of 1:20,000 levonordefrin contains 0.5 mg/ml of levonordefrin; therefore no more than two cartridges (3.6 ml) should be administered. If the patient is also being sedated, then additional epinephrine could be administered (see Table).

Maximum Allowable Vasoconstrictor for the Cardiac Patient

VASOCONSTRICTOR CONCENTRATION AND TYPE	VASOCONSTRICTOR (MG/ML)	STANDARD DENTAL CARTRIDGE (MG/1.8 CC)	MAXIMUM ALLOWED CARTRIDGES
1:20,000 levonordefrin	0.5	0.09	2
1:50,000 epinephrine	0.02	0.036	1
1:100,000 epinephrine	0.01	0.018	2
1:200,000 epinephrine	0.005	0.009	4

When treating a patient with coronary artery disease, the objective is to prevent increases in heart rate. Increases in heart rate can decrease stroke volume and thereby decrease cardiac output. A decreased cardiac output will diminish the amount of oxygenated blood flowing to poorly perfused areas of the damaged pericardium.

Electing to perform a sedation procedure on a patient with coronary artery disease for minor outpatient surgical procedures (e.g., surgical extraction of a tooth) is often good treatment planning. The idea is to sedate a cardiac patient not for anxiolytic purposes, but to control heart rate. The amount of epinephrine used can be titrated to the patient's heart rate.

15. What adverse drug effects are associated with vasoconstrictor use?

Possible adverse drug reactions exist between vasoconstrictors and tricyclic antidepressants (TCAs), beta-adrenergic antagonists, volatile anesthetics, cocaine, and other vasoconstricting products.

TCAs (e.g., amitriptyline) increase the availability of endogenous norepinephrine, which could create an exaggerated heart rate or blood pressure response with the use of sympathomimetics (e.g., epinephrine, ephedrine, phenylephrine). Additionally, TCAs block muscarinic and alpha$_1$-adrenergic receptors that directly depress the myocardium. The potential for this adverse reaction is greatest during the first 14–21 days of drug initiation, probably because of downregulation of the norepinephrine receptors as treatment continues. This same type of exaggerated response was originally thought to exist with monoamine oxidase (MAO) inhibitors, but now that appears not to be the case. This adverse reaction appears to have the greatest adverse effect with the use of levonordefrin and imipramine (Tofranil).

Epinephrine has the potential to counteract vasodilating beta$_2$ receptors thus allowing epinephrine to act vascularly as a pure alpha-adrenergic stimulant. It is therefore prudent to limit the amount of vasoconstrictors used in these patients and to aspirate to prevent any intravascular injections.

The potential for dysrhythmic effects exists between the inhalational anesthetic halothane (Fluothane) and epinephrine or levonordefrin by stimulation of both alpha$_1$ and beta receptors. It is recommended that 2 µg/kg of epinephrine be used when halothane is administered. The greatest potential exists for an adverse reaction during the first 10 minutes of halothane administration, so it is prudent to wait this amount of time before injecting the local.

Cocaine also potentiates the effects of adrenergic vasoconstrictors. The dysrhythmic results of this interaction can be life threatening. Unfortunately, obtaining a factual health history from a cocaine-user may be difficult. All suspected drug users should be made aware of these lethal side effects, especially if cocaine has been used recently.

16. What types of local anesthetics have the greatest allergic potential?

Esters have a greater allergic potential than amides do. Procaine (Novocain) was at one time the most commonly used ester local anesthetic in dentistry. Although procaine is no longer available in dental cartridges, practitioners still need to be aware of ester allergies. Patients often give a history of rapid heart rate following the administration of a local anesthetic. The vasoconstrictor in the local anesthetic or an intravascular injection is often the cause. Practitioners are often quick to attribute a history of "allergy to Novocain" to the effects of the vasoconstrictor. A careful history taking may reveal that the patient did indeed have an allergic reaction to procaine when the anesthetic was available (prior to 1996).

Other topical esters are still commonly used in the practice of dentistry. Most topical local anesthetic ointments and gels contain benzocaine (an ester). Intraoral topical sprays may contain benzocaine and tetracaine (an ester). It is not uncommon for an oral and maxillofacial surgeon to use topical cocaine solutions (4%) as topical applications to the nasal mucosa to control homeostasis.

The newest local anesthetic, articaine, is classified as an amide but has both amide and ester linkages. Therefore, it has the potential to cause an ester allergic reaction as well.

17. To what components of a local anesthetic are patients most likely to be allergic?

1. **Methylparaben**, a bacteriostatic preservative, is found in multidose vials of local anesthetics. Many oral and maxillofacial surgeons use multidose vials in their offices, the emergency room, or the operating room and need to be cautious of potential allergic reactions.

Methylparaben is no longer added to dental cartridges (since 1984) because the cartridge is intended to be used as a single-dose vial so a preservative would not be required.

2. **Bisulfites** are food and drug preservatives. They are commonly used as preservatives at salad bars and in wines. Any local anesthetic cartridge containing a vasoconstrictor will have metabisulfite added as a preservative for the vasoconstrictor. Patients with known bisulfite allergies need to be administered local anesthetics without vasoconstrictors. Interestingly, one of the new manufacturers of propofol also uses bisulfite as a preservative.

3. **Sulfa drug** allergies are common among our patient population. Articaine contains a small amount of sulfa and should not be administered to these patients.

4. **Latex** allergies should also be considered with the use of local anesthetics. The local anesthetic itself contains no latex, but its container may. The needle puncture diaphragm of dental cartridges and multidose vials contains latex. The dental plunger of a dental cartridge may also contain latex. A disposable latex-free syringe is recommended for the latex-allergic patient. The anesthetic solution may be drawn using a filtered needle or by removing the rubber diaphragm.

18. What is the significance of lipid solubility of a local anesthetic?
  The lipid solubility determines the potency of a local anesthetic. A greater lipid solubility produces a more potent local anesthetic (see Table). Bupivacaine is a more potent local anesthetic than lidocaine, for example. Therefore, only a 0.5% solution is required to obtain comparable local anesthesia instead of a 2% solution.

Properties of Local Anesthetics

AGENT	LIPID SOLUBILITY	PROTEIN BINDING	DURATION	PKA	ONSET TIME
Mepivacaine	1	75	Medium	7.6	Fast
Lidocaine	4	65	Medium	7.7	Fast
Bupivacaine	28	95	Long	8.1	Moderate
Tetracaine	80	85	Long	8.6	Slow
Etidocaine	140	95	Long	7.7	Fast

19. What is the significance of the protein-binding ability of a local anesthetic?
  The degree of protein binding will determine the duration of a local anesthetic. A greater degree of protein binding at the receptor site will create a longer duration of action (see Table in question 18). Vasoconstrictors will also determine the duration of a local anesthetic but for different reasons.

20. What does the pKa of a local anesthetic determine?
  The pKa of a local anesthetic determines its onset time. The closer the pKa of a local anesthetic is to the pH of tissue (7.4), the more rapid the onset (see Table in question 18). The pKa of a local anesthetic is the pH at which equal concentrations of ionized and unionized forms exist.

21. Why are local anesthetics often ineffective when injected into an area of infection?
  Local anesthetics exist in both and ionized (cation) and unionized (base) form. If an acidic tissue infection exists, then the unionized form may be neutralized. The base form is necessary for passage of the anesthetic into the nerve membrane.

22. Why does inflammation impede the onset of local anesthesia?
  Products of inflammation in the tissues lower the pH of the affected tissue and limit the formation of free base (the reaction shifts to the left). Inflammatory exudates also enhance nerve conduction, making the blockage of nerve impulses more difficult.

23. How does lidocaine toxicity affect the central nervous system (CNS)?
  Lidocaine usually has a sedative effect on the brain. Initially, lidocaine toxicity depresses brain function in the form of drowsiness and slurred speech. It can progress to unconsciousness and even coma.

24. What cardiovascular effects does lidocaine toxicity exhibit?

Lidocaine has a depressor effect on the myocardium. Toxic doses of lidocaine cause sinus bradycardia, because lidocaine increases the effective refractory period relative to the action potential duration and lowers cardiac automaticity. If a very high dose has been administered, impaired cardiac contractility, arteriolar dilation, and profound hypotension and circulatory collapse can result.

25. What is the mechanism of degradation epinephrine?

The action of epinephrine is terminated primarily by its reuptake by the adrenergic nerves. Epinephrine that is not taken up again is rapidly metabolized and inactivated in the blood by the enzymes catechol-O-methyltransferase (COMT) and by MAO, both of which are present in the liver. One of the final produces is vanillylmandelic acid (VMA). Only a small percentage (1%) of epinephrine is excreted unchanged in the urine.

26. How do you calculate the amount, in milligrams, of any anesthetic and vasoconstrictor in a given solution.

For local anesthetics, for every 1% solution there is 10 mg/ml. Therefore:

Total milligrams = % of the solution × 10 × total milliliters

For vasoconstriction, for every 1:100,000 there is 0.01 mg/ml. Therefore:

Total milligrams = ratio × total milliliters

27. Discuss the effect and importance of pKa of a local anesthetic.

Because only the base form can diffuse rapidly into the nerve, drugs with a high pKa tend to have a slower onset (bupivacaine: pKa 8.1) than similar agents with more favorable dissociation constants (lidocaine: pKa 7.9).

28. A healthy, afebrile 70-kg man has been referred to your office for extraction of a symptomatic, abscessed mandibular molar. You have made two attempts to anesthetize the inferior alveolar nerve, the long buccal nerve, and the lingual nerve and have given an intraligament injection. Adequate soft tissue anesthesia has been obtained, but the patient complains when you attempt to luxate the tooth. List ten ways that may help achieve adequate anesthesia.

1. Allow adequate time for the anesthetic to take affect. Sit the patient in an upright position and wait an additional 5–10 minutes. This is difficult for the oral and maxillofacial surgeon who is inherently impatient.

2. Consider readministering the local anesthetic at a higher level on the ramus.

3. Consider innervation from the mylohyoid nerve and anesthetize accordingly (lingual to the mandibular second molar).

4. Administer another cartridge of anesthetic at the highest level possible by using the Gow-Gates technique (intraoral condylar injection).

5. Administer an intraosseous injection or use an intraosseous system (e.g., Stabident).

6. Consider using a higher pH anesthetic solution (one without a vasoconstrictor) to help overcome the acidity created by the infection.

7. Alkalinize (buffer) your anesthetic by adding sodium bicarbonate to your local anesthetic just prior to injecting.

8. Use a larger amount (but do note exceed the maximum recommended dose) of local anesthetic to overcome the acidity created by the infection.

9. Sedate the patient with a small amount of narcotic or nitrous oxide and proceed.

10. Consider placing the patient on antibiotics and reschedule the procedure.

29. A healthy 60-kg woman has been referred to your office for extraction of an infected posterior molar. The patient presents with trismus and has been on antibiotics and analgesic medication for a week with little relief. What can you do to help her?

Administer local anesthesia using an extraoral approach or by using the closed-mouth mandibular block (Vazirani block, Akinosi block, or Vazirani-Akinosi block).

An **extraoral block** is performed by first preparing the epidermis (i.e., with povidone-iodine [Betadine]) adjacent to the lateral portion of the zygomatic arch. A lateral approach to the nerve can be accomplished by using a short-length needle and injecting just below the sigmoid notch of the zygomatic arch.

A **closed-mouth block** can be performed by retracting the buccal tissues away from the dentition and inserting a long needle at the medial border of the ramus and adjacent to the mucogingival junction of the maxillary posterior molars. Then insert the needle to the approximate middle portion of the ramus and deposits the local anesthetic.

30. What types of local anesthetics can be used in the pregnant and lactating patient?

Category B (see lists below) local anesthetics are recommended for the pregnant and lactating patient. Local anesthetics can cross the placental barrier but are generally not harmful unless excessive amounts are administered. A mother's normal tissue pH is 7.4 whereas the fetus has a pH of approximately 7.2. An excessive amount of local anesthetic could dangerously lower the fetus's pH (ion trapping).

Category B	*Category C*
Lidocaine	Articaine
Prilocaine	Bupivacaine
Etidocaine	Mepivacaine

31. During delivery of an inferior alveolar injection, you know that you have directly contacted the nerve (bull's-eye) because the patient jumps. Should you deliver the local anesthetic at this location?

Although definitive anesthesia will be obtained, one should never directly inject a local anesthetic within the nerve sheath to avoid traumatizing (lacerating) the nerve or causing the development of a neuroma. More importantly, the administration of a fluid bolus within the nerve sheath can physically damage the nerve and cause indefinite facial pain. Injecting anesthetic directly into a foramen (e.g., mental) also carries the risk of traumatizing the nerve. Additionally, paresthesia has been reported with the use of 4% solutions of local anesthetics. Thus, additional care should be taken when injecting prilocaine or articaine near a foramen.

32. What profession uses local anesthetics most frequently on a daily basis?

With the possible exception of the obstetric anesthesiologists, dental practitioners, specifically oral and maxillofacial surgeons, use local anesthetics most frequently. Therefore, a thorough understanding of the pharmacokinetics and pharmacodynamics of local anesthetics is essential.

BIBLIOGRAPHY

1. Bennett CR: Monheim's Local Anesthesia and Pain Control in Dental Practice, 6th ed. St. Louis, Mosby, 1978.
2. Braverman B, McCarthy RJ, Ivankovich AD: Vasopressor challenges during chronic MAOI or TCA treatment in anesthetised drugs. Life Sci 40:2587–2595, 1987.
3. Fitzpatrick K: Local anesthetics. In Duke J (ed): Anesthesia Secrets, 2nd ed. Philadelphia, Hanley & Belfus, 2000, pp 63–68.
4. Haas DA, Lennon D: A 21-year retrospective study of reports of paresthesia following local anesthetic administration. J Can Dent Assoc 61:319–330, 1995.
5. Local Anesthetics for Dentistry: Prescribing Information. Westborough, MA, Astra USA, 1995.
6. Malamed SF: Handbook of Local Anesthetics, 4th ed. St. Louis, Mosby, 1997, pp 2–302.
7. Moore PA: Preventing local anesthetic toxicity. J Am Dental Assoc 123:61–64, 1992.
8. Moore PA: Adverse drug interactions in dental practice: Interactions associated with local anesthetics, sedatives and anxiolytics. J Am Dental Assoc 130:541–554, 1999.
9. Roering DL, Kotrly KJ, Vucins EJ, et al: First pass uptake of fentanyl, meperidine, and morphine in the human lung. Anesthesiology 67:466–472, 1987.

10. Samdal F, Arctander K, Skolleborg KC, Amland PF: Alkalisation of lignocaine-adrenaline reduces the amount of pain during subcutaneous injection of local anesthetic. Scand J Plast Reconstr Hand Surg 28:33–37, 1994.
11. Stoelting RK, Miller RD: Local anesthetics. In Stoelting RK, Miller RD (eds): Basics of Anesthesia, 4th ed. New York, Churchill Livingstone, 2000, pp 80–88.
12. Wilburn-Goo D, Lloyd LM: When patients become cyanotic: Acquired methemoglobinemia. J Am Dental Assoc 130:826–831, 1999.
13. Yagiela JA: Adverse drug interactions in dental practice: Interactions associated with vasoconstrictors. J Am Dental Assoc 130:701–709, 1999.

6. INTRAVENOUS SEDATION AND ANESTHETIC AGENTS

Bradley A. Gregory, D.M.D.

1. How is an intravenous (IV) anesthetic agent used in anesthesia?

An IV anesthetic is a drug that is intravenously injected in order to induce unconsciousness at the beginning of general anesthesia. At the same time, it allows rapid recovery after termination of its effect.

2. What are the properties of an ideal induction agent?

1. The drug should be soluble in water, have IV fluid compatibility, and be stable in aqueous solution.

2. It should elicit rapid onset and recovery of anesthesia (within 1 arm-brain circulation time).

3. It should not possess any unwanted cardiovascular or neurologic side effects or produce any unwanted movements.

4. It should retain anticonvulsant, antiemetic, analgesic, and amnestic properties.

5. It should not impair renal or hepatic function or steroid synthesis.

3. What are barbiturates?

Barbiturates are a derivative of barbituric acid. They exhibit a dose-dependent central nervous system (CNS) depression with hypnosis and amnesia. Barbiturates are very lipid soluble, which results in a rapid onset of action. They are used most often for induction of anesthesia because they produce unconsciousness in less than 30 seconds.

4. Describe the pharmacologic effects of barbiturates.

Barbiturates decrease the rate of dissociation of gamma-aminobutyric acid (GABA) from its receptors. GABA, an inhibitory neurotransmitter, causes an increase in chloride concentration within the membranes of postsynaptic neurons resulting in hyperpolarization. Barbiturates are capable of depressing the reticular activating system, which is important in maintaining wakefulness and medullary ventilatory centers to decrease responsiveness to ventilatory stimulant effects of carbon dioxide. In addition, barbiturates induce depression of the medullary vasomotor center, causing decreased sympathetic nervous system impulses from autonomic ganglia. This results in decreases in blood pressure (10–20 mmHg) secondary to peripheral vasodilation. Finally, barbiturates are potent cerebral vasoconstrictors resulting in decreases in cerebral blood flow, cerebral blood volume, and intracranial pressure (ICP).

5. What are the pharmacokinetics of barbiturates?

Maximal uptake of barbiturates by the brain occurs within 30 seconds after IV administration. This accounts for the rapid (1 arm-brain circulation) induction of anesthesia. The redistribution of these drugs from the brain to inactive tissues, especially skeletal muscle and fat, results in prompt awakening. The elimination of barbiturates is dependent on hepatic function because less than 1% of the administered dose is cleared unchanged by the kidneys.

6. What are the most commonly used barbiturates for induction of anesthesia?

Thiopental sodium (Pentothal) is a thiobarbiturate usually prepared as a 2.5% solution. The pH of thiopental is 10.5. When injected intravenously, it can be irritating. An induction dose of 3–5 mg/kg produces a loss of consciousness within 30 seconds and recovery in 5–10 minutes. Because the elimination half-life is 6–12 hours, patients may experience a slow recovery. After 24 hours, approximately 28–30% may be detectable in the body. Thiopental is not used to maintain anesthesia because of accumulation in inactive tissues with repeated doses.

Methohexital (Brevital) is somewhat less lipid soluble and less ionized at physiologic pH than thiopental. The pH is 10.5. An induction dose of 1–2 mg/kg produces loss of consciousness in less than 20 seconds and recovery in 4–5 minutes. The elimination half-life of methohexital is 3 hours, which allows a clearance rate that is 3–4 times faster than that of thiopental. In addition, methohexital activates epileptic foci, facilitating their identification during surgery to ablate these sites.

7. What is propofol?
Propofol (Diprivan), a substituted isopropylphenol, is an IV sedative-hypnotic agent used for induction and maintenance of anesthesia. It can also be used during conscious sedation. Propofol is highly lipophilic, which increases its ability to cross the blood-brain barrier.

8. Describe the pharmacokinetics and pharmacologic effects of propofol.
An intravenous induction dose of 2.0–2.5 mg/kg produces unconsciousness in less than 30 seconds followed by recovery in 4–8 minutes. A rapid elimination half-life of 0.5–1.5 hours results in prompt hepatic metabolism to inactive metabolites. In addition, redistribution to inactive tissue sites plays a significant role in early awakening. Because propofol exhibits awakening with minimal residual CNS effects more quickly than any other IV anesthetic, it is the most widely used agent for ambulatory anesthesia. Anesthesia is maintained with a continuous infusion of 0.1–0.2 mg/kg/min or intermittent doses. Propofol causes a 20–30% decrease in blood pressure and heart rate. The cardiovascular effects are due to rapid arterial and venous vasodilation and mild negative inotropic effects. Propofol has a low incidence of postoperative nausea and vomiting. Pain on injection may be related to release of local kininogens, although the exact cause remains unknown. Awake patients are likely to experience pain at the injection site; the pain may be decreased with administration of lidocaine prior to injection.

9. What are the pharmacologic properties and side effects of etomidate?
Etomidate (Amidate) is a carboxylated imadazole derivative. An induction dose of 0.2–0.4 mg/kg IV produces rapid induction of anesthesia that lasts 3–12 minutes. The CNS effects are dose dependent, and recovery of psychomotor skills is equal to that of thiopental. Rapid awakening results from redistribution and nearly complete hydrolysis to inactive metabolites. Because etomidate produces no noticeable cardiovascular changes, it is used in patients with limited cardiac reserve. In addition, etomidate decreases cerebral blood flow and ICP. Like methohexital, it activates seizure foci.

Side effects include venoirritation with rapid infusion, involuntary skeletal muscle movements, and a high incidence of nausea and vomiting. Also, etomidate suppresses adrenocortical function for up to 8 hours after administration. During this time, the adrenal cortex is unresponsive to adrenocorticotropic hormone (ACTH).

10. What is ketamine and how does it exert its physiologic action?
Ketamine, a phencyclidine (PCP) derivative, is ten times more lipid soluble than thiopental, enabling it to cross the blood-brain barrier quickly. It produces dissociative anesthesia, which can be seen on electroencephalogram (EEG) as dissociation between the thalamus and limbic system. Rapid CNS depression with hypnosis, sedation, amnesia, and intense analgesia occurs in 30–60 seconds after IV administration. The anesthetic induction doses are 1–2 mg/kg IV, with effects lasting 5–10 minutes, or 10 mg/kg IM, which acts in 2–4 minutes. A ketamine dart of 4 mg/kg IM can be administered to uncooperative patients to facilitate completion of short procedures.

11. What are the pharmacologic effects and side effects of ketamine?

Ketamine is highly lipid soluble, is rapidly redistributed to muscle and fat, and undergoes extensive hepatic metabolism to a weakly active metabolite, norketamine. Ketamine stimulates the cardiovascular system, increasing the heart rate, blood pressure, and cardiac output. In patients with ischemic heart disease, ketamine may adversely increase myocardial oxygen requirements. In addition, ketamine produces bronchial smooth muscle relaxation because of sympathetic stimulation, which may be beneficial in patients with bronchospasm or asthma. Airway secretions are increased by ketamine, creating the need for anticholinergics such as glycopyrrolate in the preoperative period. Ketamine is a potent cerebral vasodilator and will increase ICP in patients with intracranial lesions. Finally, emergence from ketamine anesthesia may be associated with unpleasant auditory, visual, and out-of-body illusions that can progress to delirium. It is recommended that benzodiazepines or droperidol be administered either preoperatively or after induction to decrease the incidence of emergence delirium.

12. What are the clinical uses for benzodiazepines?

- Preoperative medication
- Intravenous sedation
- Induction of anesthesia
- Maintenance of anesthesia
- Suppression of seizure activity

Anterograde amnesia, minimal depression of ventilation and the cardiovascular system, and sedative properties make benzodiazepines favorable preoperative medications.

13. Where in the central nervous system do benzodiazepines exert their amnestic effect?

These effects occur at benzodiazepine receptors, which are found on postsynaptic nerve endings in the CNS. Benzodiazepine receptors are part of the GABA receptor complex. The GABA receptor complex consists of two alpha subunits, which benzodiazepines bind to, and two beta subunits, with which GABA binds. A chloride ion channel exists in the middle of the receptor complex. Benzodiazepines enhance the binding of GABA to beta subunits, which opens the chloride ion channel. Chloride ions flow into the neuron hyperpolarizing it and inhibiting action potentials.

14. What clinical properties make benzodiazepines good preoperative medications?

At lower doses, only anxiolysis is obtained. Anterograde amnesia, sedation, and anxiolysis are produced at higher concentrations. At this concentration, patients are conscious and can maintain their own airway but will not remember events during surgery. Finally, at even higher concentrations, benzodiazepines will produce unconsciousness, although they are not complete anesthetics. A complete general anesthetic produces the effects already mentioned plus analgesia, control of the autonomic nervous systems, and occasionally muscle relaxation. Benzodiazepines do not provide analgesia, and they should not be used alone to produce general anesthesia. They are best used in low doses to supplement inhaled or intravenous anesthetics to provide amnesia.

15. What benzodiazepines are most commonly used as amnestics in anesthesiology?

1. Midazolam (most common)
2. Lorazepam
3. Diazepam

16. What are the properties and pharmacokinetics of midazolam?

Midazolam is prepared as a water-soluble compound that is transformed into a lipid-soluble compound by exposure to the pH of blood upon injection. This unique property of midazolam improves patient comfort when administered by the IV or IM route. This prevents the need for an organic solvent such as propylene glycol, which is required for diazepam and lorazepam. Midazolam is the most lipid soluble of the three and, as a result, has a rapid onset and a relatively short duration of action. The elimination half-life is 1–4 hours. A dose of 1–2.5 mg administered intravenously is useful for anxiolysis, amnesia, and conscious sedation. Induction of anesthesia can be produced by the administration of 0.1–0.2 mg/kg IV. Unconsciousness will occur within 60–90 seconds. This is more rapid than diazepam but slower than the barbiturates. Benzodiazepines are not used often for induction because of the potential for delayed awakening, particularly with diazepam and lorazepam.

17. What are the properties and actions of diazepam?
Diazepam is a water-insoluble benzodiazepine and requires the organic solvent propylene glycol to dissolve it. Propylene glycol is most likely responsible for the venoirritation and thrombophlebitis that may occur during injection. At the same time, it is less lipid soluble than midazolam. A dose of 5–10 mg given intravenously will provide amnestic, calming, and sedative effects; however, midazolam will have a quicker onset and greater amnestic effect than diazepam. The induction dose of diazepam is 0.3–0.5 mg, and onset is slightly slower than that of midazolam. In addition, diazepam (0.1 mg/kg IV) is effective at abolishing the seizure activity that is produced by local anesthetics, alcohol withdrawal, and status epilepticus. The elimination half-life of diazepam is 21–37 hours, which may account for the delayed wakening after induction doses. Diazepam undergoes hepatic metabolism to active desmethyldiazepam and oxazepam that can produce sedation 6–8 hours after its initial administration.

18. List the properties and actions of lorazepam.
• Lorazepam is the least lipid soluble of the three main benzodiazepines, resulting in a slow onset of action but long duration of action.
• Lorazepam requires propylene glycol to dissolve it, which increases its venoirritation.
• Lorazepam is a more powerful amnestic agent than midazolam, but its slow onset and long duration of action limit its usefulness for preoperative anesthesia.

19. What is the antagonist for benzodiazepines?
Flumazenil, a competitive antagonist, given in increments of 0.2 mg IV every 60 seconds will reverse unconsciousness, sedation, respiratory depression, and anxiolysis. Flumazenil has a rapid onset with the peak effect occurring in about 1–3 minutes. The effect of flumazenil lasts for about 20 minutes, and resedation may occur.

20. What is the mechanism of action of opioids?
Opioids act as agonists through complex interactions with mu, delta, and kappa receptors in the CNS. Supraspinally, mu receptors are responsible for analgesia, euphoria, miosis, nausea and vomiting, urinary retention, depression of ventilation, and bradycardia. Delta and kappa receptors are active at the spinal level mediating spinal analgesia, sedation, and miosis. In addition, opioids may act presynaptically to interfere with the release of neurotransmitters such as acetylcholine, dopamine, norepinephrine, and substance P.

21. How are opioids used clinically?
Uses include provision of analgesia before or after surgery, synergistic effects with inhaled anesthetics being used for maintenance of anesthesia, induction and maintenance of anesthesia (particularly in patients with severe cardiac dysfunction), and inhibition of reflex sympathetic nervous system activity. Usually, opioids are administered intermittently in lower doses during maintenance of anesthesia or as continuous infusions to augment inhaled anesthetics. Often times, small doses of fentanyl, sufentanil, or alfentanil are administered just prior to direct laryngoscopy and tracheal intubation to attenuate blood pressure and heart rate responses evoked by these stimuli.

22. What are the pharmacologic effects of opioids?
Opioids are cardiac-stable drugs. In many settings, opioids are used as the principal anesthetic agent for cardiac anesthesia because of their hemodynamic stability; however, they do

lack an amnestic effect. At the same time, opioids can cause a dose-dependent bradycardia resulting from vagal stimulation in the medulla. In contrast, meperidine will cause tachycardia because it is structurally similar to atropine and elicits atropine-like effects. Opioids act on the medullary ventilatory centers to produce rapid and sustained dose-dependent depression of ventilation. This is characterized by increases in the resting $PaCO_2$ and decreased responsiveness to the ventilatory stimulant effects of carbon dioxide. In the CNS, opioids do not produce unconsciousness reliably. They do, however, stimulate dopamine receptors in the chemoreceptor trigger zone of the medulla, causing nausea and vomiting. Finally, rapidly administered high doses can cause spasm of the thoracoabdominal muscles resulting in hypoventilation.

23. What are the properties and adverse effects of the opioid IV induction agents?

Fentanyl (Sublimaze) is 100 times more potent than morphine. Its onset of action is quicker than that of morphine, its duration of action is shorter than morphine, and its elimination half-life is longer than morphine. Anesthetic doses of 30–100 µg/kg produce an onset of action in 1–2 minutes. Because it is very lipid soluble, it is rapidly redistributed to inactive tissues. Over time it is slowly released into the plasma and made available for clearance.

Sufentanil (Sufenta) is structurally similar to fentanyl but is 5–7 times more potent. It is more lipid soluble, which results in faster onset of action. Its elimination half-time (2–3 hours) is somewhat shorter than that of fentanyl, resulting in more rapid awakening and less postoperative respiratory depression. Induction doses range from 5 to 13 µg/kg.

Alfentanil (Alfenta) is one-fifth to one-third as potent as fentanyl. Because it is more lipid soluble than fentanyl, alfentanil has a rapid onset of action and short duration of action. Alfentanil often causes nausea and vomiting.

24. Which opioids stimulate the release of histamine?

Morphine, codeine, and meperidine (Demerol) cause histamine release resulting in vasodilation and possible hypotension. Fentanyl, sufentanil, and alfentanil do not stimulate histamine release.

25. What opioid antagonist is most commonly used in clinical anesthesia?

Naloxone is the pure mu-receptor antagonist that is used to reverse the effects of opioids. Naloxone will reverse overdoses and the respiratory depressant effects, however, at the same time, it reverses the analgesic effects. Normal dosages may cause abrupt reversal, which can result in tachycardia, hypertension, pulmonary edema, and cardiac dysrhythmias. To avoid these adverse effects, naloxone should be given in doses of 40 µg (0.1 ml), repeated every few minutes.

26. Why is propofol the best agent for outpatient anesthesia?

- Rapid induction and recovery
- Lower incidence of nausea and vomiting
- Patients regain cognitive function quickly, which leads to shorter recovery period

27. Which intravenous induction agents are recommended for use in major trauma or other hypovolemic states?

Etomidate is an agent that is commonly used because of its cardiac stability in patients with limited cardiac reserve. **Ketamine** is recommended for patients who are hypovolemic because of the direct stimulation of sympathetic outflow from the CNS. However, patients with depleted endogenous catecholamines may not be able to respond to the stimulation, resulting in more hypotension.

28. Which induction agents alter ICP?

Thiopental, propofol, etomidate, and fentanyl reduce ICP because they cause decreases in cerebral blood flow and cerebral metabolic consumption of oxygen. Ketamine increases cerebral blood flow, cerebral metabolism, and ICP.

29. What effect does age have on dosing of induction agents?

With increasing age, elimination time and renal clearance time increase resulting in longer lasting drug effects. Elderly patients are more sensitive to intravenous anesthetics; therefore, dose reductions are necessary in this group of patients.

BIBLIOGRAPHY

1. Hatheway J: Opioids. In Duke J (ed): Anesthesia Secrets, 2nd ed. Philadelphia, Hanley & Belfus, 2000, pp 51–55.
2. Hudson RJ, Stanski DR, Burch PG: Pharmacokinetics of methohexital and thiopental in surgical patients. Anesthesiology 59:215–219, 1983.
3. McDowell G: Intravenous induction agents. In Duke J (ed): Anesthesia Secrets, 2nd ed. Philadelphia, Hanley & Belfus, 2000, pp 47–50.
4. Reves JG, Fragen RJ, Vinik HR, Greenblatt DJ: Midazolam: Pharmacology and uses. Anesthesiology 62:310–324, 1985.
5. Stoelting RK, Miller RD: Intravenous anesthetics. In Stoelting RD, Miller RD (eds): Basics of Anesthesia. New York, Churchill Livingstone, 1999, pp 73–82.
6. Winkelmann G: Benzodiazepines. In Duke J (ed): Anesthesia Secrets, 2nd ed. Philadelphia, Hanley & Belfus, 2000, pp 56–58.

7. INHALATIONAL ANESTHESIA

Christopher L. Maestrello, D.D.S., and Matthew R. Cooke, D.D.S.

1. What inhalational anesthetics are currently available and how are they delivered in clinical use?

Five volatile liquids (desflurane, enflurane, halothane, isoflurane, and sevoflurane) and one gas (nitrous oxide) are used clinically. Enflurane is used infrequently and will not be discussed in this chapter. The volatile liquids require a vaporizer for inhalational administration. Additionally, the desflurane vaporizer has a heating component to allow delivery at room temperature.

These inhalation agents can be administered in a hospital operating room or in a clinical situation provided adequate scavenging and ventilation exists. Many oral and maxillofacial procedures require a nonsurgical field; therefore, anesthetic delivery systems can be used in an office setting. Inhalational anesthetic delivery systems exist for the delivery of one or multiple gases. These delivery systems have mandatory scavenging and fail-safe mechanisms to optimize safety.

2. How long can oxygen at 2 L/min be delivered from an E cylinder with a reading of 500 psi?

A full E cylinder of oxygen (O_2) contains approximately 600 L at a pressure of 2000 psi. At 2 L/min, a full E cylinder will deliver O_2 for approximately 300 minutes, or 5 hours. A reading of 500 psi will therefore give you approximately 1 hour and 15 minutes of O_2.

3. How long can nitrous oxide (N_2O) at 2 L/min be delivered from an E cylinder that reads 750 psi?

N_2O has a pressure of 750 psi and contains approximately 1600 L in an E cylinder. N_2O is a compressed liquid and not a compressed gas like O_2. A compressed liquid does not show a linear correlation between volume and pressure as does a compressed gas. N_2O pressure will remain at 750 psi until all the liquid has been vaporized. Therefore, an estimated time cannot be determined.

4. Why is N_2O use contraindicated in patients with conditions involving closed gas spaces?

N_2O has a low blood-to-gas partition coefficient (0.46) and therefore low solubility. It can leave the blood and enter air-filled cavities 34 times more quickly than nitrogen can leave the cavity to enter the blood. The use of N_2O can increase the expansion of compliant cavities, such as a pneumothorax, bowel gas in a bowel obstruction, and an air embolism. An increase in pressure will occur when N_2O is used with noncompliant cavities such as the middle ear or sinuses.

The oral and maxillofacial surgeon needs to be cautious when treating the recent trauma patient (e.g., motor vehicle accident victim). An asymptomatic, undiagnosed closed pneumothorax can double in size in 10 minutes after the administration of 70% N_2O. Nitrous oxide–oxygen sedation should be postponed in patients with gastrointestinal obstructions, middle ear disturbances, and, possibly, sinus infections.

5. Should a patient with an upper respiratory infection (URI) be given N_2O via a nasal hood?

Because a patient with a URI has nasal blockage, the delivery of the N_2O is limited and the potential for leakage of N_2O around the hood is more likely. In addition, patients with a URI are also more likely to have associated middle ear and sinus infections. Therefore, the use of N_2O with patients with URI is unwise.

6. Can inhalational anesthetics be administered to patients with chronic obstructive pulmonary disease (COPD)?

Administration of volatile anesthetics (desflurane, enflurane, halothane, isoflurane, and sevoflurane) is not a concern for COPD patients (asthmatic bronchitis, emphysema, and chronic bronchitis). All volatile anesthetics are bronchodilators and, therefore, are beneficial to patients with COPD.

N_2O-O_2, however, should be used cautiously. Patients with mild to moderate COPD should be administered a supplemental inspired oxygen concentration (FiO_2) of no greater than 40. N_2O-O_2 sedation without any additional intravenous sedation is generally safe. Remember, 4 L through a nasal cannula equals 36% O_2.

Nasal cannula (3–6 L/min): $FiO_2 = 20 + 4 \times L/min$
Face mask with reservoir (6–10 L/min): $FiO_2 = 10 \times L/min$

During deep sedation, keep patients breathing spontaneously and do not take away their respiratory drive. O_2 supplementation should be avoided or used only with extreme caution in patients with severe COPD. COPD patients have an increased incidence of pulmonary bullae or blebs (combined alveoli). Because of N_2O's low blood solubility, it can increase the volume and pressure of these lung defects, which could create an increased risk of barotrauma and pneumothorax.

Carbon dioxide (CO_2) is a respiratory stimulus for patients with normal respiratory physiology. Patients with COPD retain larger amounts of CO_2 in their lungs and, over time, lose this respiratory drive. COPD patients thus develop a hypoxic drive. The potential for the hypoxic drive to cease with the severe chronic patient exists when O_2 is greater than 21% room air (i.e., N_2O-O_2 at 70/30%).

Asthmatic bronchitis patients may be of any age and could easily be encountered in the office. Patients with debilitating emphysema and chronic bronchitis are often chronically ill and are not be seen commonly in an office setting. They may, however, be encountered in nursing homes and hospitals.

7. When is administration of N_2O-O_2 sedation contraindicated in an asthmatic patient?

There are no contraindications for the use of N_2O-O_2 sedation in asthmatic patients. Because anxiety is a stimulus for an asthmatic attack, N_2O-O_2 sedation is actually beneficial for these patients.

There have been no reported allergies to N_2O. The potential for an allergic reaction does exist, however, in the latex-allergic individual who receives N_2O-O_2 via a nasal hood.

8. What is the second gas effect?

This occurs when one gas speeds the rate of increase of the alveolar partial pressure of a second gas. This effect is normally associated with an inhalational induction involving a large volume of N_2O and a volatile anesthetic. N_2O's low blood solubility allows it to be absorbed quickly by the alveoli, thus causing an increase in the alveolar concentration of the volatile anesthetic. In theory, a high concentration of one gas (e.g., 70% N_2O) could speed the induction of a second, less-soluble gas (e.g., halothane).

Inhalational inductions are normally used in energetic pediatric patients. Obtaining intravenous access in children who cannot sit still is difficult, and a quick induction is desirable. The rate of induction of halothane should be increased when it is used concurrently with 70% N_2O.

9. Define minimal alveolar concentration (MAC).

MAC is the concentration of an inhaled anesthetic at 1 atm that prevents skeletal muscle movement's response to a painful stimulus (e.g., surgical skin incision) in 50% of patients. A MAC of 1.3 prevents skeletal movement in approximately 95% of individuals undergoing surgery. The potency of anesthetic gases can be compared using MAC.

MAC of Commonly Used Agents

AGENT	MAC
Nitrous oxide	104
Isoflurane	1.15
Halothane	0.77
Desflurane	6.0
Sevoflurane	1.71

10. What factors affect MAC?

Factors that *decrease* MAC:
Higher altitudes ($\downarrow$ barometric pressure)
Pregnancy
Hypothermia
Hyponatremia
Alcohol (acute use)
Barbiturates
Calcium channel blockers
Opioids

Factors that *increase* MAC:
Increased central neurotransmitter levels
 (MAOIs, cocaine, ephedrine, levodopa)
Hyperthermia
Alcohol (chronic use)
Hypernatremia

11. Explain how MAC values can be used to gauge awareness during surgery.

Intraoperative patient awareness is a concern with all patients undergoing a deep sedation or general anesthesia. Volatile anesthetics have amnestic properties at an adequate MAC. Intravenous medications are often used in conjunction with volatile anesthetics, which often causes a decrease in MAC. This decreased MAC may prevent an amnestic state. Although specific concentrations of volatile agents have not been established for the elimination of intraoperative recall, clinical studies show that awareness is eliminated between 0.4 and 0.6 MAC for isoflurane. Attaining a MAC of 0.8 has been recommended to guarantee unconsciousness.

Awareness precautions need to be taken with certain anesthetic techniques. An anesthetist may be tempted to decrease the concentration of a volatile anesthetic when a paralytic has been used because surgical stimulation has been eliminated. The addition of midazolam, an amnestic benzodiazepine, can be used in situations where MAC has been reduced below 0.8. MAC is often reduced in patients who develop intraoperative hypotension because of volatile inhalational vasodilating properties. Vasopressors, such as ephedrine and phenylephrine, may be necessary in order to maintain a MAC of 0.8 when additional amnestic medications are not being used.

12. Why are additive values of MAC for inhalational anesthetics beneficial?

Additive values are beneficial when a decrease in ventilatory and circulatory effects of volatile anesthetics is desired. MAC values are additive; therefore, the simultaneous administration of N_2O with a volatile anesthetic will decrease the MAC of both agents. For example, using 0.5 MAC N_2O (approximately 50%) with 0.5 MAC isoflurane (approximately 0.6%) results in a MAC of 1.0.

The only inhalational anesthetics that would be administered simultaneously would be a volatile anesthetic (desflurane, halothane, isoflurane, and sevoflurane) and N_2O. Fail-safe mechanisms exist on anesthetic machines to prevent the simultaneous administration of two volatile agents.

N_2O has a MAC greater than 100% and therefore cannot be used as a sole anesthetic agent because a minimum of 21% O_2 is required at 1 atm. Typically, N_2O concentrations of 20–70% are used.

13. What are the hemodynamic effects of volatile anesthetics?

Volatile anesthetics depress the cardiovascular system, and this depression results in a reduced mean arterial pressure. Halothane primarily causes a reduction in heart rate and contractility. Desflurane, isoflurane, and sevoflurane cause primarily a decrease in systemic vascular resistance, which is reflected by a reduced blood pressure.

14. What are the hemodynamic considerations of the combined use of a volatile anesthetic and the intravenous anesthetic propofol?

The inhalational anesthetics desflurane, isoflurane, and sevoflurane and the intravenous agent propofol are potent vasodilators. Additive effects causing hypotension from a decrease in systemic vascular resistance occur with simultaneous administration of these two anesthetic groups. Combining these agents should be done cautiously in elderly patients and patients taking hypertensive medications. Noting preoperative blood pressures is extremely important. Selection of an alternative intravenous anesthetic agent may be indicated. If propofol is used along with a volatile anesthetic, then vasopressors (e.g., ephedrine, phenylephrine) should be diluted properly and made readily available.

15. What are the ventilatory effects of volatile anesthetic?

Volatile anesthetics will cause a dose-dependent decrease in ventilation. Volatile anesthetics cause a decrease in tidal volume (TV) with a compensatory increase in respiratory rate (RR) but a net decrease in minute ventilation (mV).

Ventilatory effects of volatile anesthetics: net $\downarrow$mV = $\uparrow$RR × $\downarrow$TV

This decreased minute ventilation causes an increase in CO_2. An increase in CO_2 stimulates the respiratory drive in the unanesthetized patient. Inhalational anesthetics, however, shift the CO_2 response curve to the right and lessen the ventilatory response to hypercarbia and hypoxia.

Oxygenation and Ventilation

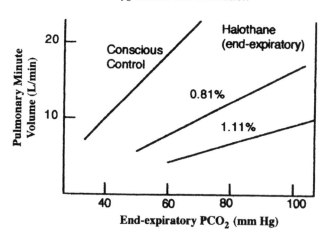

The CO_2 response curve. Note the effects of inhalational anesthetics on the pulmonary minute volume. (From Adamson DT: Oxygenation and ventilation. In Duke J (ed): Anesthesia Secrets, 2nd ed. Philadelphia, Hanley & Belfus, 2000, pp 5–10, with permission; adapted from Foltz B, Benumof J: Mechanisms of hypoxemia and hypercapnia in the perioperative period. Crit Care Clin 3:279, 1987.)

16. What adverse reaction can occur if halothane and epinephrine are combined?

The potential for life-threatening dysrhythmic effects exists between inhalational anesthetics and vasoconstrictors. The combination creating the greatest adverse effect is between halothane and epinephrine. The addition of thiopental (Pentothal), an ultra short-acting barbiturate, further enhances these dysrhythmic effects. The true mechanism of action creating these dysrhythmic disturbances is not completely understood, but it appears to involve stimulation of both alpha and beta adrenergic receptors.

The potential for this adverse reaction is greatest when anesthesia and surgery have just begun. If anesthesia is induced with thiopental and maintained with halothane, and local anesthesia involving epinephrine is used by the surgeon, then an adverse reaction may ensue. Several recommendations have been proposed to prevent such reactions. Do not inject a local anesthetic with epinephrine immediately after the induction of anesthesia with halothane or thiopental; it is prudent to wait for 10 minutes. Use 2 µg/kg of epinephrine if either halothane or thiopental is being administered and 1 µg/kg if halothane and thiopental are being used. Remember, local anesthetic with 1:100,000 epinephrine contains 10 µg/ml of epinephrine.

17. Define partition coefficient and explain how it can influence the speed of induction.

A partition coefficient is defined as a distribution ratio of a volatile anesthetic as it distributes itself between two phases at equilibrium when the temperature, pressure, and volume are the same. A blood-to-gas coefficient therefore describes the distribution of anesthetic between blood and gas. A high blood solubility requires a greater concentration of inhaled anesthetic to be dissolved in the blood before equilibrium with the gas phase can occur. The blood acts as an inactive reservoir that prevents the anesthetic from reaching the site of action, thereby slowing induction.

Partition Coefficients for Inhaled Anesthetics

	DESFLURANE	HALOTHANE	ISOFLURANE	N_2O	SEVOFLURANE
Blood:gas	0.42	2.4	1.4	0.46	0.68
Brain:blood	1.3	2.9	1.6	1.1	1.7
Muscle:blood	2.0	3.4	2.9	1.2	3.1
Fat:blood	27	51	45	2.3	48
Oil:blood	18.7	224	90.8	1.4	47.2

The difference in blood-to-gas partition coefficients between halothane and sevoflurane explains why sevoflurane is a more rapid induction agent. With all other factors being equal (e.g., alveolar concentration, cardiac output), the lower solubility of sevoflurane will make it more readily available as an anesthetic.

18. Which volatile anesthetic has the quickest wake-up potential after a long (> 5 hours) surgical procedure?

Anesthetic takes awhile to be distributed from the blood to the tissues (e.g., muscle, fat). As the length of time of a surgery increases and tissues become increasingly saturated with anesthetic, wake-up times increase. The fat-to-blood partition coefficient for desflurane is the lowest for all volatile anesthetics, and it therefore provides the quickest wake-up. A common misconception is that sevoflurane has a quick wake-up time because it has a quick onset. For short surgeries, this is true, because tissue saturation has not had time to occur. For long surgeries, however, sevoflurane does not provide a quick wake-up (check sevoflurane's tissue:blood coefficients in the table in question 17).

CONTROVERSIES

19. What is diffusion hypoxia?

Although its existence has been questioned, diffusion hypoxia is postulated to occur when the administration of N_2O has been discontinued with the spontaneous breathing of room air. The theory holds that N_2O's low blood solubility allows it to leave the blood rapidly and enter the alveoli. Excessive N_2O in the alveoli dilutes the O_2 and makes the patient hypoxic. This phenomenon has been refuted by many studies. Nonetheless, because of side effects such as headaches, nausea, vomiting, and lethargy, administering O_2 for 3–5 minutes following N_2O use is prudent.

20. What are the concerns to administration of N_2O-O_2 sedation to an obstetric patient?

N_2O crosses the placenta and therefore has the potential to cause teratogenic effects to the fetus. The greatest potential for problems exists during the first trimester when organs are forming. Significant exposure during the first 6 weeks can inhibit DNA synthesis. Consequently, female surgeons and staff who aren't aware that they are pregnant may be at greater risk than patients.

Recent research has refuted the claim that N_2O is dangerous to the fetus. Although N_2O has been used safely for years in obstetrics, it would be wise to obtain a medical consult prior to its administration in pregnant women who are in their second and third trimester. Even if N_2O-O_2 sedation is approved by the patient's obstetrician, it should be used only for short procedures, and no more than 50% N_2O should be administered.

BIBLIOGRAPHY

1. Adamson DT: Oxygenation and ventilation. In Duke J (ed): Anesthesia Secrets, 2nd ed. Philadelphia, Hanley & Belfus, 2000, pp 5–10.
2. Cahalan MK, Lurz FW, Eger EI 2d, et al: Narcotics decrease heart rate during inhalation anesthesia. Anesth Analg 66:166-170, 1987.
3. Christensen LQ, Bonde J, Kampmann JP: Drug interactions with inhalational anaesthetics. Acta Anesthesiol Scand 37:231–244, 1993.
4. Clark MS, Brunick AL: Handbook of Nitrous Oxide Sedation. St. Louis, Mosby, 1999.
5. Eger EI 2d, Saidman LJ: Hazards of nitrous oxide anesthesia in bowel obstruction and pneumothorax. Anesthesiology 26:61–66, 1965.
6. Fiedler SO: Volatile anesthetics. In Duke J (ed): Anesthesia Secrets, 2nd ed. Philadelphia, Hanley & Belfus, 2000, pp 43–47.
7. Foltz B, Benumof J: Mechanisms of hypoxia and hypercarbia in the perioperative period. Crit Care Clin 3:279, 1987.
8. Hayashi Y, Kamibayashi T, Sumikawa K, et al: Adrenoreceptor mechanism involved in thiopental-epinephrine-induced arrhythmias in dogs. Am J Physiol 265:H1380–H1385, 1993.
9. Johnston RR, Eger EI 2d, Wilson C: A comparative interaction of epinephrine with enflurane, isoflurane, and halothane in man. Anesth Analg 55:709–712, 1976.
10. Kamibayashi T, Hayashi Y, Takada K, et al: Adrenoreceptor mechanism involved in thiopental-induced potentiation of halothane-epinephrine arrhythmias in dogs. Res Comm Mol Pathol Pharmacol 93:225–234, 1996.
11. Katz RL, Matteo RS, Papper EM: The injection of epinephrine during general anesthesia with halogenated hydrocarbons and cyclopropane in man. 2. Halothane. Anesthesiology 23:597–600, 1962.
12. Malamed SF: Sedation: A Guide to Patient Management, 3rd ed. St. Louis, Mosby, 1995.
13. Miller HJ: Chronic obstructive pulmonary disease. In Duke J (ed): Anesthesia Secrets, 2nd ed. Philadelphia, Hanley & Belfus, 2000, pp 220–228.
14. Ottevaere JA: Awareness during anesthesia. In Duke J (ed): Anesthesia Secrets, 2nd ed. Philadelphia, Hanley & Belfus, 2000, pp 165–168.
15. Rosen MA: Management of anesthesia for the pregnant surgical patient. Anesthesiology 91:1159–1163, 1999.
16. Stoelting RK, Miller RD: Effects of inhaled anesthetics on ventilation and circulation. In Stoelting RK, Miller RD (eds): Basics of Anesthesia, 3rd ed. New York, Churchill Livingstone, 1994, pp 47–57.

III. Postoperative Care

8. FLUID AND ELECTROLYTE MANAGEMENT

Lubor Hlousek, D.M.D., M.D., and Hamid Hajarian, M.S., D.D.S., M.D.

1. The postoperative basic metabolic panel (BMP) received for a patient who just underwent lengthy composite resection of intraoral malignant tumor reveals a potassium level of 6.5 mEq/L. What is the sequence of further management of this patient?

First, repeat the study to rule out an artifact. Then, obtain a 12-lead electrocardiogram (ECG) and look for peaked T waves, prolonged PR interval, decreased P wave, or widened QRS complex. If positive for ECG changes, give 10 ml of 10% calcium gluconate intravenously to stabilize myocardial membranes and prevent ventricular fibrillation. Also administer 10–15 units of regular insulin (which drives potassium intracellulary) in 50–100 ml of $D_{50}W$ intravenously and 20–60 gm of potassium trapping resin (Kayexalate) in 100–150 gm of sorbitol orally or as an enema. If the ECG is normal, stop administration of potassium and repeat the study in several hours.

2. What electrolyte disturbance can occur during massive rapid blood transfusion (2 L over 30 minutes) and how can you prevent it?

Acute hypocalcemia can occur during massive rapid transfusion of whole blood (more than 500 ml every 5–10 minutes). Therefore, it is best to infuse 0.2 gm of calcium chloride via a separate intravenous access for each 500 ml of whole blood. Ionized calcium should be monitored as should the QT interval on the ECG. In a hypocalcemic patient under general anesthesia, a prolonged QT interval would precede spontaneous tetany. Tingling and hyperactive reflexes cannot be assessed.

3. Which electrolyte disturbance mimics hypocalcemia? How can this be prevented in patients hospitalized for severe facial trauma or infection?

Symptoms of magnesium depletion include hyperactive deep tendon reflexes and positive Chvostek's sign (hyperactive facial muscle contracture upon a tap over facial nerve). It is often coupled with hypocalcemia, and both deficiencies should be corrected together. Anticipation of the problem and close monitoring of intravenous magnesium levels in a patient on intravenous fluid support is appropriate. The normal serum level of magnesium is 1.3–2.1 mEq. Symptomatic patients with normal renal function can be given 80 mEq of magnesium sulfate per liter of intravenous fluids over 4–6 hours. Asymptomatic patients should receive the same amount over 24 hours.

4. Which commonly used parenteral fluid most closely resembles extracellular fluid? How does its composition differ from 5% dextrose in half normal saline (D_5-$\frac{1}{2}$ NS)?

	ELECTROLYTE CONTENT (mEq/L)						OSMOLARITY
	SODIUM	POTASSIUM	CALCIUM	MAGNESIUM	CHLORIDE	HCO_3	(in Osm)
Lactated Ringer's	130	4	3	—	109	28 (as lactate)	273
Extracellular fluid	142	4	5	3	103	27	280–310
D_5-$\frac{1}{2}$ NS	77	—	—	—	77	—	407

5. In which condition is fluid resuscitation preferable with 5% dextrose in water (D_5W) over lactated Ringer's solution?

Symptomatic hypernatremia. Otherwise D_5W is rarely indicated because the glucose load may induce osmotic diuresis.

6. What are the critical levels of hyponatremia and how can this condition be corrected?

Symptoms usually occur during an acute, sudden decrease of sodium levels to < 130 mEq/L or during a chronic, gradual decrease to < 120 mEq/L. Treat the underlying cause or restrict free water intake first. Treat only acutely hyponatremic and profoundly symptomatic patients and raise serum sodium levels by 2 mEq/L/hr, but no higher than 125 mEq/L, with 3% NaCl.

$$\frac{2 \text{ mEq/L} \times 0.6 \times (\text{body weight in kg}) \times 1000}{513 \text{ mEq/L}} = \text{ml/hr of 3\% NaCl}$$

For example, for a 70-kg patient:

$$\frac{2 \times 0.6 \times 70 \times 1000}{513} \cong 160 \text{ ml/hr of 3\% NaCl}$$

7. What are the risks of rapid correction of hyponatremia or hypernatremia?

Rapid correction of hyponatremia with hypertonic solution may lead to permanent brain damage, seizures, and pontine myelinolysis. Rapid expansion of the extracellular fluid compartment can also worsen preexisting conditions, such as congestive heart failure. Rapid correction of hypernatremia and a severe decrease in serum osmolarity can cause convulsions, coma, and death.

8. What is the difference between the syndrome of inappropriate antidiuretic hormone production (SIADH) and diabetes insipidus?

In SIADH, there is increased production of ADH (as in a paraneoplastic syndrome), which may result in excessive retention of water and dilutional hyponatremia. In the opposite situation of diabetes insipidus (DI) there is insufficient secretion of ADH (as in a trauma to the hypophysis) with a resultant water loss and hypernatremia.

9. How is water deficit in hypernatremia calculated and replaced?

Slowly replace the lost water after calculating the water deficit.

Water deficit = $0.6 \times (\text{body weight in kg}) \times [(Na/140) - 1]$

For example, in a 70-kg patient with a serum sodium of 150 mEq/L:

Water deficit = $0.6 \times 70 \times [(150/140) - 1] = 42$ liters of body water $\times (1.07 - 1) = 3$ L

10. What is the maintenance fluid requirement of a healthy 72-kg adult who is restricted from oral intake (NPO) while awaiting surgery?

Maintenance fluid should be replaced with lactated Ringer's solution or D_5-$\frac{1}{2}$ NS with 20 mEq KCl/L in the following amount:

40 ml/hr for the 1st 10 kg of body weight + 20 ml/hr for 2nd 10 kg + 10 ml/hr for each additional 10 kg

Therefore, for a 72-kg patient, the fluid requirement is:

40 ml/hr + 20 ml/hr + 52 ml/hr = 112 ml/hr (for practical purposes 115 ml/hr)

11. How will the same situation be managed in a patient with end stage renal disease?

Intravenous fluids will be restricted to minimal level, usually 30 ml/hr of D_5-$\frac{1}{2}$ NS regardless of weight. Potassium will be usually avoided.

12. What is the drug therapy for an unconscious patient who develops diabetes insipidus after extensive panfacial and cranial fractures? How does therapy differ in a patient who is conscious and alert?

Unconscious patients may receive 5 units of the ADH analogue desmopressin (1-deamino-8-D-arginine vasopressin; DDAVP) subcutaneously every 4 hours along with slow replacement of free water. Patients who are alert and have sufficient oral intake of water may receive 2–4 μg of intranasal DDAVP twice a day.

13. How is the true serum calcium level calculated in a patient with a laboratory calcium concentration of 7.5 mg/dl and an albumin level of 2.0 gm/dl? What other laboratory value might be helpful?

Most serum calcium is bound to albumin, and therefore hypoalbuminemia will give false reading of hypocalcemia. The minimal normal albumin level is 3.5 gm/dl, and the corrected calcium level is calculated as follows:

(3.5 gm/dl – albumin level) × 0.8 + calcium level (mg/dl)
(3.5 – 2.0) × 0.8 + 7.5 = 8.7 mg/dl of corrected calcium level

The measurement of ionized calcium (iCa) in serum will give a true level of available calcium in serum.

14. What is normal plasma osmolarity and how is it calculated?

Normal plasma osmolarity is 290–310 mOsm/L. It can be calculated as follows:

$$\text{Plasma osmolarity} = 2[Na^+] + (\text{glucose}/18) + (BUN/2.8)$$

Discrepancies between measured and calculated plasma osmolarity may indicate presence of other osmotically active substances, such as ketone bodies.

15. An 11-month-old child who underwent palatoplasty had minimal blood-loss but is refusing any type of feeding and will be temporarily started on parenteral fluids. She weighs 22 pounds. What is her total body water? What is her minimal acceptable urine output? What maintenance parenteral fluids should be prescribed?

Total body water in infants represents 75–80% of the kilogram body mass (in comparison to 50–60% in adults). Adequate urinary output in children younger than 1 year is 2.0 ml/kg/hr (in comparison to 0.5–1.0 ml/kg/hr in adults).

Maintenance intravenous fluids would be D_5-$\frac{1}{4}$ NS + 20 mEq KCl/L in the amount of 40 ml/hr. The amount of fluids is calculated the same way as in adults. The sodium and potassium intake requirements for infants are 3 mEq/kg/day and 2 mEq/kg/day, respectively.

16. A young, healthy woman who was hospitalized and treated for Ludwig's angina is unable to have any oral intake and is currently running a fever of 39.4°C. She weighs 60 kg, and her electrolytes are within normal limits. How should her parenteral fluids be managed?

Two to 2.5 ml/kg/day per each degree above 37.0°C are added to the appropriate maintenance fluid requirement to compensate for insensible losses due to fever. This patient's baseline would be 100 ml/hr of lactated Ringer's solution, and 12 ml/hr would be added according to the formula:

$$\frac{2 \times 60 \ (kg)}{24 \ (hr)} \times 2.4 \ (°C) = 12 \ ml/hr$$

17. Explain how low serum sodium concentration can be an artifact of measurement.

Hyperlipidemia and hyperproteinemia cause exclusion of sodium from a water-free space in the plasma sample. Therefore, apparent hyponatremia can be an artifact in the presence of either one of these conditions.

18. A 65-year-old man sustained severe facial trauma and underwent reconstructive surgery that lasted 12 hours. His medical history reveals chronic renal disease, and his preoperative chest radiograph is suggestive of left ventricular hypertrophy (LVH). The patient is managed on parenteral fluids in the intensive care unit. On the third postoperative day, his SaO_2 is difficult to maintain above 90% on 35% oxygen (O_2) administered via endotracheal tube. What is the possible cause? What diagnostic and therapeutic measures can you take?

This patient is manifesting symptoms of pulmonary edema, possibly due to fluid overload. It can be escalated by mobilization of fluid from the third space, which frequently starts on the third postoperative day. Therefore, lung auscultation, chest radiograph, and BMP with electrolyte level would be appropriate. Fluid restriction and possible administration of a loop diuretic (e.g., 10 mg of furosemide intravenously) would be the first line of action. Some patients with severely compromised cardiac function may require placement of a Swan-Ganz catheter to monitor extracellular fluids and central venous pressure.

19. What is the significance of anion gap and how is it calculated?

Anion gap can be calculated quickly from results of the basic metabolic panel (BMP). Concentration of two major cations in extracellular fluid (and plasma) approximately equals the concentration of the three major anions:

$$[Na+] + [K+] = [Cl^-] + [HCO_3^-] + [anion\ gap]$$

Anion gap normally ranges from 8 to 12 mmol/L. It becomes significant in the presence of metabolic acidosis, which can be due to an increase in anion gap (anion gap acidosis) or due to a drop in bicarbonate with normal anion gap (non-anion gap acidosis). The quick estimate may help differentiate the two.

20. What are the most common causes of anion gap acidosis?

The anion gap will increase in renal failure, lactic acidosis (decreased perfusion or intense exercise), or ketoacidosis (diabetes mellitus or starvation) and following ingestion of ethylene glycol, salicylates, methanol, and paraldehyde.

21. A patient has hyposmolar, hypervolemic hyponatremia 24 hours after surgery. What is the initial treatment?

Restrict oral fluid intake (usually to about 1000 cc/24 hours). This patient most likely has been overhydrated with hypotonic IV fluid. If the sodium level is not in the range that needs emergent correction, the patient will mobilize the fluid, and the sodium level will be corrected slowly on its own.

22. A trauma patient who has undergone repair of maxillofacial fractures develops oliguria with a serum osmolarity of 1000 mOsm/dl. What is the most likely diagnosis?

SIADH, probably due to trauma.

23. A patient who has been on IV antibiotics for 7 days develops diarrhea. The patient is hemodynamically stable. What is the most appropriate fluid to administer initially?

This patient is suffering from insult to normal intestinal function. Thus, the patient is losing sodium, potassium, and, to a lesser extent, other ions (e.g., calcium, magnesium). Lactated Ringer's solution is the best fluid for this situation, because it contains sodium, potassium, calcium, lactic acid, and sodium bicarbonate, which resemble the fluid lost from small intestine.

24. A patient with history of congestive heart failure is on loop diuretics and digoxin. He is admitted for maxillofacial surgery. Perioperatively, what is the most important electrolyte to check and adjust?

Potassium. Loop diuretics (e.g., furosemide) are potassium-wasting drugs. Digoxin is an inotrope, which blocks Na/K channels. The serum potassium level of patients who take digoxin and loop diuretics should be safely above 4.0 mEq/L in order to prevent arrhythmia. This patient has the potential to develop hypokalemia because of the loop diuretic. Thus, paying close attention to serum potassium level is critical for prevention of cardiac dysfunction.

25. A patient manifests signs and symptoms of muscle twitching and prolonged QT on ECG. What electrolyte should be checked?

Calcium. Hypocalcemia increases excitation of the neuromuscular system, causing cramps and tetany. Chvostek's sign and Trousseau's sign (carpopedal spasm following occlusion of arterial blood supply to the arm for 3 minutes) are clinically important indications of hypocalcemia. Prolonged QT may lead to arrythmias and subsequent heart failure if not treated.

26. A trauma patient develops polyuria with low osmolarity on day 1 of hospital admission. What is the most likely diagnosis and what is the initial management?

Diabetes insipidus is the most likely diagnosis. The initial management would be intravenous $\frac{1}{2}$ NS and DDAVP. In diabetes insipidus, ADH is not adequately released from the posterior pituitary. In this patient, trauma to the stalk in the pituitary gland is probably the cause. Therefore, the patient is losing free water. The patient requires IV fluid to keep him or her hemodynamically stable and also to prevent hyperosmolar hypovolemic hypernatremia. This is best accomplished with a hypotonic solution such as $\frac{1}{2}$ or $\frac{1}{4}$ normal saline. Patient also needs exogenous replacement of ADH. Thus, DDAVP needs to be administered intravenously to prevent free water loss.

27. Following a motor vehicle accident, a patient is on a ventilator, receives appropriate fluid, has a Foley catheter, and has no oral intake. What is the source of his insensible fluid loss?

Perspiration. Sensible losses are through the kidneys and feces. Insensible losses are through the skin and lungs. When a patient is on a closed-system ventilator, there is really no insensible loss through the lungs. Thus, the only insensible loss that needs to be replaced is the evaporated sweat.

28. A patient, who has a past medical history significant for chronic renal failure, is put on a regular diet. The next day, the patient develops flaccid muscles and decreased urine output. His magnesium is normal. Which electrolyte is the most likely cause?

Potassium. Hyperkalemia is characterized by flaccid muscle, fatigue, and ECG abnormalities in severe cases. Considering the patient's history, he might have hypermagnesemia or hyperkalemia, but the magnesium is reported as normal. Therefore, the potassium level must be checked and treated accordingly.

29. A patient with a history of insulin-dependent diabetes mellitus and buccal space infection has a fever of 38°C and is responding to treatment very slowly. She progresses into diabetic ketoacidosis. Her potassium is 6.2 in a nonhemolyzed serum, and her glucose is 400 mg/dl. How should her potassium be corrected?

Intravenous insulin in D_5-$\frac{1}{2}$ NS. True severe hyperkalemia is a serious condition that needs to be treated urgently. Initial treatment is administration of insulin with glucose to force the potassium ions into intracellular compartments. This could be followed by administration of calcium gluconate to protect myocardium against hyperpolarization, intravenous administration of appropriate sodium bicarbonate and an oral chelating agent (EDTA). In life-threatening situations or if the patient is refractory to the above treatment, plasmapheresis is the treatment of choice.

30. Twenty-four hours after an elderly patient underwent oral maxillofacial surgery, she develops tonic-clonic seizures. Her laboratory results indicate that her serum sodium is 119 mEq/L and her serum osmolarity is 250 Osm. The patient is euvolemic with stable vital signs. What is the appropriate fluid management of the patient?

Fluid restriction and very slow replacement with hypertonic saline solution (usually 3% NaCl). Many conditions can cause hypotonic, euvolemic hyponatremia. This patient is symptomatic (seizure), which should be treated first (i.e., with Valium). Sodium must be replaced very slowly to prevent central nervous system damage.

BIBLIOGRAPHY

1. Arieff AL, Ayus JC: Treatment of symptomatic hyponatremia: Neither haste nor waste [editorial]. Crit Care Med 19:748, 1991.

2. Lyerly HK, Gaynor JW (eds): Handbook of Surgical Intensive Care: Practices of the Surgical Residents of the Duke University Medical Center, 3rd ed. St. Louis, Mosby, 1992.
3. Narins EG (ed): Maxwell and Kleemnan's Clinical Disorders of Fluid and Electrolyte Metabolism, 5th ed. New York, McGraw-Hill, 1994.
4. Oh MS, Carroll HJ: Disorders of sodium metabolism: Hypernatremia and hyponatremia. Crit Care Med 20:94–103, 1992.
5. Roberts JP, Roberts JD, Skinner C, et al: Extracellular fluid deficiency following operation and its correction with Ringer's lactate: A reassessment. Ann Surg 202:1–8, 1985.
6. Shires GT, Canizaro PC, Shires GT III, et al: Fluid, electrolyte, and nutritional management of the surgical patient. In Schwartz SI (ed): Principles of Surgery, 5th ed. New York, McGraw-Hill, 1989.
7. Tierney ML Jr, McPhe SJ, Papadakis MA: Current Medical Diagnosis and Treatment, 3rd ed. Stamford, CT, Appleton & Lange, 1995.
8. Whang R, Ryder KW: Frequency of hypomagnesemia and hypermagnesemia: Requested vs. routine. JAMA 263:3063–3064, 1990.
9. Wrenn KD, Slovis CM, Slovis BS: The ability of physicians to predict hyperkalemia from the ECG. Ann Emerg Med 20:1229–1232, 1991.

9. NUTRITIONAL SUPPORT

Sonia Francioni, D.M.D., and Vincent B. Ziccardi, M.D., D.D.S.

1. What is enteral nutrition?

Enteral nutrition is nutritional support consisting of a liquid formula administered via a tube into the gastrointestinal (GI) tract where the nutrients are absorbed. When the gut is functional, enteral nutrition is the preferred approach to nutritional support because it offers major advantages over parenteral nutrition.

2. When is enteral feeding/nutrition indicated?

Inability to ingest food normally due to maxillofacial trauma
Protein-energy malnutrition
Normal functioning bowel

3. When is enteral nutrition contraindicated?

- Complete gastric or intestinal obstruction when access cannot be placed distal to the obstruction
- Ileus
- High-output enteric fistulas (> 500 ml/day)
- Acute pancreatitis (moderate to severe)
- Refusal of nutritional support by the patient or the patient's legal guardian
- Severe diarrhea or vomiting

4. What are the physical properties of enteral nutrition?

- **Osmolality:** Most enteral formulas are well tolerated and range from 300 to 700 mOsm/kg.
- **Renal solute load:** If the renal solute load of a formula is high, a large quantity of water must be administered to excrete it.
- **Viscosity:** Formulas containing larger molecules and formulas with a high caloric content per unit volume tend to be more viscous.

5. Name the three routes of administration for short-term feedings.

1. Nasogastric tube (NGT)
2. Nasoduodenal tube (NDT)
3. Nasojejunal tube (NJT)

6. If a patient is at risk for aspiration, which short-term feeding route is indicated?

If a patient is at risk for aspiration, the nasoduodenal and nasojejunal (postpyloric) routes are best. The technique of nasoduodenal feeding can overcome problems of gastric retention. There are fewer problems with gastroesophageal reflux and subsequent risk of tracheobronchial aspiration. The technique of nasojejunal feeding bypasses an obstructive lesion or motor abnormalities involving the GI tract proximal to the jejunum.

7. What route of administration is indicated for long-term enteral feedings?

For long-term enteral feeding, enterostomies are the preferred access route. Percutaneous endoscopic gastrostomy (PEG) involves placement of a 16- to 18-gauge latex or silicone catheter through the abdominal wall and directly into the stomach.

8. Which feeding route is preferred when a patient is at risk for aspiration?

If a patient is at risk for aspiration, the feeding tube should be placed in the small intestine either surgically via a jejunostomy or nonsurgically via a percutaneous jejunostomy tube.

9. Where does a nasogastric tube extend and what are some advantages to its use?

The NGT extends from the nose into the stomach. NGTs are advantageous because:
- The NGT tolerates high osmotic loads without cramping, distention, vomiting, diarrhea, or fluid and electrolyte shifts.
- It allows intermittent or bolus feedings because the stomach has a large reservoir capacity.
- It is easier to position a tube into the stomach than into the jejunum.
- The presence of hydrochloric acid in the stomach may help prevent infection.

10. Where does a nasoduodenal tube extend and when is it indicated?

The nasoduodenal tube extends from the nose through the pylorus and into the duodenum. NDT feedings are indicated in:
- Patients at risk for aspiration
- Patients who are debilitated, demented, stuporous, or unconscious
- Patients with gastroparesis or delayed gastric emptying

11. What is meant by continuous feeding and what are its advantages and disadvantages?

Continuous feeding allows a patient to receive a constant infusion of enteral feedings. The advantages of continuous feeding are decreased risk of aspiration, bloating, distention, and osmotic diarrhea with improved patient tolerance. The disadvantages of continuous feeding are that it requires the patient to be physically connected to the apparatus during infusion and the expense associated with the purchase of volumetric infusion pumps.

12. What is parenteral nutrition?

Parenteral nutrition is a sterile and nutrient-dense solution that is infused intravenously by a peripheral or a central venous access, thereby entirely bypassing the digestive tract.

13. Name the two types of parenteral nutrition and describe the differences between the two.

1. **Peripheral parenteral nutrition** (PPN) is a means of nutritional support in which the parenteral nutrition is administered directly into the peripheral vein. PPN must have a lower osmolarity to prevent phlebitis. PPN is indicated for anticipated short-term use (< 10 days) because PPN usually does not meet all the nutritional needs of the patient.

2. **Total parenteral nutrition** (TPN) is a means of nutritional support in which a parenteral solution is administered directly into a central vein (usually the superior vena cava). It is indicated for anticipated long-term use (> 10 days). TPN provides total caloric, protein, lipid and nutrient supplementation for patients who cannot tolerate oral or enteral feedings.

14. When is TPN indicated?

Mechanical intestinal obstruction
Severe malabsorption
Active inflammatory bowel disease
Small bowel fistula

15. What three macronutrients are required when infusing TPN?

Glucose, protein, and lipids.

16. What parameters should be monitored in patients receiving TPN?

- Metabolic parameters: sodium, potassium, chloride, CO_2, blood urea nitrogen (BUN), creatinine, glucose, hematocrit, hemoglobin, white blood cell count (WBC), calcium, magnesium, phosphorus, and platelets

- Nutrition: daily weight evaluations, albumin, and prealbumin
- Fluid status
- Infection: If WBC count is increasing or the patient is febrile, a blood culture should be obtained and consideration given to changing the central line.

17. Which complications are associated with parenteral nutrition?
- Venous thrombosis with increased risk for pulmonary embolism
- Catheter-related sepsis usually caused by staphylococcal, fungal, and gram-negative organism infection
- Metabolic complications such as hyperglycemia, which may be associated with glycosuria, osmotic diuresis, diabetic ketoacidosis (DKA), fatty infiltration of the liver, and acalculous cholecystitis

BIBLIOGRAPHY

1. Bickston SJ: Nutritional therapy. In Ewald GA, McKenzie CR (eds): The Washington Manual of Medical Therapeutics. Boston, Little, Brown, 1995, pp 34–42.
2. Morrison G, Hark L (eds): Medical Nutrition and Disease. Cambridge, MA, Blackwell Science, 1996.
3. Rombeau JL, Caldwell MD (eds): Enteral and Tube Feeding, 2nd ed. Philadelphia, W.B. Saunders, 1990.
4. Rombeau JL, Caldwell MD (eds): Parenteral Nutrition. Vol. 2, 2nd ed. Philadelphia. W.B. Saunders, 1993.
5. Torosian MH (ed): Nutrition for the Hospitalized Patient. New York, Marcel Dekker, 1995.
6. Ziccardi VB, Bergen-Shapiro M: Metabolic and nutritional aspects of facial trauma. Oral Maxillofac Clin North Am 10:507–518, 1998.

10. POSTOPERATIVE COMPLICATIONS

Robert E. Doriot, D.D.S.

1. What are the most common causes of fever in the first 24 hours after surgery?
Atelectasis
Aspiration pneumonia
An ill-defined response to the surgery itself

2. What are the most common causes of postoperative fever in the first 24–72 hours?
Atelectasis
Bacterial pneumonia
Thrombophlebitis

3. What are the most common causes of fever 72 hours after surgery?
Pneumonia
Pulmonary emboli
Intravenous (IV) catheter infection
Wound infection
Urinary tract infection

4. What are the "five W's" of postoperative fever?
The "five W's" are the possible causes of any postoperative fever: *w*ind, *w*ater, *w*ound, *w*alking, and *w*onder drugs.

5. When can the surgical site be considered the source of postoperative fever?
The surgical site should not be considered the primary source of postoperative fever until at least 48–72 hours after surgery.

6. How often should IV catheter sites be changed to avoid infection?
In general, IV access sites should be changed every 72 hours.

7. What are the common signs and symptoms of phlebitis?
Pain
Tenderness
Edema
Erythema
Streaking of the limb

8. What is the treatment for phlebitis?
1. Remove the intravenous catheter.
2. Elevate the affected limb.
3. Apply warm, moist packs to the infected site.
4. Initiate IV antibiotics (preferably cefazolin [Ancef], 1 gm IV bolus push every 8 hours), for appropriate staphylococcus coverage.

9. What are the most frequent respiratory complications following oral and maxillofacial surgery?
Pulmonary atelectasis
Aspiration pneumonia
Pulmonary embolus

10. Which group of patients is predisposed to the development of postoperative atelectasis?

Postoperative atelectasis occurs more often in smokers than in any other subset of patients.

11. Where is the most common site for aspiration pneumonia to develop?

If aspiration pneumonia occurs, it is most likely to manifest itself initially in the patient's right lung.

12. Where do most postoperative pulmonary emboli originate?

The deep venous systems of the lower extremities, especially in nonambulatory patients.

13. What is Virchow's triad?

Virchow's triad is the name given to the three chief causes of deep venous thrombosis (DVT): (1) damage to the endothelial lining of the vessel, (2) venous stasis, and (3) a change in blood constituents attributable to postoperative increase in the number and adhesiveness of the patient's platelets.

14. What are the classical clinical features of DVT?

Calf swelling and tenderness
Fever
Chest pain
Sudden dyspnea
Tachypnea

15. What is Homans' sign?

Homans' sign is pain in the calf that is elicited by forced dorsiflexion of the foot. It was once considered pathognomonic for the presence of DVT, but it is no longer taught because performing this maneuver can increase the risk of movement of an existing thrombus.

16. What is the immediate treatment of DVT?

A patient who has developed a DVT should be started immediately on systemic anticoagulation with elevation of the affected limb. Subcutaneous heparin and low–molecular-weight heparin are choices to consider.

17. How are the development of fever and the patient's heart rate interrelated?

For every 1°C rise in body temperature, there is a corresponding 9–10 beat per minute increase in the patient's heart rate.

18. What are some common causes of postoperative bleeding?

Incompletely ligated or cauterized vessels
Wound infection
Coagulopathy
Rebound effect of hypotensive anesthesia

19. What are some common causes of postoperative hypotension?

A good differential diagnosis for the development of hypotension should include intravascular hypovolemia, rewarming vasodilation, myocardial depression, and hypothyroidism.

20. Name the most common causes of the development of postoperative hypertension.

Pain and anxiety
Overdistention of the bladder
Hypoxia
Hypercapnia

21. What are some possible treatment options for postoperative hypotension?
- Elevation of the lower extremities
- Administration of carefully monitored fluid boluses
- Administration of vasopressors (e.g., ephedrine)

22. What is the most common cardiac arrhythmia observed in the postoperative period? Why?
The most common postoperative arrhythmia is the development of ventricular complexes or premature ventricular contractions (PVCs). Hypoxia, pain, or fluid overload, all of which are common in the postoperative period, can precipitate PVCs.

23. What is the most common cause of dysuria in the immediate postoperative period?
The agents incorporated in the administration of general anesthesia can inhibit the micturitic reflex, and the patient can suffer bladder distention, which itself may inhibit the ability to micturate.

24. What are some other causes of dysuria in the postoperative period?
- "Positional inhibition" (many patients find it difficult to pass urine while supine)
- Preexisting prostatism
- Inadequate fluid replacement during surgery, which creates a hypovolemic state

25. Describe the treatment options for postoperative dysuria in a patient with suprapubic pain and an obviously distended bladder elicited by palpation in the first 4–6 hours after surgery.
Treatment of postoperative dysuria should begin simply by having the patient stand by or sit on the toilet while running water in the sink. If this does not help and there is no evidence a of hypovolemic state, then the patient should be catheterized. If the residual measures > 300 cc then the catheter should be left in overnight.

26. What are some common causes of postoperative nausea and vomiting?
Hypoxia, hypotension, and narcotics.

27. What types of patients are more likely to develop postoperative nausea and vomiting?
Postoperative nausea and vomiting occurs more frequently in children than in adults and more commonly in women than in men.

28. What is a seroma and how can it be prevented?
A seroma is fluid (other than pus or blood) that has collected in the wound. Seromas often appear after surgical procedures that involve elevation of skin flaps and transection of numerous lymphatic channels. The incidence of seromas can be decreased if proper pressure dressing is applied to the wound after surgery.

29. What is the treatment of seroma?
Seromas should be evacuated either by needle aspiration or by incision and drainage because they can delay healing and provide an excellent medium for bacterial growth. A pressure dressing should be placed immediately after drainage to help seal lymphatic leaks and prevent additional accumulation of fluids.

30. How can aspiration be prevented?
Aspiration can be prevented by avoiding general anesthesia in patients who have recently eaten, positioning the patient correctly before endotracheal intubation, and using high-volume, low-pressure cuffs on the endotracheal tube. If the risk of aspiration is high, metoclopramide should be administered before surgery to minimize the incidence of aspiration pneumonia.

31. Which surgical patients are predisposed to aspiration?

Tracheostomy patients. Incidence has been reported as high as 80%.

32. Why does postoperative pneumonia develop?

After surgery, a patient's host defense against pneumonia is compromised. This impairment is likely caused by several factors: the cough mechanism may be impaired and may not effectively clear the bronchial tree, the mucociliary transport mechanism may be damaged by endotracheal intubation, and the alveolar macrophage may be compromised by a number of factors that may be present during and after surgery (e.g., hypoxia, pulmonary edema, aspiration, or corticosteroid therapy). All of these factors may decrease the patient immune response to infection with pneumonia and increase the incidence of postoperative pneumonia.

33. What is the primary pathogen for postoperative pneumonia?

Approximately half of the pulmonary infections that follow surgery are caused by gram-negative bacilli, which are usually acquired by aspiration of oropharyngeal secretions.

34. What is the treatment for postoperative pneumonia?

Appropriate antibiotic therapy, which can be determined through sputum culture, and sensitivity and clearing of secretions through aggressive suctioning and chest physical therapy.

35. What are the common causes of postoperative cardiac arrhythmias?

Postoperative arrhythmias are generally related to reversible factors such as hypokalemia, hypoxemia, alkalosis, and digitalis toxicity, but they could be the first sign of postoperative myocardial infarction. Postoperative myocardial infarction is rare with an incidence of 0.7% for patients without preexisting cardiac disease. However, incidence increases to 6% for patients with preexisting cardiac disease.

36. Why is postoperative myocardial infarction difficult to diagnose?

Over one-third of postoperative myocardial infarctions are asymptomatic secondary to the residual effects of anesthesia and analgesics administered postoperatively.

BIBLIOGRAPHY

1. Leigh JM: Postoperative care. In Rowe NL, Williams IL (eds): Maxillofacial Injuries, Vol. II. New York, Churchill-Livingstone, 1985, pp 695–708.
2. Meyer LE: Postoperative problems. In Kwan PH, Laskin DM (eds): Clinical Manual of Oral and Maxillofacial Surgery, 2nd ed. Carol Stream, IL, Quintessence, 1997, pp 215–225.
3. Pellegrini CA: Postoperative complications. In Way L (ed): Current Surgical Diagnosis and Treatment, 6th ed. Los Altos, CA, Lange, 1983, pp 23–38.

IV. *Management of Medical Emergencies*

11. BASIC LIFE SUPPORT

Mark A. Oghalai, D.D.S.

1. What maneuver should the rescuer first use to open the airway in an otherwise un-injured patient?
Head-tilt with chin-lift.

2. What is the most frequent cause of airway obstruction in an unconscious person?
The tongue.

3. What are the ABCs of cardiopulmonary resuscitation (CPR)?
Airway, breathing, and circulation.

4. A victim whose heart and breathing have stopped has the best chance for survival if emergency medical services (EMS) are activated and CPR is begun within how many minutes?
Four minutes.

5. At what point should the EMS be activated with adult victims?
Immediately when an adult is found to be unresponsive.

6. At what point should the EMS be activated with infant and children victims in a one person rescue?
After 1 minute of CPR.

7. What is the length of time recommended to deliver each breath to an adult victim?
1.5–2 seconds/breath.

8. What is the length of time recommended to deliver each breath to an infant or child victim?
1–1.5 seconds/breath.

9. What is the best indicator of effective ventilation?
Seeing the chest rise when delivering breaths.

10. What is the minimum length of time used when assessing for a pulse?
5 seconds.

11. When an adult victim has a pulse but is breathless, what is the recommended rate of rescue breathing?
Once every 5–6 seconds (10–12 breaths/minute).

12. When a child has a pulse but is breathless, what is the recommended rate of rescue breathing?
Once every 3 seconds (20 breaths/minute).

13. What should be done after each rescue breath?
Watch the victim's chest fall as you allow time for the lungs to empty.

14. In a victim with a pulse, how often should the pulse be checked during rescue breathing?
Once every minute.

15. What happens if chest compressions are interrupted?
Blood flow and blood pressure will drop to zero.

16. In a pulseless victim, how often should the pulse be checked during CPR?
After the first minute and every few minutes thereafter.

17. Name the two primary indicators of effective CPR.
1. Seeing the chest rise when rescue breathing is delivered
2. Presence of a pulse during chest compressions

18. What are the three main categories of airway obstructions?
1. Partial airway obstruction with good air exchange
2. Partial airway obstruction with poor air exchange
3. Complete airway obstruction

19. In the initial assessment, how is the presence or absence of breathing determined?
Watch for movement of the chest while listening and feeling for air movement at the nose and mouth.

20. Where is the correct location for applying pressure for external chest compressions in adult and children victims?
The lower half of the sternum, two fingerwidths superior to the xiphoid process.

21. Where is the ideal location for applying pressure for external chest compressions in infants?
One fingerwidth below the nipple line.

22. What is the depth of external chest compressions in adults?
1.5–2 inches.

23. What is the depth of external chest compressions in children?
1–1.5 inches.

24. What is the depth of external chest compressions in infants?
0.5–1 inch.

25. What is the rate of external chest compressions for adults?
80–100/minute.

26. What is the rate of external chest compressions for children?
100/minute.

27. What is the rate of external chest compressions for infants?
At least 100/minute.

28. What is the ratio of external chest compressions to breaths for one rescuer with an adult victim?

Fifteen compressions for every two breaths.

29. What is the rate of external chest compressions to breaths for one or two rescuers with a pediatric victim?

Five compressions for each breath.

30. What is the rate of external chest compressions to breaths for one or two rescuers with an infant victim?

Five compressions for each breath.

31. What is the recommended method of clearing foreign body airway obstructions in infants?

A combination of back blows and chest thrusts.

32. What is the recommended method of clearing foreign body airway obstructions in children and adults?

The Heimlich maneuver.

33. Why should blind finger sweeps not be used in children and infants?

The object may be pushed deeper in the airway.

BIBLIOGRAPHY

1. Efferon DM: Cardiopulmonary Resuscitation, 4th ed. Tulsa, OK, CPR Publishers, 1993.
2. Malmed SF: Handbook of Medical Emergencies in the Dental Office, 5th ed. St. Louis, Mosby, 1999.
3. Strauss RA: Managing medical emergencies. In Kwon P, Laskin D (eds): Clinical Manual of Oral and Maxillofacial Surgery, 2nd ed. Chicago, Quintessence, 1997, pp 141–142.

12. ADVANCED CARDIAC LIFE SUPPORT

Kathy A. Banks, D.M.D., and Sonia Francioni, D.M.D.

1. How is the diagnosis of cardiac arrest established?
By definition, the patient is in full cardiac arrest if he or she:
Is not responsive
Is not breathing
Has no pulse

2. What are the three mechanisms of cardiac arrest?
1. Ventricular fibrillation/pulseless ventricular tachycardia
2. Pulseless electrical activity
3. Asystole
Ventricular fibrillation is most commonly present during the first minute following the onset of cardiac arrest.

3. Which types of chest pain suggest ischemia?
 • Uncomfortable squeezing pressure, fullness, or pain in the center of the chest lasting >
   15 minutes
 • Pain that radiates to the shoulder, neck, arm, and jaws
 • Pain between the shoulder blades
 • Chest discomfort with light-headedness, fainting, sweating, and nausea
 • A feeling of distress, anxiety, or impending doom

4. What is the recommended initial management for a stable patient with chest pain that is suggestive of ischemia?
1. Call for help
2. Perform immediate assessment including:
      Vital signs and SaO_2 monitoring
      IV access and electrocardiogram (ECG)
      Targeted history and physical examination
      Initial serum cardiac marker levels, electrolytes, and coagulation studies
      Portable chest x-ray
3. Immediate general treatment:
      Oxygen at 4 L/minute
      Aspirin (160–325 mg)
      Nitroglycerin (sublingual or spray)
      Morphine (IV) if pain is not relieved by nitroglycerin

5. What is the most common arrhythmia following electrical shock?
The most common arrhythmia caused by electrocution is **ventricular fibrillation**; hence cardiac arrest is the primary cause of death from electrical shock. Other rhythms that may occur following electrical shock are ventricular tachycardia progressing to ventricular fibrillation and asystole.
Electrical shock is the cause of over 1000 deaths per year in the United States. Electrical shock results in injuries ranging from unpleasant sensation to instant cardiac death. Exposure to high-tension current (greater than 1000 V) is more likely to produce serious injury. However, death can result from exposure to relatively low voltage (100 V) household currents. Alternating currents are more dangerous than direct currents. Alternating currents

produce muscle tetany, which may prevent the victim from releasing the electrical source and thus prolong the contact.

6. What is ventricular fibrillation?

Ventricular fibrillation (V-fib) is a cardiac dysrhythmia that occurs when multiple areas within the ventricles display unsynchronized depolarization and repolarization. As a result, the ventricles do not contract as a unit. Instead, the ventricles appear to quiver, or fibrillate, as multiple areas of the ventricle are contracting and relaxing in a disorganized fashion. The net result is no cardiac output and no pulse.

7. How is ventricular fibrillation treated initially according to the American Heart Association (AHA) recommendations?

- The initial treatment for ventricular fibrillation is always **defibrillation**.
- Begin with the universal algorithm:
    Assess the airway, breathing, and circulation (ABCs).
    Ascertain that the patient is in cardiac arrest.
    Begin cardiopulmonary resuscitation (CPR) until defibrillator is attached, and confirm V-fib.
- Countershock up to three times
    First shock = 200 joules
    Second shock = 200–300 joules
    Third shock = 360 joules
- If V-fib persists:
    Continue CPR, intubate, and establish IV access.
    Administer epinephrine (1.0 mg IV).
    Within 30 seconds of epinephrine bolus, shock with 360 joules.

8. What two medications are used in the treatment of refractory V-fib?

1. **Lidocaine** is generally accepted as the initial antifibrillatory agent in the treatment of V-fib at a recommended dose of 1–1.5 mg/kg (about 50–150 mg for an average adult patient). The drug should be circulated for about 30–60 seconds as CPR is performed, and then a countershock of 360 joules should be given. The bolus of lidocaine may be repeated in 3–5 minutes up to a total dose of 3 mg/kg. Upon return of spontaneous circulation, infusion of lidocaine is started at a rate of 2–4 mg/min.

2. **Bretylium** is used in V-fib that is refractory to defibrillation and lidocaine. The initial bolus dose is 5 mg/kg. The drug should be circulated for about 30–60 seconds by performing CPR. Then defibrillate. A second dose of 10 mg/kg can be given in 5 minutes. The maximum dose is 30 mg/kg.

9. Define tachycardia.

Tachycardia means that there is a rapid heart rate. Normal heart rate is considered by most to be between 60 and 100 beats per minute (bpm). Thus a heart rate of greater than 100 bpm can be classified as tachycardia. Not all patients with a heart rate of 100 bpm or more will require treatment. The following cardiac rhythms are considered tachyarrhythmias:

Atrial flutter
Atrial fibrillation
Paroxysmal supraventricular tachycardia (PSVT)
Ventricular tachycardia
Wide complex tachycardia of uncertain type

A patient with tachycardia or tachyarrhythmia needs treatment when there are signs and symptoms associated with the rapid heart rate. The following signs and symptoms indicate that the patient is already or is becoming hemodynamically unstable:

Chest pain	Pulmonary congestion
Shortness of breath	Congestive heart failure
Decreased level of consciousness	Premature ventricular contractions
Hypotension	Acute myocardial infarction (MI)
Shock	Ventricular rate > 150 bpm

10. Which tachyarrhythmias are supraventricular?

If the QRS complex is narrow, then the tachyarrhythmia is **supraventricular**. This means the arrhythmia is originating at or above the level of the atrioventricular (AV) node:

Sinus tachycardia
Atrial fibrillation
Atrial flutter
PSVT

If the QRS complex is wide, then the tachycardia is of **ventricular** origin:

Wide complex tachycardia of uncertain type
Ventricular tachycardia

11. How is the decision made whether to cardiovert a patient with tachycardia?

According to the AHA algorithm for tachycardia (with pulse):

1. Assess the patient.
   - ABCs
   - Oxygen, monitors, IV, and pulse oximetry
   - Brief history and targeted physical examination
   - 12-lead ECG
2. Determine if the patient is hemodynamically stable.
   - If there are *no* serious signs or symptoms of hemodynamic instability, treatment begins with diagnosis of the specific tachyarrhythmia and specific treatment for the particular tachyarrhythmia.
   - If there *are* serious signs and symptoms of hemodynamic instability:
     Synchronized cardioversion is performed.
     Synchronized cardioversion is not performed when tachycardia is a reflection of another underlying condition. For example, tachycardia that develops in response to severe hypotension, MI, or pulmonary edema.

12. Explain the pathophysiology of PSVT.

PSVT is a distinct clinical syndrome characterized by repeated episodes of tachycardia with abrupt onset lasting a few seconds to many hours. PSVT is due to a reentry mechanism involving the AV node alone or the AV node and an extranodal bypass tract.

13. According to AHA protocol, what is the treatment of PSVT in a stable patient?

1. Consider vagal maneuver (carotid body massage or Valsalva)
2. Treatment with adenosine:
   - Begin with 6 mg rapid IV push
   - Second dose of 12 mg
   - Third dose of 12 mg
3. Treatment with verapamil:
   - 2.5–5 mg IV slow push
   - Second dose of 5–10 ng IV
4. Consider other drugs:
   - Diltiazem
   - Digoxin
   - Beta-blocker

14. What are the signs and symptoms of atrial fibrillation and atrial flutter?

Atrial fibrillation (A-fib) may result from multiple areas of reentry within the atria or from multiple ectopic foci. A-fib may be associated with sick sinus syndrome, hypoxia, increased atrial pressure, and pericarditis. Because there is no uniform atrial depolarization, no P-wave will be seen on ECG. Hypotension may result from A-fib.

Atrial flutter (A-flutter) is the result of reentry circuit within the atria. Atrial flutter rarely occurs in the absence of organic disease. It is seen in association with mitral or tricuspid valvular disease, acute cor pulmonale, and coronary artery disease. Signs and symptoms include hypotension, ischemic pain, and severe congestive heart failure.

15. According to AHA protocol, how is A-fib treated?
1. Rule out precipitating causes for A-fib and A-flutter:

Heart failure	Pulmonary embolism
Acute MI	Substance abuse
Hyperthyroidism	Hypokalemia
Hypoxia	Hypomagnesemia

2. Administer rate-slowing drugs:
   Diltiazem
   Verapamil
   Beta-blockers
   Digoxin
3. Anticoagulation: consider heparin
4. Chemical cardioversion
   Procainamide
   Quinidine
5. Electrical cardioversion if drug therapy is unsuccessful

16. What is bradycardia?

The term *bradycardia* simply means that the heart rate is slow. Normal heart rate is considered by most to be 60–100 bpm. According to this definition, every patient with a heart rate less than 60 bpm is bradycardic. Not all patients with a heart rate less than 60 bpm will need treatment. Autonomic influence or intrinsic disease affecting the cardiac conduction system most often causes bradycardia.

A patient may have a relative bradycardia. An example is the patient with severe hypotension but with a heart rate of 70 bpm; the heart rate of 70 in a hypotensive patient may not sustain the cardiac output.

17. Name the principal bradyarrhythmias.
Sinus bradycardia
Atrial fibrillation with slow ventricular response
Atrioventricular block:
   First degree heart block
   Second degree heart block, types I and II
   Third degree heart block
Relative bradycardia
Other rhythms that may also be considered bradyarrhythmias are:
Pulseless electrical activity
Asystole

18. When does sinus bradycardia need treatment?

A patient with slow heart rate needs treatment only if there are serious signs or symptoms associated with the slow heart rate that indicate the patient is already or is becoming hemodynamically unstable. These signs and symptoms include:

Chest pain   Shock
Shortness of breath   Pulmonary congestion
Decreased level of consciousness   Congestive heart failure
Hypotension   Acute MI

19. How is a patient with a bradyarrhythmia initially managed according to AHA protocol?
1. Supportive actions:
   - Assess ABCs
   - Oxygen, IV, monitors, and pulse oximetry
   - Brief history and targeted physical examination
   - 12-lead ECG
2. Determine if bradycardia is hemodynamically significant.
   - If the patient is *not* hemodynamically unstable:
     Determine if there is severe conduction disturbance (Mobitz II second degree heart block, third degree heart block).
     Monitor patient.
     Be prepared to begin transcutaneous pacing (TCP) on standby.
   - If the patient *is* hemodynamically unstable:
     Atropine, 0.5–1.0 mg IV
     Transcutaneous pacing
     Dopamine infusion beginning with 5 µg/kg/min
     Epinephrine infusion, 1–2 µg/min
     Fluid challenge

20. What is meant by the term "heart block"?
Heart block is used interchangeably with the correct term *atrioventricular block*. Atrioventricular block describes a delay or interruption in conduction between the atria and the ventricles, which may be caused by one or more of the following causes:
- Lesion in the conduction pathway
- Prolonged refractory period along the conduction pathway
- Supraventricular heart rates that surpass the refractory period of the atrioventricular node

21. What is first degree heart block?
First degree heart block is the prolonged delay in conduction at the AV node or the bundle of His. The diagnosis of first degree heart block is based on the PR interval. First degree heart block exists when the PR interval is longer than 0.2 seconds.

22. According to AHA protocol, how is first degree heart block treated?
First degree heart block requires no treatment unless there are associated symptoms.

23. What is second degree heart block?
In second degree heart block, not every atrial impulse is able to pass through the AV node into the ventricles. The atrial impulses that are conducted to the ventricle will stimulate ventricular contraction. Therefore, the ratio of P to QRS will be greater than 1:1.
Type I second degree heart block (Wenckebach):
- Occurs at the level of the AV node
- Usually due to increased parasympathetic tone or drug effects
- Characterized by progressive elongation of the PR interval
- Conduction velocity through AV node gradually decreases until impulse is blocked, resulting in skipped ventricular beat

Type II second degree heart block:
- Occurs below the level of the AV node, uncommonly at the bundle of His
- Usually due to lesion along pathway
- The PR interval does not lengthen before skipped ventricular beat
- May have more than one skipped ventricular beat in a row
- Poorer prognosis than type I second degree heart block
- More likely to progress to complete heart block than type I

24. According to AHA protocol, how is type I second degree heart block treated?

Type I second degree heart block rarely requires treatment unless symptoms associated with bradycardia develop. Treatment should be directed at addressing the underlying cause of the block:

Decreased parasympathetic tone
Digitalis toxicity
Propranolol toxicity/overdose
Verapamil toxicity/overdose
If serious symptoms occur then the following treatment is recommended:
Atropine, 0.5–1.0 mg
TCP
Dopamine infusion beginning with 5 µg/kg/min
Epinephrine infusion, 1-2 µg/min
Fluid challenge if appropriate

25. According to AHA protocol, how is type II second degree heart block treated?

Type II second degree heart block requires no treatment unless symptoms associated with bradycardia develop. If serious symptoms develop, then the following treatment is recommended:

Atropine, 0.5–1.0 mg
TCP
Dopamine beginning with 5 µg/kg/min
Epinephrine infusion, 1–2 µg/min
Fluid challenge if appropriate

26. What is third degree heart block?

Third degree heart block occurs when no atrial impulses are transmitted to the ventricles. The atrial rate will be equal to or greater than the ventricular rate. If block occurs at the AV node, a junctional pacemaker may initiate ventricular depolarizations at a regular rate of 40–60 bpm. If the block is infranodal, usually both bundle branches are blocked and there is significant disease of the conduction pathway.

27. According to AHA protocol, how is third degree heart block treated?

Third degree heart block is treated only if there are signs and symptoms that the patient is or is becoming hemodynamically unstable. Recommended treatment for third degree heart block is:

Atropine, 0.5–1.0 mg
TCP
Dopamine infusion beginning with 5 µg/kg/min
Epinephrine infusion, 1-2 µg/min
Fluid challenge if appropriate

28. What is pulseless electrical activity (PEA)?

The term is used to describe a group of diverse ECG rhythms that manifest electrical activity but are similar in that the patient will be without a pulse. Therefore, the PEA is a non-perfusing rhythm.

The types of rhythms included in the PEA group are:

EMD: organized ECG rhythm present, no pulse

Pseudo-EMD: as above, but with some meaningful cardiac contraction

Idioventricular, ventricular escape: wide QRS, no atrial activity, and no pulse

Bradyasystolic: profound bradycardia with periods of asystole, no pulse

PEA is almost always a secondary disorder resulting from some underlying condition.

29. What are the causes of PEA?

The underlying causes of PEA can easily be remembered using the mnemonic "Drug PATCH":

Drug: ABCDs—*a*ntidepressants, *b*eta blockers, *c*alcium channel blocker, *d*igitalis

Pulmonary embolism

Acidosis, acute MI

Tension pneumothorax

Cardiac tamponade

Hypovolemia, hypoxia, hypothermia, hyperkalemia

Alternatively, the causes of PEA can be divided into three basic categories:

1. **Inadequate ventilation:**
   Intubation of right mainstem bronchus
   Tension pneumothorax
   Bilateral pneumothorax
2. **Inadequate circulation:**
   Pericardial effusion with tamponade
   Myocardial rupture
   Ruptured aortic aneurysm
   Massive pulmonary embolus
   Hypovolemia
3. **Metabolic disorder:**
   Electrolyte disturbances (hyper- or hypokalemia, hypomagnesemia)
   Persistent severe acidosis (diabetic ketoacidosis or lactic acidosis)
   Tricyclic overdose
   Hypothermia

30. According to AHA protocol, how is PEA treated?

1. Continue CPR.
2. Intubate/establish IV access.
3. Assess blood flow using Doppler.
4. Consider and treat underlying causes.
5. Epinephrine, 1 mg IV push. Repeat every 3–5 minutes.
6. Atropine, 1 mg push, if pulse is present and absolute bradycardia (< 60 bpm). Repeat every 3–5 minutes.

31. What is asystole?

The term *asystole* indicates the absence of ventricular activity. The patient will be without pulse. ECG will show characteristic flat line tracing without P-waves and QRS complexes. The underlying causes of asystole can be remembered using the mnemonic PHD:

Preexisting acidosis

Hypoxia, hyperkalemia, hypokalemia, hypothermia

Drug overdose

32. How is a flat line rhythm verified to be asystole?

- The patient will be pulseless.
- The patient will be unresponsive.

- The monitoring leads are correctly hooked up.
- There will be flat line recording in more than one lead.

33. What four conditions other than asystole can lead to a flat line tracing on ECG?
1. Fine V-fib
2. Loose electrode leads
3. No power
4. Signal gain is turned down

34. What four conditions are pulseless?
There are four conditions in which the patient will present without a pulse and are therefore considered nonperfusing conditions:
1. Ventricular fibrillation
2. Pulseless ventricular tachycardia
3. PEA:
   Electromechanical dissociation
   Pseudo-EMD (pulse will be very faint and evident only by Doppler)
   Ventricular escape rhythms
   Post defibrillation idioventricular rhythms
4. Asystole

35. According to AHA protocol, what is the treatment for asystole?
The treatment sequence for asystole is virtually the same algorithm for PEA:
1. Continue CPR.
2. Intubate/establish IV access.
3. Confirm asystole.
4. Consider and treat underlying causes.
5. TCP only if started early.
6. Epinephrine, 1 mg IV push. Repeat every 3–5 minutes.
7. Atropine, 1 mg IV, if pulse and absolute bradycardia (< 60 bpm). Repeat every 3–5 minutes.

36. What is shock?
The term *shock* denotes a clinical syndrome in which there is inadequate cellular perfusion and inadequate oxygen delivery for the metabolic demands of the tissues. Types of shock include:
Cardiogenic shock
Hypovolemic shock
Septic shock
Neurogenic shock
Flow disruption shock
Anaphylactic shock

In general, shock is characterized by:
Increased vascular resistance
   Cool mottled skin
   Oliguria
Tachycardia
Adrenergic response
   Diaphoresis
   Anxiety
   Vomiting
   Diarrhea
Myocardial ischemia
Mental status changes

37. What is the pathophysiology of acute cardiogenic pulmonary edema?
Acute cardiogenic pulmonary edema results from an increase in pulmonary venous pressure that leads to engorgement of the pulmonary vasculature. Lung compliance will decrease, and small airway resistance will increase. Lymphatic flow increases, presumably to maintain the pulmonary extravascular liquid volume. The net result is dyspnea and hypoxia, followed by shock.

38. What drugs are useful in the treatment of acute pulmonary edema?
Norepinephrine
Dopamine
Dobutamine
Nitroglycerin
Nitroprusside
Furosemide
Amrinone
Aminophylline
Thrombolytic agents
Digoxin

39 When is synchronized cardioversion used?
Tachycardia
PSVT
Atrial fibrillation
Atrial flutter

40. What are the signs and symptoms of cardiac tamponade?
Persistent tachycardia with falling blood pressure
Pulsus paradoxus
Pulsatile neck veins
Enlarging heart shadow on chest x-ray

41. What are the signs and symptoms of hypovolemic shock?
1. Cardiac output will be low due to inadequate left ventricular filling.
2. Hypotension may lead to changes in the ECG.

42. How is hypovolemic shock treated?
• Volume loss can be diagnosed through history and clinical evaluation.
• Replace volume with crystalloid or colloid solution when the hematocrit is normal.
• With active bleeding, hemostasis must be achieved first. If the hematocrit is dangerously low, transfusion of whole blood or packed red blood cells is indicated.

43. What drugs are used in the treatment of a patient with ventricular tachycardia who is hemodynamically stable?
Lidocaine
Procainamide
Bretylium
Magnesium

44. What are the four life-threatening conditions that may mimic acute MI and that may lead to cardiovascular collapse?
1. Massive pulmonary embolism
2. Hypovolemic and septic shock

3. Cardiac tamponade
4. Aortic dissection

45. What drugs can be administered via an endotracheal tube?
Naloxone
Atropine
Diazepam (Valium)
Epinephrine
Lidocaine

BIBLIOGRAPHY

1. Cohn E, Gilroy-Doohan M: Flip and See ECG. Philadelphia, W.B. Saunders, 1996.
2. Cummins RO (ed): Advanced Cardiac Life Support. Dallas, American Heart Association, 1997.
3. Grauer K, Caballaro D: ACLS: Rapid Reference. St. Louis, Mosby, 1997.
4. Thaler MS: The Only EKG Book You'll Ever Need. Philadelphia, Lippincott-Raven, 1997.

13. ADVANCED TRAUMA LIFE SUPPORT

Richard Long, D.D.S., and Vincent B. Ziccardi, M.D., D.D.S.

1. What is the correct sequence of evaluation and intervention that should be followed in all injured patients?

The mnemonic ABCDE defines the order of evaluation and intervention that should be followed in all injured patients:

Airway with cervical spine control
Breathing
Circulation
Disability or neurologic status
Exposure (undress) with temperature control

2. What determines the maximum rate of fluid administration through a catheter?

The maximum rate of fluid administration is determined by the internal diameter of the catheter and inversely by its length. The flow is not determined by the size of the vein in which the catheter is placed.

3. Which spinal cord tracts can be readily assessed clinically?

- The **corticospinal tract** is in the posterolateral aspect of the cord and controls motor function on the ipsilateral side and is tested by voluntary muscle contractions or involuntary response to painful stimulus.
- The **spinothalamic tract** is in the anterolateral aspect of the cord that transmits pain and temperature sensation from the contralateral side of the body.
- The **posterior columns** carry proprioceptive impulses from the ipsilateral side of the body and are tested by position sense of the fingers and toes or tuning fork vibratory sense.

4. Describe neurogenic shock.

Neurogenic shock results from impairment of the descending sympathetic pathways in the spinal cord. This results in loss of vasomotor tone and loss of sympathetic innervation to the heart. Loss of vasomotor tone causes vasodilatation of visceral and lower extremity vessels, pooling of blood intravascularly, and subsequent hypotension. Loss of sympathetic innervation to the heart will decrease the patient's ability to become tachycardic and may even cause the patient to become bradycardic. Fluid administration alone may cause fluid overload and congestive failure. Vasopressors and atropine are used in the treatment of neurogenic shock.

5. Which three radiographs should be obtained in a blunt trauma patient during a trauma resuscitation?

At the very least, the patient with blunt trauma should have cervical spine, anteroposterior chest, and anteroposterior pelvis radiographs. These films should be taken by portable means, in the resuscitation area if necessary, but should not interfere with the resuscitation process.

6. What is the optimal urinary output for adult and pediatric trauma patients?

A urinary output of at least 0.5 ml/kg/hr (50 ml/hr) in an adult patient and 1.0 ml/kg/hr in a pediatric patient older than 1 year should be maintained.

86

7. What are the benefits of endotracheal intubation?

Endotracheal intubation provides:

A secure airway

A means of delivering supplementary oxygen

A way to support ventilation

Prevention against aspiration

A means of providing pulmonary care

8. What O_2 saturation level corresponds with a PaO_2 of 27 mmHg? Of 30 mmHg? Of 60 mmHg? Of 90 mmHg?

PaO$_2$ LEVEL	O$_2$ SATURATION LEVEL
27 mmHg	50%
30 mmHg	60%
60 mmHg	90%
90 mmHg	100%

9. What is the most common cause of shock in a trauma patient?

Hemorrhage.

10. Describe the four classes of hemorrhage.

Class I is a loss of up to 15% of circulating blood volume. The clinical symptoms are minimal with mild tachycardia and no measurable changes in blood pressure, pulse pressure, or respiratory rate.

Class II is a loss of 15–30% of blood volume. Clinical symptoms include tachycardia, tachypnea, and a decrease in pulse pressure.

Class III results from a loss of 30–40% of blood volume. This equals about 2 L of blood in the average adult. Patients will have inadequate perfusion, marked tachycardia, tachypnea, significant changes in mental status, and a measurable fall in systolic pressure.

Class IV hemorrhagic shock occurs with a more than 40% blood volume loss. This is an immediate life-threatening event. Marked tachycardia, significant depression in systolic blood pressure, and very narrow pulse pressure will result. Diastolic pressure may be unobtainable in class IV hemorrhage.

11. What is the initial fluid of choice in resuscitation and why?

Lactated Ringer's solution is the initial choice for fluid resuscitation because it is an isotonic electrolyte solution, provides transient intravascular expansion, and further stabilizes vascular volume by replacing accompanying fluid losses into the interstitial and intercellular spaces.

12. What is a tension pneumothorax?

A tension pneumothorax develops when a one-way valve air leak occurs either from the lung or through the chest wall. Air is forced into the thoracic cavity without any means of escape, causing collapse of the affected lung. The mediastinum and trachea are displaced to the opposite side, decreasing venous return and compressing the opposite lung.

13. How is tension pneumothorax diagnosed and treated?

The diagnosis of tension pneumothorax should be made clinically and not radiographically because it is a medical emergency. It is characterized by respiratory distress, tachycardia, hypotension, tracheal deviation, unilateral absence of breath sounds, neck vein distention, and cyanosis as a late manifestation. Tension pneumothorax requires immediate decompression and is managed initially by rapidly inserting a needle into the second intercostal space in the midclavicular line of the affected hemithorax. Definitive treatment requires the insertion of a chest tube into the fifth intercostal space, usually anterior to the midaxillary line.

14. What is diagnostic peritoneal lavage (DPL)?

DPL is an operative procedure used for evaluating intra-abdominal trauma and is 98% sensitive for intraperitoneal bleeding. DPL is performed by making a 3–4-cm midline vertical incision in the abdominal skin inferior to the umbilicus. Some surgeons vary the position of the incision and some use a horizontal incision just below and to the right or left of midline. The incision is carried to fascia, and the peritoneum is incised allowing a peritoneal dialysis catheter to be inserted into the peritoneal cavity. Ten milliliters per kilogram of warm Ringer's lactate/normal saline (up to 1 L) are then instilled into the peritoneum, which is then drained by gravity after sitting for 5–10 minutes. A sample of the fluid is sent for erythrocyte and leukocyte counts (unspun). A grossly bloody lavage is immediately positive and no further testing is needed. A rule of thumb for a positive DPL is the inability to read newsprint through the lavage fluid. Laboratory testing identifying the need for surgical intervention is indicated by 100,000 red blood cells/mm^3 or more and greater than 500 white blood cells/mm^3.

15. For a patient with suspected abdominal trauma, does computed tomography (CT) or diagnostic peritoneal lavage provide a better initial exam?

DPL is the best initial exam for a patient with suspected abdominal trauma because it is faster than CT, requires no transport time, is more sensitive than CT, and is safe for all patients.

16. What is the Glasgow coma scale?

The Glasgow coma scale (GCS) provides a quantitative measure of a patient's level of consciousness. The GCS is the sum of scores for three areas of assessment: (1) eye opening, (2) verbal response, and (3) best motor response. The minimum GCS score that can be obtained is 3, and the maximum GCS is 15.

The eye opening response (E score) is graded as follows:
• Spontaneous—already open with blinking (E = 4 points)
• To speech—not necessarily to a request for eye opening (E = 3 points)
• To pain—stimulus should not be applied to the face (E = 2 points)
• None (E = 1 point)

The verbal response (V score) is graded in the following manner:
• Oriented—knows name, age, etc. (V = 5 points)
• Confused conversation—still answers questions (V = 4 points)
• Inappropriate words—speech is either exclamatory or random, but recognizable words are produced (V = 3 points)
• Incomprehensible sounds—grunts and groans are produced, but no actual words are uttered (V = 2 points)
• None (V = 1 point)

Best motor response (M score) is graded as follows:
• Obeys—moves limb to command and pain is not required (M = 6 points)
• Localizes—changing the location of the pain stimulus causes purposeful motion toward the stimulus (M = 5 points)
• Withdraws—pulls away from painful stimulus (M = 4 points)
• Abnormal flexion—decorticate posture (M = 3 points)
• Extensor response—decerebrate posture (M = 2 points)
• No movement (M = 1 point)

17. What are the signs and symptoms of an epidural hematoma?

Loss of consciousness followed by an intervening lucid interval
Secondary depression of consciousness
Development of hemiparesis on the contralateral side
A dilated and fixed pupil on the ipsilateral side as the impact area is also a hallmark of this injury.

18. What are the goals when assessing a trauma patient's extremities?
1. Identification of life-threatening injury
2. Identification of limb-threatening injury
3. Systematic review to avoid missing any other extremity injury

19. Define compartment syndrome and its treatment.

Compartment syndrome occurs when increased pressure in a confined anatomical area prevents capillary perfusion, thus threatening the function and viability of the perfused tissues. Unless mean arterial pressure is 30–40 mmHg above compartmental tissue pressure, neuromuscular survival is threatened. When symptoms or suspicion of a compartmental syndrome is present, all potentially constricting materials must be released. If symptoms do not respond, prompt fasciotomy may be required unless compartmental pressure measurements exclude the compartment syndrome definitively.

20. How are thermal burns classified?

The depth of burn is the key to evaluating severity, planning treatment, and determining outcomes for thermal burns. **First-degree** burns are characterized by erythema, pain, and the absence of blisters. Sunburn is an example of a first-degree burn. **Second-degree** burns are partial-thickness burns and are characterized by a red or mottled appearance with associated swelling and blister formation. The surface may appear wet and weeping and is painful and hypersensitive to touch. **Third-degree** or full-thickness burns are dark and leathery in appearance. The skin may appear translucent, mottled, or waxy-white. The surface is painless and generally dry.

21. What is the most common acid-base disturbance that develops during pediatric resuscitation?

Respiratory acidosis secondary to hypoventilation and hypoxia.

22. Describe the hemodynamic changes during pregnancy and their importance in managing the pregnant trauma patient and fetus.

Cardiac output is increased 1.0–1.5 L/min after the 10th week of pregnancy. As maternal blood volume is decreased during trauma, placental blood flow is preferentially reduced. Heart rate increases throughout pregnancy. This must be considered in interpreting the tachycardic response to hypovolemia. Blood pressure decreases 5–15 mmHg (systolic and diastolic) during the second trimester. This usually returns to near normal at term. Some pregnant women may exhibit profound hypotension when placed in the supine position. This supine hypotensive syndrome is relieved by turning the patient to the left lateral decubitus position.

BIBLIOGRAPHY

1. Advanced Trauma Life Support Student Manual. Chicago, American College of Surgeons, 1995.
2. Berry MJ, McMurray RG, Katz VL: Pulmonary and ventilatory responses to pregnancy, immersion, and exercise. J Appl Physiol 66:857–862, 1989.
3. Blow O, Bassam D, Butler K, et al: Speed and efficiency in the resuscitation of blunt trauma patients with multiple injuries: The advantage of diagnostic peritoneal lavage over abdominal computerized tomography. J Trauma 44:287–290, 1998.
4. Chiquito PE: Blunt abdominal injuries: Diagnostic peritoneal lavage, ultrasonography, and computed tomography scanning. Injury 27:117–124, 1996.
5. Gennarelli TA: Emergency department management of head injuries. Emerg Med Clin North Am 2:749–760, 1984.
6. Heppenstall RB, Sapega AA, Scott R, et al: The compartment syndrome: An experimental and clinical study of muscular energy metabolism using phosphorus nuclear magnetic resonance spectroscopy. Clin Orthop 226:138–155, 1988.
7. Servadei F, Vergoni G, Staffa G, et al: Extradural haematomas: How many deaths can be avoided? Protocol for early detection of haematoma in minor head injuries. Acta Neurochir 133(1–2):50–55, 1995.

14. CRICOTHYROTOMY AND TRACHEOSTOMY

Timothy S. Bartholomew, D.D.S., and A. Omar Abubaker, D.M.D., Ph.D.

1. What are the different methods of achieving and securing an airway in an emergency?

Simple maneuvers for airway management include head tilt and chin lift or jaw-thrust in the noninjured patients. Other adjunctive methods of airway management include the use of oral and nasal airways. The definitive method for airway control is by oral and nasal intubation. However, there may be situations in which this is difficult, impossible, or contraindicated, such as in severe panfacial trauma, massive upper airway bleeding, spasm of facial muscles, and laryngeal stenosis or deformities of the oronasopharynx. In such instances, if nonsurgical airway is unsuccessful, cricothyrotomy, whether by needle or surgical technique, may be the quickest, easiest, safest, and most effective way to obtain a patent airway.

2. What is the advantage of cricothyrotomy?

Cricothyrotomy should be viewed as the method of choice in procuring a patent airway in patients with acute obstruction of the airway, making it a very versatile procedure. Cricothyrotomy has the following advantages over the standard tracheostomy:

- It is faster.
- It is technically easier to perform with minimal instrumentation inside and outside an operating room setting.
- The incidence of operative and postoperative complications is low.
- It is safer to perform in patients with definite or suspected cervical spine injury or pharyngeal pathology.

3. When should cricothyrotomy be replaced with tracheostomy?

Unless the plan is to discontinue the access altogether, cricothyrotomy should be converted to tracheostomy within a maximum of 5–7 days.

4. Describe the anatomy pertinent to cricothyrotomy.

The thyroid cartilage consists of two quadrilateral-shaped laminae of hyaline cartilage that fuse anteriorly. The anterosuperior edge of the thyroid cartilage, the laryngeal prominence, is known as the Adam's apple. The angle at which these laminae converge is more acute in men than in women and therefore is more easily located in men. The thyroid prominence is the most important landmark in the neck when performing a cricothyrotomy. The next cartilaginous ring below the larynx (and the only complete ring) is the cricoid cartilage. It helps to maintain the laryngeal lumen and forms the inferior border of the cricothyroid membrane. This membrane, another important landmark, is a dense fibroelastic membrane located between the thyroid cartilage superiorly and the cricoid cartilage inferiorly and bounded laterally by the cricothyroid muscles. It is approximately 22–30 mm wide, 9–10 mm high, and 13 mm inferior to the vocal cords. This membrane can be identified by palpating a notch (a slight indentation or dip) in the skin inferior to the laryngeal prominence in an adult. Although the right and left cricothyroid arteries (branches of the right and left superior thyroid arteries, respectively) traverse the superior part of the cricothyroid membrane, these vessels are not of clinical significance or the cause of problems when performing a cricothyrotomy.

The tissue layers involved in cricothyrotomy include the subcutaneous tissue, cervical fascia, cricothyroid membrane, and tracheal mucosa. The distance from skin to tracheal lumen is only 10 mm in most adult patients. In contrast to the main body of the trachea, the posterior wall at this level of the upper airway is rigidly separated from the esophagus by the tall posterior cricoid cartilage shield, making esophageal perforation unlikely during cricothyrotomy.

The highly vascular thyroid gland lies over the trachea at the level of the second and third tracheal rings. If the tracheal rings or the thyroid gland is encountered when performing a cricothyrotomy, the incision is too low in the neck and must be redirected more superiorly.

5. Describe the technique of cricothyrotomy.

If there are no known or suspected cervical spine injuries, the patient's head may be hyperextended. Identify and palpate the notch or dip in the neck below the laryngeal prominence. Once the pertinent landmarks are identified, the right-handed surgeon then stabilizes the thyroid cartilage between the thumb and middle finger of his left hand and identifies the cricothyroid space with his left index finger. If local anesthetic is used, it should also be injected into the tracheal lumen to diminish the cough reflex during tube placement. A 3–4-cm transverse or vertical skin incision is made. A vertical incision is preferred in an emergency situation because, if the skin incision is too high or too low, it may be extended easily, saving time and avoiding a second incision. A short, horizontal stab incision (about 1 cm long) is made with a number 11 blade in the lower part of the cricothyroid membrane (nearer the cricoid ring) to avoid the cricothyroid arteries. Mayo scissors are spread horizontally in the incision to widen the space. Alternatively, the handle of the scalpel may be inserted and twisted 90°. Next, the opening is enlarged with Trousseau dilators or a curved hemostat. After stabilization of the larynx, the tracheostomy tube is inserted, the dilator or hemostat is removed, and the cuff of the tracheostomy tube is inflated (see Figure).

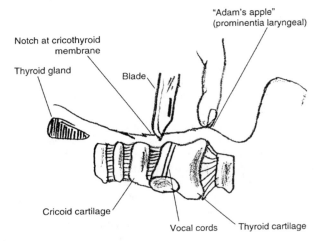

Landmark and incision for cricothyrotomy. (From Braun RJ, Cutilli BJ: Cricothyrotomy. In Braun RJ, Cutilli BJ (eds): Manual of Emergency Medical Treatment for the Dental Team. Baltimore, William & Wilkins, 1999, p 35, with permission.)

6. When is a tracheostomy the preferred emergency surgical airway?

In pediatric patients younger than 10–12 years. The small 3-mm-wide cricothyroid membrane and poorly defined anatomic landmarks make cricothyrotomy all but impossible in children.

7. What are the indications for a tracheostomy?

- Airway obstruction—e.g., from trauma, foreign bodies, irritants, anomalies, vasomotor incidents, laryngeal dysfunction, tumors, and obstructive sleep apnea syndrome
- For control of mucous secretion retention caused by inability to cough or expectorate— e.g., as in comatose and trauma patients
- Mechanical respiratory support—e.g., acute or chronic respiratory or central nervous system (CNS) diseases, multiple trauma patients
- Elective—e.g., for major head and neck procedures

8. Describe the surface anatomy landmarks for tracheostomy.

The most important anatomic landmarks for the tracheostomy procedure are the thyroid notch, cricoid ring, sternal notch, and innominate artery, which is above the sternal notch in approximately 25% of patients. The location for skin incision (approximately 4–6 cm long) for tracheostomy should be about 2 cm below the cricoid ring or midway between this ring and the sternal notch.

9. From skin to the trachea, list the layers encountered during the dissection for a tracheostomy.

Skin
Subcutaneous connective tissue
Platysma
Investing fascia
Linea alba of the infrahyoid muscles
Thyroid isthmus
Pretracheal fascia
Tracheal rings

10. What are the important principles in tracheostomy?
- Hyperextension of the neck, except in patients with suspected cervical spine injuries, facilitates the procedure.
- Always suture the flange of the tracheostomy tube to the skin.
- Never suture the skin incision tightly around the tube; leave the wound open to allow air to leak out.
- Upon decannulation, place tape across the stoma; do not suture the stoma closed.
- The cricoid cartilage and first tracheal ring must not be injured.
- The incision must not extend below the fourth ring (usually at rings 2 and 3).

11. Describe the technique for performing a tracheostomy.

A 4–6-cm incision is carried through skin, subcutaneous tissue, and platysma. Flaps are retracted superiorly, and a vertical incision in the fascia overlying the strap muscles is made. After the cricoid cartilage is identified, the thyroid isthmus may be retracted superiorly or divided and tied off. This exposes the second, third, and fourth tracheal rings. Using a hypodermic needle and a syringe, aspirate air from the trachea and inject 1–2 cc of local anesthetic to minimize coughing when entering the trachea. Make a 1-cm horizontal incision into the trachea above and below the ring of choice. This ring is cut so that a small rectangular window into the trachea is made. Place sutures in each side of the trachea to facilitate locating the tracheal stoma should the tube become dislodged. Insert the tracheostomy tube into the opening, taking care not to tear the cuff and not to insert the tube in the space anterior or lateral to the trachea. Once the tube is in place, inflate the cuff and check the chest for breath sounds. Leave the skin edges around the tube open or only partially closed with nonresorbable sutures, leaving a small space to minimize the danger of air escape into the subcutaneous tissue. Suture the tube to the skin, and secure it with a tape tied in a square knot around the neck (see Figure, next page).

12. What major vessels may be encountered during tracheostomy?

The anterior jugular vein and the jugular venous arch are found in the suprasternal space of Burns. The infrahyoid vein and artery and thyroid artery all lie in the space between the pretracheal and infrahyoid fascia.

13. Which tracheal rings are covered by the thyroid isthmus?

Second through fourth rings.

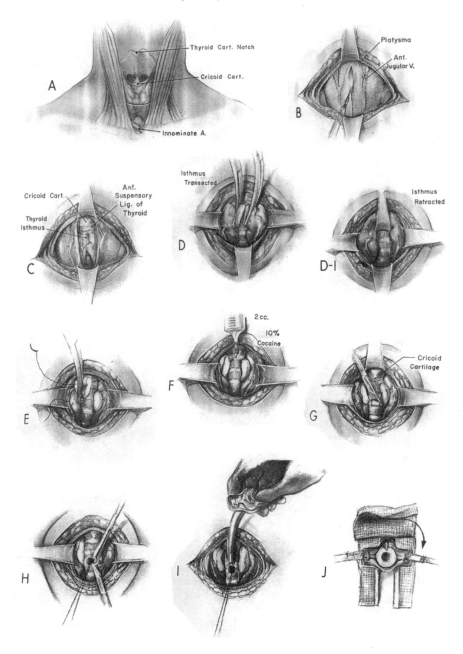

A, Surface anatomy landmarks for tracheostomy. *B*, After skin and platysma incisions are completed, a vertical incision is made in the fascia at midline between the strap muscles. *C*, The cricoid cartilage and thyroid isthmus exposed. *D* and *E*, The thyroid isthmus transected, retracted, and secured with ligature. *F*, Using a smaller gauge needle, air is aspirated into the syringe, and 2% lidocaine (Xylocaine) is injected into the lumen of the trachea. *G* and *H*, A window is cut into the second, third, or fourth ring of the trachea. Alternatively, the ring is left pedicle inferiorly and sutured to the skin. *I* and *J*, The tracheostomy tube is inserted into the trachea and secured in place. (From Lore JM: Emergency procedure. In Lore JM (ed): An Atlas of Head and Neck Surgery. Philadelphia, W.B. Saunders, 1988, p 31, with permission.)

14. What are the advantages of an inverted-U entrance incision into the trachea?

This incision prevents the cannula from being inserted anterior to the trachea. In addition, the patient can breath more easily through the stoma if the cannula is lost, and changing the cannula is easier.

15. What instrument is used to assist with insertion of the tracheostomy tube?

Trousseau dilator.

16. Why are high-volume, low-pressure tracheostomy tube cuffs preferable?

High-volume, low-pressure tracheostomy tube cuffs prevent occlusion of submucosal capillaries of the tracheostomy and, therefore, decrease the risk of tracheal stenosis (submucosal capillaries are occluded at pressures > 25 cm H_2O).

17. List the possible intraoperative complications associated with tracheostomy.

- **Hemorrhage**. The anterior jugular system and its anastomoses, thyroid isthmus, high aortic arch (in children and the elderly) may be elevated into the surgical field by neck hyperextension, thyroid veins and arteries, left innominate or brachiocephalic veins, or erosion of tracheostomy tube through the anterior tracheal wall.
- **Subcutaneous emphysema**. This can result from a wound that has been closed too tightly around the tracheostomy tube or sutures that are placed after decannulation.
- **Recurrent laryngeal nerve injury**. The laryngeal nerve innervates the trachea, esophagus, and all the intrinsic muscles of the larynx except the cricothyroid. Damage to this nerve produces vocal cord paralysis.
- **Pneumothorax** or **pneumomediastinum**. These are more common in pediatrics where the lung apex extends further into the lower neck. It can also result from false passage of a tracheostomy tube between the anterior tracheal surface and the mediastinal tissues.

18. What are the possible postoperative complications associated with tracheostomy?

- **Atelectasis**. This is caused if blood or foreign material is aspirated into the tube or if the tracheostomy tube is directed into one main stem bronchus resulting in collapse of the opposite lung.
- **Tracheoesophageal fistula**. This rarely occurs in an orderly tracheostomy. It may accompany emergency stab-type tracheotomy or if an ill-fitting tracheostomy tube rubs against the posterior tracheal wall.
- **Subglottic edema and tracheal stenosis**. These are preventable by entering the trachea below the second tracheal ring. The most common symptom is increasing stridor.
- **Pneumonia**
- **Difficult decannulation**
- **Persistent fistula after decannulation**. Vertical incisions heal more rapidly than horizontal ones. This may require operative closure with resection of the tracheotomy tract.
- **Tracheo-innominate fistula**. Minor bleeding from tracheostomy tube may herald this. Overinflating the tracheostomy cuff or endotracheal tube while attempting to compress the innominate artery anteriorly against the sternum with a finger inserted through the tracheostomy wound usually treats such bleeding. This is usually associated with an anomalous, superiorly placed artery crossing the trachea or use of a tracheal ring below the four rings.

19. Describe the steps involved in the decannulation of the tracheotomy.

Once the problem that required tracheostomy has been resolved, the process of removing the tracheostomy tube should begin. The initial step in this process is to change to a smaller size tube. Then, a capping trial can be attempted: the cuff is deflated for progressively longer periods of time until the patient can tolerate this with good oxygenation and phonation. If the patient tolerates this, remove the tube altogether. Reapproximate the wound edges, and place additional pressure dressing. Instruct the patient to apply pressure on the dressing when talking and coughing for the first 3–5 days. Change the pressure dressing as needed. Occasionally, rigid endoscopy may be done to assess the patency of the aerodigestive tract.

20. What is the postoperative care for a tracheostomy?

Once the tracheostomy procedure is completed, diligent postoperative care and observation are essential to prevent postoperative complication associated with this procedure. Both the surgeons and the nursing staff should supply this care, including:

- Performing a chest x-ray in the recovery room to check tube position
- Changing the tube on the third or fourth postoperative day
- Using humidified air to keep tracheal mucosa moist
- Frequently suctioning the tracheostomy tube because the tracheotomy reduces the efficiency of coughing and initially there are more secretions from the trachea
- Performing routine wound care and changing the tracheostomy tube

BIBLIOGRAPHY

1. Braun RF, Cutilli BJ: Cricothyrotomy. In Braun RF, Cutilli BJ (eds): Manual of Emergency Medical Treatment for the Dental Team. Baltimore, William & Wilkins, 1999, pp 35–37.
2. Bradley PJ: Management of airway and tracheostomy. In Hibbert J (ed): Otolaryngology: Laryngology and Head and Neck Surgery, 6th ed. Bath, England, Butterworth-Heinemann, 1997 pp 5.7.1–.5.7.20
3. Demas PN, Sotereanos GC: The use of tracheotomy in oral and maxillofacial surgery. J Oral Maxillofac Surg 46:483–486, 1988.
4. Feinberg SE, Peterson LJ: Use of cricothyrotomy in oral and maxillofacial surgery. J Oral Maxillofac Surg 45:873–878, 1987.
5. Lewis RJ: Tracheostomy. Indications, timing and complications. Clinic Chest Med 13:137–149, 1992.
6. Lore JM: Emergency procedures. In Lore JM (ed): An Atlas of Head and Neck Surgery, 3rd ed. Philadelphia, W.B. Saunders, 1988, pp 31–47.
7. Montgomery WW: Surgery of the Upper Respiratory System, 2nd ed. Philadelphia, Lea & Febiger, 1989.
8. Parsons DS, Smith WC: Difficult tracheostomy decannulation. In Gates GA (ed): Current Therapy in Otolaryngology—Head and Neck Surgery, 5th ed. St. Louis, Mosby, 1994, pp 444–448.
9. Weissler MC: Tracheostomy and intubation. In Head and Neck Surgery—Otolaryngology. Philadelphia, J.B. Lippincott, 1993, pp 711–724.

15. MALIGNANT HYPERTHERMIA

Kathy A. Banks, D.M.D., and Jennifer Lamphier, D.M.D.

1. What is malignant hyperthermia (MH)?

A hypermetabolic state involving skeletal muscle that is precipitated by certain anesthetic agents in genetically susceptible individuals.

2. Which patients are at risk of developing MH?

Patients at risk of developing MH include those with:
- Diagnosis of MH (see question 6)
- A first-degree relative with diagnosis of MH
- An elevated resting creatine kinase (CK) and family with suspected MH tendency
- Central core disease
- Musculoskeletal disease associated with MH (see question 5)

3. How is MH inherited?

MH is an autosomal dominant disease that is thought to be caused by a defect on chromosome 19. Chromosome 7q and chromosome 17 have also been implicated. It has also been postulated that MH and central core disease may be allelic and thus can be coinherited.

4. What is the incidence of MH?

Less than 0.5% of all patients who are exposed to anesthetic agents.

5. With which muscle diseases has MH been associated?

- Dystrophinopthy
- Phosphorylase deficiency
- Minicore disease
- Myotonia
- King-Denborough and Barnes myopathies

6. How are susceptible patients diagnosed?

The diagnosis of MH in susceptible patients is made by muscle contracture test. Muscle fibers from MH-positive patients will produce an exaggerated response to electrical stimulation when exposed to halothane and caffeine. When a muscle contracture test is not possible, muscle biopsy may be performed. Characteristic findings on muscle biopsy include variable muscle fiber size, increased number of internalized nuclei, and the presence of "moth-eaten" fibers. These findings are nonspecific and cannot be used alone to establish diagnosis. Patients with MH may also have elevated baseline CK levels.

7. Which anesthetic drugs are known to trigger MH?

Inhalation anesthetics:
Halothane
Enflurane
Isoflurane
Desflurane
Sevoflurane

Depolarizing neuromuscular blockade agents:
Succinylcholine
Decamethonium
Suxamethonium

8. Which other drugs are suspected of causing MH?
Ketamine
Catecholamines
Phenothiazines
Monoamine oxidase (MAO) inhibitors

9. What are the five major clinical characteristics of MH?
1. Acidosis
2. Rigidity
3. Fever
4. Hypermetabolism
5. Myoglobinuria

10. What are the three early presenting signs and symptoms of MH during an anesthetic procedure?
1. Early masseter contracture following administration of succinylcholine
2. An unexplained rise in end-tidal CO_2 following induction of anesthesia
3. An unexplained tachycardia following induction of anesthesia

11. What are the other clinical findings in MH?
• Cyanosis and skin mottling
• Hypertension
• Tachypnea
• Elevated CK and potassium
• Cardiac dysrhythmias
• Cardiac arrest

12. What is the pathogenesis of MH?
Abnormal calcium channels of the sarcoplasmic reticulum impair the ability to sequester calcium, which leads to decreased control of cytosolic calcium levels. The defect causes a calcium-induced calcium release (positive feedback) that is abnormal in skeletal muscle. Exposure to certain "MH-triggering" anesthetics causes a sudden, prolonged release of calcium. This excessive release of calcium leads to excessive muscle contraction and oxygen consumption, elevated temperature, and depletion of high-energy phosphate compounds. Energy exhaustion limits calcium reuptake by the sarcoplasmic reticulum, ultimately leading to cell lysis. Glycogenolysis and leakage of organic acids into the blood result in acidosis. The hypermetabolic state manifests as muscle rigidity, acidosis, hypercarbia, hypertension, and tachypnea. Potassium and myoglobin released from the lysed cells cause hyperkalemia and myoglobinuria. Hyperkalemia, hypercarbia, and acidosis lead to cardiac dysrhythmia or arrest. Myoglobinuria leads to renal failure. Proteins released from lysed myocytes such as CK can be measured.

13. What are the effects of myoglobinuria associated with MH on the kidneys?
Rhabdomyolysis results in release of excessive amounts of heme protein myoglobin in the urine. The urine becomes cola colored. Acute tubular obstruction with myoglobin and free chelatable iron leads to necrosis and renal failure.

14. What is the initial management of an acute attack of MH in the adult patient?
1. Discontinue the anesthetic agent.
2. Hyperventilate with 100% oxygen.
3. Administer dantrolene sodium intravenously until heart rate and end-tidal CO_2 decrease.
4. Begin infusion of iced intravenous fluids (avoid lactated Ringer's).

5. Cool patient with iced saline lavage of stomach, bladder, and rectum; cooling blankets; and ice packs.

6. Draw blood for serum electrolytes, arterial blood gases, prothrombin time (PT), partial thromboplastin time (PTT), and myoglobin studies.

7. Monitor vital signs, electrocardiogram (ECG), end-tidal CO_2, blood gases, temperature, and urine output.

8. Treat metabolic acidosis with sodium bicarbonate.

9. Treat arrythmias with antiarrhythmic drugs (avoid calcium channel blockers).

10. Treat hyperkalemia with glucose and insulin.

11. Maintain urinary output of greater than 2 ml/kg/hr with hydration and diuretics (furosemide or mannitol).

15. How is cardiac arrest managed in children during an acute MH attack?
Treat hyperkalemia first.

16. What is the postoperative management of a patient who has experienced an acute attack of MH?
- Continual monitoring in the intensive care unit (ICU) setting for a minimum of 24 hours
- Follow-up measurements of blood gases, potassium, calcium, and urine myoglobin
- Administration of intravenous dantrolene sodium

17. What is dantrolene sodium and how does it work?
Dantrolene sodium is a hydantoin derivative muscle relaxant that exerts its muscle-relaxant effect by interfering with excitation-contraction coupling in the muscle fiber. Dantrolene sodium is used in the treatment of MH because it blocks calcium release from the sarcoplasmic reticulum calcium channels.

18. What is the recommended dose of dantrolene sodium for treatment of MH?
- 2–3 mg/kg IV every 5 minutes up to a total dose of 10 mg/kg
- 1 mg/kg IV every 6 hours for 24–48 hours in recovery
- Then oral dantrolene for an additional 24 hours

19. What is the mortality associated with MH?
The mortality rate is greater than 40% when dantrolene is not administered. The mortality rate approaches 0% with the administration of dantrolene and appropriate treatment.

20. How can MH be prevented?
- Those at risk for MH should not be given triggering agents.
- Identify patients at risk for development of MH in the preoperative phase.

21. How do you manage a known or suspected MH patient?
When a known or suspected MH patient is about to undergo a procedure that requires the use of an anesthetic agent, a series of steps can be taken to prevent the occurrence of MH:
1. **Preoperative Preparations**
   - Ensure that the anesthetic vaporizers on the anesthesia machine are disabled by removing, draining, or taping in the "off" position.
   - Flow 10 L/m O_2 through the circuit via the ventilator for at least 20 minutes. If the fresh gas hose is replaced, 10 minutes is adequate. During this time, a disposable, unused breathing bag should be attached to the Y-piece of the circle system, and the ventilator should be set to inflate the bag periodically.
   - Use a new or disposable breathing circuit.
   - Place a cooling blanket on the table.

- Dantrolene prophylaxis should be considered on an individual basis but is not recommended for most MH-susceptible patients. When used, dosage is 2.5 mg/kg IV starting immediately prior to anesthesia. Dantrolene can worsen muscle weakness in patients with muscle disease and should be used with caution. For most procedures, even those requiring general anesthesia, dantrolene prophylaxis may be omitted.

2. **Intraoperative Considerations**
   - Consider an alternative anesthetic technique such as spinal, epidural, regional, or local anesthesia. Local anesthetics do not trigger MH; thus any type of regional anesthesia is safe for MH-susceptible patients.
   - Safe general anesthesia agents include benzodiazepines, opioids, barbiturates, protocol, ketamine, nitrous oxide, and etomidate. Pancuronium, atracurium, vecuronium, doxacurium, or curare may be used for relaxation. Neostigmine and atropine are used for reversal without problems.
   - Avoid using unsafe drugs and MH triggers, such as halothane, enflurane, isoflurane, desflurane, sevoflurane, ether, methoxyflurane, cyclopropane, and succinylcholine.
   - Use adequate monitoring techniques to check blood pressure, central temperature, ECG, pulse oximeter, and capnograph. Monitoring respiratory rate and volume is strongly suggested if general anesthetic is used. Use an arterial line, central venous pressure (CVP), or other invasive monitor when appropriate for the surgical procedure and underlying medical condition.

22. Is there a hotline or Web site to obtain more information on MH?

Yes. The telephone hotline is in operation 24 hours a day, 7 days a week to help in the management of ongoing MH. Within the U.S., the number is (800) MH-HYPER. Outside the U.S., call (800) 644-9737 or (315) 464-7079. In addition, information can be faxed free of charge by calling (800) 440-9990. The Web site URL is http://www.mhaus.org.

BIBLIOGRAPHY

1. Bertorini TE: Myoglobinuria, malignant hyperthermia, neuroleptic malignant syndrome and serotonin syndrome. Neurol Clin 15:649–671, 1977.
2. Carr AS, Lerman J, Cunliffe M, et al: Incidence of malignant hyperthermia reactions in 2,214 patients undergoing muscle biopsy. Can J Anesth 42:281–286, 1995.
3. Gronert GA, Mott J, Lee J: Aetiology of malignant hyperthermia. Br J Anaesth 60:253–267, 1988.
4. Malignant Hyperthermia Association of the United States: Preventing Malignant Hyperthermia: An Anesthesia Protocol [brochure]. Sherburne, NY, MHAUS, 1999.
5. Murphy F: Hazards of anesthesia. In Longnecker DE, Murphy FL (eds): Dripps, Eckenhoff, Vandam Introduction to Anesthesia, 9th ed. Philadelphia, W.B. Saunders, 1997, pp 477-480.

V. Management Considerations in the Medically Compromised Patient

16. MANAGEMENT OF SURGICAL PATIENTS WITH CARDIOVASCULAR DISEASES

A. Omar Abubaker, D.M.D., Ph.D., and James A. Giglio, D.D.S., M.Ed.

ISCHEMIC HEART DISEASE, MYOCARDIAL INFARCTION, AND VALVULAR DISEASE

1. Name the known risk factors for the development of ischemic heart disease (IHD).
Age, male gender, positive family history, hypertension, smoking, hypercholesterolemia, and diabetes mellitus. Sedentary lifestyle and obesity are often associated factors.

2. Explain the determinants of myocardial oxygen supply and demand.
Oxygen (O_2) supply to the myocardium is determined by oxygen content and coronary blood flow. Oxygen content can be calculated by the following equation:

$$O_2 \text{ content} = [1.39 \text{ ml } O_2/\text{g of hemoglobin} \times \text{hemoglobin (g/dl)} \times \% \text{ saturation}] + [0.003 \times PaO_2]$$

Coronary blood flow occurs mainly during diastole, especially to the ventricular endocardium. Coronary perfusion pressure is determined by the difference between diastolic blood pressure and left ventricular end-diastolic pressure (LVEDP). Anemia, hypoxemia, tachycardia, diastolic hypotension, hypocapnia (coronary vasoconstriction), coronary occlusion (IHD), vasospasm, increased LVEDP, and hypertrophied myocardium all may adversely affect myocardial O_2 supply.

Myocardial O_2 demand is determined by heart rate, contractility, and wall tension. Increases in heart rate increase myocardial work and decrease the relative time spent in diastole (decreased supply). Contractility increases in response to sympathetic stimulation, which increases O_2 demand. Wall tension is the product of intraventricular pressure and radius. Increased ventricular volume (preload) and increased blood pressure (afterload) both increase wall tension and O_2 demand.

3. What is the pathophysiology of myocardial ischemia?
Ischemia occurs when coronary blood flow is inadequate to meet the needs of the myocardium. Atherosclerotic lesions that occlude 50–75% of the vessel lumen are considered hemodynamically significant. Nonstenotic causes of ischemia include aortic valve disease, left ventricular hypertrophy, ostial occlusion, coronary embolism, coronary arteritis, and vasospasm.

The right coronary artery system is dominant in 80–90% of people and supplies the sinoatrial node, atrioventricular node, and right ventricle. Right-sided coronary artery disease often manifests as heart block and dysrhythmias. The left main coronary artery gives rise to the circumflex artery and left anterior descending artery, which supply the majority of the interventricular septum and left ventricular wall. Significant stenosis of the left main coronary artery (left main disease) or the proximal circumflex and left anterior descending arteries (left main equivalent) may cause severely depressed myocardial function during ischemia.

4. Describe the pathogenesis of a perioperative myocardial infarction.

A myocardial infarction (MI) is usually caused by platelet aggregation, vasoconstriction, and thrombus formation at the site of an atheromatous plaque in a coronary artery. Sudden increases in myocardial O_2 demand (tachycardia, hypertension) or decreases in O_2 supply (hypotension, hypoxemia, anemia), can precipitate MI in patients with IHD. Complications of MI include dysrhythmias, hypotension, congestive heart failure, acute mitral regurgitation, pericarditis, ventricular thrombus formation, ventricular rupture, and death.

5. What clinical factors increase the risk of a perioperative MI following noncardiac surgery?

IHD (prior MI or angina) and congestive heart failure are historically the strongest predictors of an increased risk for perioperative MI. Other risk factors include valvular heart disease (particularly aortic stenosis), arrhythmias due to underlying heart disease, advanced age, type of surgical procedure, and poor general medical status. Hypertension alone does not place a patient at increased risk for perioperative MI, but these patients are at increased risk for IHD, congestive heart failure, and stroke.

6. How can cardiac function be evaluated on history and physical examination?

If a patient's exercise capacity is excellent, even in the presence of IHD, then chances are good that the patient will be able to tolerate the stresses of surgery. Poor exercise tolerance in the absence of pulmonary or other systemic disease indicates an inadequate cardiac reserve. All patients should be questioned about their ability to perform daily activities, such as cleaning, yard work, shopping, and golfing, for example. The ability to climb two to three flights of stairs without significant symptoms (angina, dyspnea, syncope) is usually an indication of adequate cardiac reserve. Signs and symptoms of congestive heart failure including dyspnea, orthopnea, paroxysmal nocturnal dyspnea, peripheral edema, jugular venous distension, a third heart sound, rales, and hepatomegaly must be recognized preoperatively.

7. What is the significance of a history of angina pectoris?

Angina is the symptom of myocardial ischemia, and nearly all patients with angina have coronary artery disease. Stable angina is defined as no change in the onset, severity, and duration of chest pain for at least 60 days. Syncope, shortness of breath, or dizziness that accompanies angina may indicate severe myocardial dysfunction due to ischemia. Patients with unstable angina are at high risk for developing an MI and should be referred for medical evaluation immediately. Patients with diabetes mellitus and hypertension have a much higher incidence of silent ischemia. Perioperatively, most ischemic episodes are silent (as determined by ambulatory and postoperative electrocardiogram [ECG]) but probably significant in the final outcome of surgery.

8. Should all cardiac medications be continued throughout the perioperative period?

Patients with a history of IHD are usually taking medications intended to decrease myocardial oxygen demand by decreasing the heart rate, preload, or contractile state (beta-blockers, calcium channel antagonists, nitrates) and to increase the oxygen supply by causing coronary vasodilation (nitrates). These drugs are generally continued throughout the perioperative period. Abrupt withdrawal of beta-blockers can cause rebound increases in heart rate and blood pressure. Calcium channel blockers can exaggerate the myocardial depressant effects of inhaled anesthetics but should be continued perioperatively.

9. What ECG findings support the diagnosis of IHD?

The resting 12-lead ECG remains a low cost, effective screening tool in the detection of IHD. It should be evaluated for the presence of ST-segment depression or elevation, T-wave inversion, old MI as demonstrated by Q waves, disturbances in conduction and rhythm, and left ventricular hypertrophy. Ischemic changes in leads II, III, and aVF suggest right coronary artery disease, leads I and aVL monitor circumflex artery distribution, and leads V_3–V_5 look at the distribution of the left anterior descending artery. Poor progression of anterior forces suggests significant left ventricular dysfunction, possibly related to IHD.

10. What tests performed by medical consultants can help further evaluate patients with known or suspected IHD?

Exercise ECG is a noninvasive test, that attempts to produce ischemic changes on ECG (ST depression ≥ 1 mm from baseline) or symptoms by having the patient exercise to maximum capacity. Information obtained relates to the thresholds of heart rate and blood pressure that can be tolerated. Maximal heart rates and blood pressure response, as well as symptoms, guide interpretation of results.

Exercise thallium scintigraphy increases the sensitivity and specificity of the exercise ECG. The isotope thallium is almost completely taken up from the coronary circulation by the myocardium and can then be visualized radiographically. Poorly perfused areas that later refill with constrast delineate areas of myocardium at risk for ischemia. Fixed perfusion defects indicate infarcted myocardium.

Dipyridamole thallium imaging is useful in patients who are unable to exercise. This testing is frequently required in patients with peripheral vascular disease who are at high risk for IHD and limited by claudication. Dipyridamole is a potent coronary vasodilator that causes differential flow between normal and diseased coronary arteries detectable by thallium imaging.

Echocardiography can be used to evaluate left ventricular and valvular function and to measure ejection fraction. Stress echocardiography (dobutamine echo) can be used to evaluate new or worsened regional wall motion abnormalities in the pharmacologically stressed heart. Areas of wall motion abnormality are considered at risk for ischemia.

Coronary angiography is the gold standard for defining the coronary anatomy. Valvular and ventricular function can be evaluated and measurements of hemodynamic indices taken. Because angiography is invasive, it is reserved for patients who require further evaluation based on previous tests or who have a high probability of severe coronary disease.

11. Based on the initial evaluation, which patients should be referred for further testing?

Patients at risk for IHD but with good exercise tolerance may not require further workup, especially if they are undergoing procedures with a low to moderate risk of perioperative MI. Patients with decreased exercise tolerance for unclear reasons or with unreliable histories should be evaluated with dipyridamole thallium testing.

Patients with documented IHD (prior MI or chronic stable angina) with good exercise tolerance can sometimes proceed with low-risk surgery without further evaluation. Patients with known IHD and poor exercise tolerance should be referred for dipyridamole thallium testing or coronary angiography prior to all but the most minor surgical procedures.

12. Which surgical procedures carry the highest risk of perioperative MI?

In general, major abdominal, thoracic, and emergency surgery carry the highest risk of perioperative MI. The highest risk noncardiac procedure is aortic aneurysm repair. These patients have a high incidence of IHD, and cross-clamping of the aorta during surgery and postoperative complications can place great stress on the heart.

13. How long should a patient with a recent MI wait before undergoing elective noncardiac surgery?

The risk of reinfarction during surgery after a prior MI has traditionally depended on the time interval between the MI and the procedure. The highest risk of reinfarction is between 0 and 3 months post-MI, lower risk is from 3 to 6 months, and a baseline risk level is reached after 6 months (approximately 5% in most studies).

14. What if surgery cannot safely be delayed for 6 months?

The patient's functional status following rehabilitation from an MI is probably more important than the absolute time interval. Patients with ongoing symptoms may be candidates for coronary revascularization prior to their noncardiac procedure. Patients who quickly return to good functional status following an MI can be considered for necessary noncardiac surgery between 6 weeks and 3 months without undue added risk.

15. How is premedication useful in the setting of IHD and surgery?

Patient anxiety can lead to catecholamine secretion and increased oxygen demand. In this regard, the goal of premedication is to produce sedation and amnesia without causing deleterious myocardial depression, hypotension, or hypoxemia. Morphine, scopolamine, and benzodiazepines, alone or in combination, are popular choices to achieve these goals. All premedicated patients should receive supplemental oxygen. Patients who use sublingual nitroglycerin should have access to their medication. Transdermal nitroglycerin can be applied in the perioperative period as well.

16. Outline the hemodynamic goals of induction and maintenance of general anesthesia in patients with IHD.

The anesthesiologist's goal must be to maintain the balance between myocardial O_2 supply and demand throughout the perioperative period. During induction, wide swings in heart rate and blood pressure should be avoided. Ketamine should be avoided because of the resultant tachycardia and hypertension. Prolonged laryngoscopy should be avoided, and the anesthesiologist may wish to blunt the stimulation of laryngoscopy and intubation by the addition of opiates, beta-blockers, or laryngotracheal or intravenous lidocaine.

Maintenance drugs are chosen with knowledge of the patient's ventricular function. In patients with good left ventricular function, the cardiac depressant and vasodilatory effects of inhaled anesthetics may reduce myocardial O_2 demand. A narcotic-based technique may be chosen to avoid undue myocardial depression in patients with poor left ventricular function. Muscle relaxants with minimal cardiovascular effects are usually preferred.

Blood pressure and heart rate should be maintained near baseline values. This can be accomplished by blunting sympathetic stimulation with adequate analgesia and aggressively treating hypertension (anesthetics, nitroglycerin, nitroprusside, beta-blockers), hypotension (fluids, sympathomimetics, inotropic drugs), and tachycardia (fluids, anesthetics, beta-blockers).

17. What monitors are useful for detecting ischemia intraoperatively?

The V_5 precordial lead is the most sensitive single ECG lead for detecting ischemia and should be monitored routinely in patients at risk for IHD. Lead II can detect ischemia of the right coronary artery distribution and is the most useful lead for monitoring P waves and cardiac rhythm.

Transesophageal echocardiography can provide continuous intraoperative monitoring of left ventricular function. Detection of regional wall motion abnormalities with this technique is the most sensitive for myocardial ischemia.

The pulmonary artery occlusion (wedge) pressure gives an indirect measurement of left ventricular volume and is a useful guide to optimizing intravascular fluid therapy. Sudden increases in the wedge pressure may indicate acute left ventricular dysfunction due to ischemia. The routine use of pulmonary artery catheters in patients with IHD has not been shown to improve outcome. However, close hemodynamic monitoring (including pulmonary artery catheter data) may be beneficial depending on the patient's condition and the nature of the surgical procedure.

18. Discuss the basic pathophysiology of cardiac valvular disease.

Mitral and aortic stenosis cause pressure overload of the left ventricle, which produces hypertrophy with a cardiac chamber of normal size. Mitral and aortic regurgitation cause volume overload, which leads to hypertrophy with a dilated chamber. The net effect of left-sided valvular lesions is an impedance to forward flow of blood into the systemic circulation. Although right-sided valvular lesions occur, left-sided lesions are more common and usually more hemodynamically significant. This chapter deals only with left-sided lesions.

19. Describe common findings of the history and physical exam in patients with valvular disease.

A history of rheumatic fever, intravenous drug abuse, or heart murmur should alert the examiner to the possibility of valvular disease. Exercise tolerance is frequently decreased. Patients may exhibit signs and symptoms of congestive heart failure, including dyspnea, orthopnea, fatigue, pulmonary rales, jugular venous congestion, hepatic congestion, and dependent edema. Compensatory increases in sympathetic nervous system tone manifest as resting tachycardia, anxiety, and diaphoresis. Angina may occur in patients with hypertrophied left ventricle even in the absence of coronary artery disease. Atrial fibrillation frequently accompanies diseases of the mitral valve.

20. Which tests are useful in the evaluation of valvular disease?

The **electrocardiogram** (EGC) should be examined for evidence of ischemia, arrhythmias, atrial enlargement, and ventricular hypertrophy. The **chest radiograph** may show enlargement of cardiac chambers, suggest pulmonary hypertension, or reveal pulmonary edema and pleural effusions. **Cardiac catheterization** is the gold standard in the evaluation of such patients and determines pressures in various heart chambers as well as pressure gradients across valves. **Cardiac angiography** allows visualization of the coronary arteries and heart chambers.

21. How is echocardiography helpful?

Doppler echocardiography characterizes ventricular function and valve function. It can be used to measure the valve orifice area and transvalvular pressure gradients, which are measures of the severity of valvular dysfunction. The function of prosthetic valves is also measured echocardiographically.

22. Which invasive monitors aid the anesthesiologist in the perioperative period?

An arterial catheter provides beat-to-beat blood pressure measurement and continuous access to the bloodstream for sampling. Pulmonary artery catheters enable the anesthetist to measure cardiac output and provide central access for the infusion of vasoactive drugs. The pulmonary capillary wedge pressure is an index of left ventricular filling and is useful for guiding intravenous fluid therapy. Transesophageal echocardiography can be used intraoperatively to evaluate left ventricular volume and function, to detect ischemia (segmental wall motion abnormalities), and intracardiac air, and to examine valve function before and after repair.

23. What is a pressure-volume loop?

A pressure-volume loop plots left ventricular pressure against volume through one complete cardiac cycle. Each valvular lesion has a unique profile that suggests compensatory physiologic changes by the left ventricle.

24. Discuss the pathophysiology of aortic stenosis.

Aortic stenosis is a fixed outlet obstruction to left ventricular ejection. Concentric hypertrophy (thickened ventricular wall with normal chamber size) develops in response to the increased intraventricular systolic pressure and increased wall tension necessary to maintain forward flow. Ventricular compliance decreases, and end-diastolic pressures increase. Contractility and ejection fraction are usually maintained until late in the disease process. Atrial contraction may account for up to 40% of ventricular filling (normally 20%). Aortic stenosis is usually secondary to calcification of a congenital bicuspid valve or rheumatic heart disease. Patients often present with angina, dyspnea, syncope, or sudden death. Angina occurs in the absence of coronary artery disease because the thickened myocardium is susceptible to ischemia (increased oxygen demand) and elevated end-diastolic pressure reduces coronary perfusion pressure (decreased oxygen supply).

25. Discuss the pathophysiology of aortic insufficiency.

Chronic aortic insufficiency is usually rheumatic in origin. Acute aortic insufficiency may be secondary to trauma, endocarditis, or dissection of a thoracic aortic aneurysm. The left ventricle experiences volume overload, because part of the stroke volume regurgitates across the incompetent aortic valve in diastole. Eccentric hypertrophy (dilated and thickened chamber) develops. A dilated orifice, slower heart rate (relatively more time spent in diastole), and increased systemic vascular resistance increase the amount of regurgitant flow. Compliance and stroke volume may be markedly increased in chronic aortic insufficiency, whereas contractility gradually diminishes. Ideally, such patients should have valve replacement surgery before the onset of irreversible myocardial damage. In acute aortic insufficiency, the left ventricle is subjected to rapid, massive volume overload with elevated end-diastolic pressures and displays poor contractility. Hypotension and pulmonary edema may necessitate emergent valvular replacement.

26. What is the pathophysiology of mitral stenosis?

Mitral stenosis is usually secondary to rheumatic disease. Critical stenosis of the valve occurs 10–20 years after the initial infection. As the orifice of the valve narrows, the left atrium experiences pressure overload. In contrast to other valvular lesions, the left ventricle shows relative volume underload due to the obstruction of forward blood flow from the atrium. The elevated atrial pressure may be transmitted to the pulmonary circuit and thus lead to pulmonary hypertension and right-heart failure. The overdistended atrium is susceptible to fibrillation with resultant loss of atrial systole, leading to reduced ventricular filling and cardiac output. Symptoms (fatigue, dyspnea on exertion, hemoptysis) may be worsened when increased cardiac output is needed, as with pregnancy, illness, anemia, and exercise. Blood stasis in the left atrium is a risk for thrombus formation and systemic embolization.

27. Describe the pathophysiology of mitral regurgitation.

Chronic mitral regurgitation is usually due to rheumatic heart disease, ischemia, or mitral valve prolapse. Acute mitral regurgitation may occur in the setting of myocardial ischemia and infarction with papillary muscle dysfunction or chordae tendineae rupture. In chronic mitral regurgitation, the left ventricle and atrium show volume overload, which leads to eccentric hypertrophy. Left ventricular systolic pressures decrease as part of the stroke volume escapes through the incompetent valve into the left atrium, leading to elevated left atrial pressure, pulmonary hypertension, and eventually right-heart failure. As in aortic insufficiency, regurgitant flow depends on valve orifice size, time available for regurgitant flow, and transvalvular pressure gradient. The valve orifice increases in size as the left ventricle increases in size. In acute mitral regurgitation, the pulmonary circuit and right heart are subjected to sudden increases in pressure and volume in the absence of compensatory ventricular dilatation, which may precipitate acute pulmonary hypertension, pulmonary edema, and right-heart failure.

PERIOPERATIVE CONSIDERATIONS IN VALVULAR DISEASE

28. What are the surgical risks for patients with valvular disease?

Patients with valvular heart disease present varying degrees of surgical risk depending on the nature and severity of the valvular disease. The risk is generally one of three types: **hemodynamic** risks, risks associated with **medications** taken for this disease, and risk of **bacterial endocarditis**.

29. True or false: Patients with valvular stenosis are at greater surgical risk than those with valvular regurgitation.

True. Among patients with valvular heart disease, valvular stenosis poses higher risks intraoperatively than valvular regurgitation, although careful fluid management is important in both entities. Such management prevents increases in afterload and possibly pulmonary edema. In addition, patients with valvular stenosis are poorly tolerant of tachyarrhythmias, and care should be taken to avoid them.

30. Discuss the perioperative management of medications for valvular disease.

Patients with valvular heart disease, especially with mechanical valves, and patients with mitral stenosis often receive anticoagulation therapy to render the prothrombin time at 1.3 to 1.5 times control, or an international normalized ratio (INR) of 2 to 3. When oral surgical procedures are to be performed on these patients, the risk of thromboembolism has to be weighed against the risks of postoperative hemorrhage. A decision should be made, in consultation with the patient's cardiologist, on stopping such medications.

In general, if the risk of thromboembolism is moderate, Coumadin can be stopped for 72 hours preoperatively and resumed the same or following day postoperatively. If the patient is at high risk for thromboembolic phenomena, then heparin can be started intravenously after Coumadin has been discontinued; heparin is discontinued 6 hours before surgery. Once hemostasis of the surgical site is assured, heparin and Coumadin can be resumed postoperatively, but close monitoring for evidence of hemorrhage is continued.

31. Which cardiac conditions require preoperative antibiotic prophylaxis for prevention of bacterial endocarditis?

Cardiac Conditions Stratification for Risk of Endocarditis

ENDOCARDITIS PROPHYLAXIS RECOMMENDED	ENDOCARDITIS PROPHYLAXIS NOT RECOMMENDED
High Risk	Negligible Risk
Prosthetic heart valves	Isolated secundum atrial septal defect
Prior bacterial endocarditis	Surgical repair of atrial septal defect, ven-
Complex cyanotic congenital heart disease	tricular septal defect, or patent ductus
Surgically constructed systemic pulmonary	arteriosus (without residua beyond 6
shunts or conduits	months)
Moderate Risk	Prior coronary artery bypass graft
Most other congenital cardiac malformations	Mitral valve prolapse without regurgitation
Acquired valvular dysfunction	Physiologic, functional, or innocent heart
Hypertrophic cardiomyopathy	murmurs
Mitral valve prolapse with regurgitations	Previous Kawasaki disease without valvular
and/or thickened leaflets	dysfunction
	Previous rheumatic fever without valvular
	dysfunction
	Cardiac pacemakers and implanted
	defibrillators

Adapted from Dajani AS, Taubert KA, Wilson W, et al: Prevention of bacterial endocarditis. Recommendations by the American Heart Association. JAMA 277:1794–1801, 1997.

32. Which dental and oral surgical procedures require preoperative antibiotic prophylaxis for prevention of bacterial endocarditis?

Dental Procedures and Endocarditis Prophylaxis

RECOMMENDED IN HIGH- AND MODERATE-RISK CARDIAC CONDITIONS	ENDOCARDITIS PROPHYLAXIS NOT RECOMMENDED
Exodontia	Restorative dentistry
Periodontal procedures	Nonintraligamentary local anesthetic injections
Incision and drainage of abscesses	Postoperative suture removal
Dental implant placement and uncovering	Placement of removable orthodontic or prostho-
Reimplantation of avulsed teeth	dontic appliances
Endodontic therapy or apical surgery	Taking oral impressions
Placement of intermaxillary fixation	Shedding (naturally) of primary teeth

(Table continued on next page.)

Dental Procedures and Endocarditis Prophylaxis (cont.)

RECOMMENDED IN HIGH- AND MODERATE-RISK CARDIAC CONDITIONS	ENDOCARDITIS PROPHYLAXIS NOT RECOMMENDED
Reduction of contaminated maxillofacial fractures	
Osteotomies	
Subgingival placement of antibiotic fibers or strips	
Intraligamentary local anesthetic injections	
Prophylactic dental or implant cleaning	
Intraoral biopsies	

Adapted from Dajani AS, Taubert KA, Wilson W, et al: Prevention of bacterial endocarditis. Recommendations by the American Heart Association. JAMA 277:1794–1801, 1997.

33. List the different antibiotic prophylactic regimens for dental and oral surgical procedures.

Antibiotic Prophylactic Regimens for Dental and Oral Surgical Procedures

	ANTIBIOTIC	REGIMEN*
Standard prophylaxis	Amoxicillin	Adults: 2 g po; children: 50 mg/kg po 1 hour before procedure
Unable to take oral medications	Ampicillin	Adults: 2 g IM or IV; children: 50 mg/kg IM or IV within 30 min of procedure
Penicillin allergy	Clindamycin or	Adults: 600 mg po; children: 20 mg/kg po 1 hour before procedure
	+ cephalexin or cefadroxil	Adults: 2 g po; children: 50 mg/kg po 1 hour before procedure
	Azithromycin or clarithromycin	Adults: 500 mg po; children: 15 mg/kg po 1 hour before procedure
Penicillin allergy and unable to take oral medications	Clindamycin or	Adults: 600 mg IM or IV; children: 20 mg/kg IM or IV within 30 min of procedure
	+ cefazolin	Adults: 1 g IM or IV; children: 25 mg/kg IM or IV within 30 min of surgery

* Total children's dose should not exceed adult dose.
Note: do not use cephalosporins in individuals with immediate-type hypersensitivity reaction to penicillin.
Adapted from Dajani AS, Taubert KA, Wilson W, et al: Prevention of bacterial endocarditis. Recommendations by the American Heart Association. JAMA 277:1794–1801, 1997.

HYPERTENSION

34. What is hypertension?

Hypertension is a sustained, elevated arterial blood pressure resulting from increased peripheral vascular resistance. An adult patient with a blood pressure (BP) reading above 140/90 mmHg is generally considered to be hypertensive.

35. List the general categories of hypertension, based on the presentation and level of need for treatment.

Hypertension clinically presents in one of four generally recognized settings: hypertensive emergencies, hypertensive urgencies, mild uncomplicated hypertension, and transient hypertensive episodes.

36. Differentiate hypertensive emergency and hypertensive urgency. How are these conditions managed?

A hypertensive *emergency* is an increased BP **with end-organ damage or dysfunction**. The brain, heart, or kidneys may be affected. BP can be as high as systolic > 210 mmHg, diastolic > 120 mmHg. Treatments for a hypertensive emergency should be rapid and aggressive, attempting to lower the BP within 60 minutes in a controlled fashion.

Hypertensive *urgency* is an elevation of BP to a potentially harmful level **without end-organ dysfunction**. Hypertensive urgency should be treated over a longer period (1–2 days).

37. What is the difference between primary and secondary hypertension?

Primary or essential hypertension is a sustained, elevated BP of unknown etiology. *Secondary* hypertension is an elevated BP that results from an identifiable cause, such as: renal artery stenosis, chronic renal parenchymal disease, aldosteronism/Cushing's syndrome, acromegaly, hypercalcemia, coarctation of the aorta, pheochromocytoma, or oral contraceptives.

38. During the perioperative period, when are the highest mean arterial pressure (MAP) readings typically recorded?

The highest MAP is typically observed in response to laryngoscopy and intubation. A single dose of a beta-adrenergic blocker 90 minutes before induction in a patient with hypertension has been shown to reduce intraoperative BP, myocardial ischemia, and postoperative morbidity.

39. How is hypertension classified?

There are different systems for classifying hypertension. For example, hypertension can be classified as high normal, mild, moderate, or severe based on the diastolic pressure alone (85–89, 90–104, 105–114, and > 115, respectively). However, hypertension typically is classified based on both the systolic and diastolic pressures into four stages. BP readings below these stages are considered either normal (< 130 for systolic, and < 85 for diastolic), or high normal, (130–139 for systolic, and 85–89 for diastolic). The four stages of hypertension are:

Stage I (mild) 140–159 systolic and 90–99 diastolic
Stage II (moderate) 160–179 systolic, and 100–119 diastolic
Stage III (severe) 180–209 systolic and 110–119 diastolic
Stage IV (very severe) > 210 systolic > 120 diastolic

40. What behavior modifications can help treat hypertension?

Patients with hypertension are encouraged to modify their lifestyle. Weight loss (10 lbs. or more in overweight people), limitation of alcohol intake to < 1 oz /day for men and 0.5 oz. for women, and aerobic physical activity for 30–45 minutes 3–5 times/week are recommended. Patients are also encouraged to maintain adequate intake of potassium, calcium, and magnesium; reduce sodium, fat, and cholesterol; and quit smoking. All of these measures been shown to lower blood pressure.

Classification of Adult Blood Pressure and Treatment Modifications

CATEGORY	SYSTOLIC (mmHg)	DIASTOLIC (mmHg)	TREATMENT
Normal	< 130	< 85	No modification
High normal	130–139	85–89	No modification
Hypertension			
Stage I	140–159	90–99	No modification, medical referral, inform patient
Stage II	160–179	100–109	Selective care*, medical referral

(*Table continued on next page.*)

Classification of Adult Blood Pressure and Treatment Modifications (cont.)

CATEGORY	SYSTOLIC (mmHg)	DIASTOLIC (mmHg)	TREATMENT
Hypertension (cont.)			
Stage III	180–209	110–119	Emergent nonstressful procedures‡ Immediate medical referral or consultation
Stage IV	≥ 210	≥ 120	Emergent nonstressful procedures‡ Immediate medical referral

* Selective may include, but is not limited to, atraumatic removal of teeth, biopsies, etc.
‡ Emergent nonstressful procedures may include, but are not limited to, procedures that alleviate pain, infection, or masticatory dysfunction. These procedures should have limited physiologic and psychological effects (e.g., incision and drainage of an abscess). In all cases the medical benefit of the procedure should outweigh the risk of complications secondary to the patient's hypertensive state.

41. Discuss pharmacologic therapy of hypertension.

Drug therapy for hypertension is based on the individual's needs and condition. For example, initial drug therapy for uncomplicated hypertension consists of diuretics and beta-blockers. **Beta-blockers** may also be prescribed for patients with hypertension after experiencing a myocardial infarction (MI). **Diuretics** can be used when there is concomitant congestive heart failure. **Calcium channel blockers** are recommended for older patients with ischemic heart disease. **Angiotensin-converting enzyme (ACE) inhibitors** benefit hypertensive patients who have diabetes and proteinuria.

Note: NSAIDs may reduce the efficacy of ACE inhibitors, diuretics, and beta-blockers. However, the reduction appears to be more likely in the NSAID class, dose, and duration not commonly prescribed for oral and maxillofacial surgery procedures. In addition, calcium channel blockers may cause gingival hyperplasia similar to the hyperplasia associated with Dilantin used to treat epilepsy.

42. Is it safe to administer local anesthesia with epinephrine to a hypertensive patient?

Cartridges of local anesthestic as used in dentistry contain epinephrine concentrations of 1:50,000 (.02 mg/ml), 1:100,000 (.01 mg/ml), or 1:200,000 (.005 mg/ml). One cartridge contains 1.8 ml solution of local anesthetic and epinephrine; therefore, one cartridge with an epinephrine concentration of 1:100,000 contains 1.8 ml × .01 mg/ml or 0.018 mg of epinephrine. According to American Dentistry Association/American Heart Association guidelines, a patient with cardiovascular disease can receive up to .04 mg of epinephrine, or up to two cartridges of agent.

If, however, the patient has poorly controlled hypertension or an otherwise significant medical risk, then the use of epinephrine becomes a clinical judgement of risk to benefits and is performed on a case-by-case basis. These patients are medical risks, not only concerning epinephrine, but also because of their overall poor medical status.

43. What is the Goldman Cardiac Risk Index? Which factors are most important in assigning risk?

Goldman's Cardiac Risk Index was established based on study of more than 1000 patients undergoing noncardiac surgery who were evaluated preoperatively. The evaluation examined certain variables obtained from the history, physical examination, ECG, and general status (pulmonary, kidney, or liver disease) and factored in the type of operation to determine the risk factors that predispose a patient to a cardiac event.

The cardiac risk index is based on a point system, and patients are assigned to four different cardiac risk index classes. According to this study, the presence of an S3 heart sound, indicating heart failure or myocardial infarction within the last 6 months, poses the greatest risk for a significant perioperative event.

Points Awarded for Cardiac Risk Factors

RISK FACTOR	POINTS
Third heart sound or jugular venous distention	11
Recent myocardial infarction	10
Rhythm other than sinus or premature atrial contractions on last ECG	7
> 5 premature ventricular contractions per minute at any time	7
Intraperitoneal, intrathoracic, or aortic operation	3
Age > 70 years	5
Important aortic stenosis	3
Emergent operation	4

Poor general medical condition
  $Po_2 < 60$ or $Pco_2 > 50$ mmHg
  $K^+ < 30$ mEq/L
  $HCO_3^- < 20$ mEq/L
  creatinine > 3 mg/dL or BUN > 50 mg/dL
  chronic liver disease
  bedridden from noncardiac causes
	3

Adapted from Goldman L: Multifactorial index of cardiac risk in noncardiac procedures. N Engl J Med 297:945–950, 1977.

Goldman's Cardiac Risk Index

CLASS	POINT TOTAL	NO OR ONLY MINOR COMPLICATION ($n = 943$) (%)	LIFE-THREATENING COMPLICATIONS* ($n = 39$) (%)	CARDIAC DEATHS ($n = 19$) (%)
I (N = 537)	0–5	532 (99)	4 (0.7)	1 (0.2)
II (N = 316)	6–12	295 (93)	16 (5)	5 (2)
III (N = 130)	13–25	112 (86)	15 (11)	3 (2)
IV (N = 18)	> 26	4 (22)	4 (22)	10 (56)

* Documented intraoperative or postoperative MI, pulmonary edema, or VT.
Adapted from Goldman L: Multifactorial index of cardiac risk in noncardiac procedures. N Engl J Med 297:945–950, 1977.

44. What are the different sympathetic nervous system receptors relative to hypertension and antihypertensive agents?
   These receptors are classified into two major categories: **alpha and beta receptors**. Each of these is further divided into two subdivisions: alpha 1 and alpha 2, and beta 1 and beta 2 receptors.
   • Alpha 1 site stimulation causes constriction of vascular smooth muscles and thus increases peripheral vascular resistance.
   • Alpha 2 stimulation inhibits the release of norepinephrine (the negative feedback to sympathetic neurons).
   • Beta 1 stimulation increases heart rate and the strength of cardiac contraction.
   • Beta 2 stimulation causes dilatation of smooth muscles of the blood vessels and airway, relaxation of uterine smooth muscle, and a variety of endocrine effects, including secretion of renin.

45. True or false: There are six different categories of oral antihypertensive agents.
   False. Antihypertensive agents are generally classified into three major categories based on their mechanisms of action: diuretics, sympatholytics, and vasodilators.

Categories and Classes of Oral Antihypertensive Agents

CATEGORY	CLASS	SUBCLASS	AGENT
Diuretics	Thiazide-type		Chlorothiazide, chlorthalidone, hydrochlorothiazide, indapamide, metolazone
	Potassium-sparing		Spironolactone, triamterene, amiloride
	Loop		Bumetanide, ethacrynic acid, furosemide, torasemide
Sympatholytics	Adrenergic-receptor blockers	Beta	Acebutolol, atenolol, betaxolol, bisoprolol, cateolol, metoprolol, nadolol, penbutolol, pindolol, propranolol, timolol
		Alpha α_1	Doxazosin, prazosin, terazosin
		$\alpha_1 + \alpha_2$	Phenoxybenzamine
		Alpha and beta	Labetalol
	Central α_2 agonists		Clonidine, guanabenz, guanfacine, methyldopa
	Postganglionic blockers		Bethanidine, guanadrel, guanethidine, reserpine
Vasodilators	Calcium channel blockers	Benzothiazepine Phenylalkylamines Dihydropyridines	Diltiazem, verapamil, amlodipine, felodipine, isradipine, nicardipine, nifedipine
	ACE inhibitors		Benazepril, captopril, enalapril, fosinopril, lisinopril, quinapril, ramipril
	Direct vasodilators		Hydralazine, minoxidil

Adapted from Dym H: The hypertensive patient. Therapeutic modalities. Oral Maxillofac Clin North Am 10:349, 1998.

46. What are the doses, mechanisms of action, and possible complications of commonly used antihypertensive agents?

Doses, Mechanisms of Action, and Possible Complications of Antihypertensive Drugs

AGENT AND DOSE	MECHANISM OF ACTION	POSSIBLE COMPLICATIONS
Diuretics		
Thiazide 25–50 mg/d	Increases urinary excretion of sodium (Na) and water by inhibiting Na reabsorption in cortical diluting tubule in nephron; exact mechanism of antihypertension is unknown; may be partially from direct ateriolar vasodilation	Hypokalemia, dehydration, hyperglycemia, hyperuricemia, decreased lithium clearance
Loop diuretics 40–240 mg/d	Inhibits Na and chloride reabsorption in promimal ascending loop of Henle; also has renal and peripheral vasodilatory effects	Hypokalemia, dehydration, hypochloremic alkalosis
Spironolactone 50–100 mg/d	Potassium-sparing; competitively inhibits aldosterone effects on distal renal tubules (increases Na and water excretion); also may block aldosterone effect on vascular smooth muscle	Hyperkalemia, gynecomastia, dehydration

(Table continued on next page.)

Doses, Mechanisms of Action, and Possible Complications of Antihypertensive Drugs (cont.)

AGENT AND DOSE	MECHANISM OF ACTION	POSSIBLE COMPLICATIONS
Central antiadrenergics		
Alpha-methyldopa PO 500–2000 mg/d IV 250–500 mg over 30–60 min every 6 h	Metabolite (alpha methylnorepine- phrine) stimulates inhibitory alpha-adrenergic receptors and inhibits sympathetic nervous system outflow, thus decreasing total peripheral resistance	Sedation, hepatic dysfunction, lupus-like symptoms, re- bound hypertension, positive Coombs' test
Clonidine PO 0.1–2.4 mg/d topical transdermal patch every 7 days	Stimulates inhibitory alpha$_2$ re- ceptors and inhibits sympa- thetic outflow	Sedation, xerostomia, rebound HTN, 50% decrease in mini- mal alveolar concentrations of volatile anesthetic
Peripheral antiadrenergics		
Prazosin (Minipress) 2–20 mg/d	Selective and competitive post- synaptic alpha receptor block- ade leads to arterioles and vasodilation	Alters test results for pheo- chromocytoma, false-positive test results for ANA, in- creased liver function tests
Terazosin (Hytrin) 1–5 mg/PO/d	Selectively inhibits alpha-recep- tors in vascular smooth mus- cles; dilates both arteriolar and venules	Decreases hematocrit, hemo- globin, albumin, leukocytes, and total protein
Guanethidine (Ismelin) 100–300 mg/d	Peripherally inhibits alpha-recep- tors and release of norepine- phrine (NE); depletes stores of NE in adrenergic nerve endings	Use with direct-acting sym- pathomimetics may precipi- tate a hypertensive crisis
Labetalol 100–400 mg PO twice daily 10–80 IV every 10 min	Competitive antagonist at beta- and alpha-adrenergic receptors	Contraindicated in asthmatic, 2nd or 3rd degree AV block, congestive heart failure, or "brittle" diabetes
Vasodilators		
Hydralazine 10–50 mg PO 4 times/d 5–10 mg IV every 20 min	Direct relaxing effect on vascular smooth muscle (arterioles > veins	Lupus-like syndrome in 1– 20% of patients on chronic therapy, decreases DBP > SBP, increases heart rate
Minoxidil 5–10 mg/d PO		Fluid retention, pericardial effusion, and hypertrichosis
Angiotensin-converting enzyme (ACE) inhibitors		
Benazepril (Lotensin) 10–40 mg/d PO) Captopril (Capoten) 6.25–150 mg PO 3 times/d Enalapril (Vasotec) 5–40 mg/d PO 1.25 mg/IV every 6 h Lisinopril (Zestril) 10–40 mg/d PO	Competes with ACE, prevents pulmonary conversion of angio- tensin I to angiotensin II (a potent vasoconstrictor); de- creases peripheral arterial resis- tance; leads to decreased aldo- sterone secretion, thereby reducing Na and water retention	10% get rash with fever and joint pain proteinuria, neu- tropenia, and cough
Calcium channel blockers		
Diltiazem (Cardizem) 30–90 mg PO 4 times/d 0.25 mg/kg IV over 2 min 5–15 mg/h IV drip	Blocks calcium movement across cell membranes, causing arterial vasodilation; nifedipine is the most potent peripheral and	Congestive heart failure, nodal changes, edema, headaches, hyperkalemia, flushing, tach- ycardia (with nifedipine only)

(*Table continued on next page.*)

Doses, Mechanisms of Action, and Possible Complications of Antihypertensive Drugs (cont.)

AGENT AND DOSE	MECHANISM OF ACTION	POSSIBLE COMPLICATIONS
Calcium channel blockers (cont)		
Isradipine (DynaCirc) 2.5–5 mg PO twice daily Nifedipine (Procardia) 10–30 mg PO 3 times/d Verapamil (Calan, Isoptin) 0.075–0.3 mg/kg IV over 2 min 80–120 PO 3 times/d	coronary artery vasodilator of calcium channel blockers; diltiazem has less negative inotropic effects than verapamil and has some selective coronary vasodilatory effects	

ANA = antinuclear antibody, AV = atrioventricular, DBP = diastolic blood pressure, HTN = hypertension, IV = intravenously, PO = orally, SBP = systolic blood pressure.
Adapted from Dym H: The hypertensive patient. Therapeutic modalities. Oral Maxillofac Clin North Am 10:349, 1998.

47. What are the commonly used *parenteral* agents used for treatment of hypertensive emergencies?

Parenteral Drugs Used for Treatment of Hypertensive Emergencies

DRUG	DOSAGE	ONSET OF ACTION	ADVERSE EFFECTS
Vasodilators			
Nitroprusside (Nipride, Nitropress)	0.25–10 µg/kg/min as IV infusion	Instantaneous	Nausea, vomiting, muscle twitching, sweating, thiocyanate, intoxication
Nitroglycerin	5–100 g/min as IV infusion	2–5 min	Tachycardia, flushing, headache, vomiting, methemoglobinemia
Diazoxide (Hyperstat)	50–100 mg/IV bolus repeated or 15–30 mg/min by IV infusion	2–4 min	Nausea, hypotension, flushing, tachycardia, chest pain
Hydralazine (Apresoline)	10–20 mg IV bolus	10–20 min	Tachycardia, flushing, headache, vomiting, aggravation of angina
Enalapril (Vasotec IV)	1.25–5 mg/Q6 h IV bolus every 6 h	15 min	Precipitious fall in blood pressure in high renin states; response variable
Nicardipine	5–10 mg/h IV infusion	10 min	Tachycardia, headache, flushing, local phlebitis
Adrenergic inhibitors			
Phentolamine (Regitine)	5–15 mg IV bolus	1–2 min	Tachycardia, flushing
Trimethaphan (Arfonad)	0.5–5 mg/min as IV infusion	1–5 min	Paresis of bowel and bladder, orthostatic hypotension, blurred vision, dry mouth
Esmolol (Brevibloc)	500 µg/kg/min for first 4 min then 150–300 µg/kg/min IV infusion	1–2 min	Hypotension
Propranolol (Inderal)	1–10 mg load; 3 mg/h	1–2 min	Beta-blocker side effect, e.g., bronchospasm, decreased cardiac output
Labetalol (Normodyne, Trandate)	10–80 mg IV bolus every 10 min 0.5–2 mg/min IV infusion	5–10 min	Vomiting, scalp tingling, burning in throat, postural hypotension, dizziness, nausea

Adapted from Dym H: The hypertensive patient. Therapeutic modalities. Oral Maxillofac Clin North Am 10:349, 1998.

48. List the commonly used *oral* drugs for treatment of hypertensive *urgencies*.

Oral Drugs Used for Hypertensive Urgencies

DRUG	CLASS	DOSAGE	ONSET	DURATION
Nifedipine (Procardia)	Calcium entry blocker	5–10 mg sublingual	5–15 min	3–5 h
Clonidine (Catapres)	Central sympatholytic	0.2 mg initial then 0.1 mg/h up to 0.7 mg total	0.5–2 h	6–8 h

Adapted from Dym H: The hypertensive patient. Therapeutic modalities. Oral Maxillofac Clin North Am 10:349, 1998.

CONGESTIVE HEART FAILURE

49. What is congestive heart failure?

Congestive heart failure (CHF) results from impaired pumping ability by the heart. A ventricular ejection fraction below 50% is indicative of CHF. Causes of CHF include MI, ischemic heart disease, poorly controlled hypertension, structural heart defects, and cardiomyopathy.

50. Describe the potential effects of long-term hypertension on end organs.

Chronically elevated BP often leads to serious consequences for the heart, CNS, and kidneys. Persistent hypertension may lead to left ventricular hypertrophy, angina pectoris with the potential for MI, CHF, and cardiomyopathy. Neurologic complications of hypertension include retinal damage with focal spasm, narrowing of arterioles and/or papilledema, cerebral infarction or hemorrhage, cerebral vascular microaneurysms (Charcot-Bouchard aneurysms), hypertensive encephalopathy, and stroke. Renal complications include renal insufficiency and renal failure.

51. What are the clinical signs and symptoms of congestive heart failure?

Fatigue and dyspnea on exertion are often the primary symptoms of CHF. Patients may also report ankle edema and 2- to 3-pillow orthopnea. Palpitation, nocturia, cough, nausea, and vomiting are associated findings. Physical findings include gallop rhythm (S_3 or an S_4), murmurs, and jugular venous distention. Pulmonary examination may reveal rales over the lung bases and decreased breath sounds. Cyanosis is often present in severe CHF.

52. What are the different classifications of heart failure?

There are different methods of classification of heart failure, such as left-sided versus right-sided, high output versus low output, backward versus forward, acute versus chronic, and compensated versus decompensated.

53. List the causes of heart failure.

Cardiac
Ischemia
• Cardiomyopathy
• Toxic
• Metabolic
• Infectious, inflammatory
• Infiltrative
• Genetic
• Idiopathic
Valvular heart diseases
• Aortic stenosis, regurgitation
• Mitral stenosis, regurgitation

Noncardiac
Hypertension
Pulmonary embolus
High-output states
Thyrotoxicosis

Cardiac (cont.)

Restrictive disease
• Pericardial
• Myocardial

Congenital disease

Electrical abnormalities
• Tachydysrhythmias
• Ventricular dyssynergy

54. What are the major physiologic alterations in patients with heart failure?
• Loss of artery compliance
• Arteriolar narrowing
• Vascular smooth muscle hypertrophy
• Enhanced vasoconstrictor activity secondary to elevated sympathetic nervous system activity
• Activation of the renin-angiotensin system resulting in sodium and water retention
• Increased levels of argentine vasopressin and endothelin
• Possibly a decrease in the local release of endothelium-derived relaxing factor (nitric oxide).

55. Which laboratory studies are useful in evaluating the patient with CHF?
Chest x-ray, electrocardiogram (ECG), echocardiogram, and radionuclear ventriculography are all useful in the evaluation of patients with heart failure. **Chest x-ray** may show cardiomegaly or evidence of pulmonary vascular congestion, including perihilar engorgement of the pulmonary veins, cephalization of the pulmonary vascular markings, or pleural effusions. The **ECG** in these patients is often nonspecific, although 70–90% of patients demonstrate ventricular or supraventricular dysrhythmias. **Echocardiography** is used to demonstrate chamber size, wall motion, valvular function, and left ventricular wall thickness. **Radionuclear ventriculography** is helpful in providing an assessment of left ventricular ejection fraction.

56. How is the severity of heart failure classified?
The status of patients with CHF is typically classified on the basis of symptoms, impairment of lifestyle, or severity of cardiac dysfunction. The New York Heart Association uses four categories that describe the symptomatic limitations of the patient with heart failure. These classifications are:

Class I—ordinary physical activity does not cause symptoms.
Class II—ordinary physical activity causes symptoms.
Class III—less than ordinary activity results in symptoms.
Class IV—symptoms occur at rest.

57. What are the principles of management for CHF?
The mnemonic MOIST 'N DAMP is helpful in listing the methods generally used in combination for the management of CHF:

Morphine
Oxygen
Inotropes (digitalis)
Sit-em-up
Tourniquets

Nitrates

Diuretics
ACE inhibitors and afterload reduction (aminophylline)
Mechanical ventilator
Phlebotomy

58. What are the different classes of drugs used in the treatment of heart failure?

Drugs used in the treatment of CHF typically fall into one of five categories: diuretics, ACE inhibitors, calcium channel blockers, digitalis, and beta-blockers.

Diuretics are used when patients with CHF exhibit signs or symptoms of circulatory congestion. *Thiazide* diuretics are often used for mild fluid retention. *Loop* diuretics such as furosemide may be substituted when thiazides fail to produce an adequate response. Addition of a second diuretic, such as metolazone, may induce an effective diuresis in patients resistant to loop diuretics alone.

ACE inhibitors are effective therapy for patients who can tolerate them. They improve LV function and exercise tolerance, and may prolong life. Hypotension and azotemia are the major side effects. A dry cough is fairly common, but rarely necessitates discontinuation of therapy. A combination of the vasodilators hydralazine and isosorbide dinitrate also has been shown to be effective in improving exercise tolerance and life span.

Calcium channel blockers may produce favorable hemodynamic responses, but negative inotropic effects. These agents are used in patients with concurrent myocardial ischemia.

Digitalis is effective in patients with underlying arterial fibrillation or a dilated LV with poor systolic function.

Beta-blockers may produce favorable long-term effects in patients with ischemic heart disease.

59. Describe the signs and symptoms of digitalis toxicity.

Patients with digitalis toxicity may present with any of the following signs and symptoms: anorexia, nausea, vomiting, abdominal pain, confusion, paresthesias, amblyopia, and scotomata. ECG findings are usually nonspecific and include atrial or ventricular dysrhythmias such as premature ventricular contractions, bigeminy, trigeminy, ventricular tachycardia, delayed atrioventricular node conduction, and complete heart block. Older patients and patients with hypothyroidism, decreased renal function, hypokalemia, hypercalcemia, and/or hypomagnesemia are more predisposed to digitalis toxicity.

60. What are the important elements of postoperative care for patients with CHF?

The peak evidence of postoperative MI occurs about 72 hours postoperatively; therefore, closely monitor the patient's cardiac status during this period. Improve pulmonary function with incentive spirometry, pulmonary toilet, and bronchodilators when appropriate. Observation of renal function and urine output is also important in these patients because postoperative renal failure has ominous implications. Pain must be well controlled to minimize physiologic stress.

Other possible postoperative complications to avoid include gastrointestinal ischemia, bleeding, stroke, graft infection, distal arterial thrombosis, and pulmonary embolism.

BIBLIOGRAPHY

1. Abbott RD: Congestive heart failure. In Duke J (ed): Anesthesia Secrets, 2nd ed. Philadelphia, Hanley & Belfus, 2000, p 193
2. Dajani AS, Taubert KA, Wilson W, et al: Prevention of bacterial endocarditis. Recommendations by the American Heart Association. JAMA 277:1794–1801, 1997.
3. Dym H: The hypertensive patient. Therapeutic modalities. Oral Maxillofac Surg Clin North Am 10:349, 1998.
4. Eagle KA, Coley CM, Nussbaum SR, et al: Combining clinical and thallium data optimizes preoperative assessment of cardiac risk before major vascular surgery. Ann Intern Med 110:859–866, 1989.
5. Glick M: New guidelines for prevention, detection, evaluation, and treatment of high blood pressure. J Am Dent Assoc 129:1588–1594, 1998.
6. Goldman L, Caldera DL, Nussbaum SR, et al: Multifactorial index of cardiac risk in patients in noncardiac surgical procedures. N Engl J Med 297:945–950, 1977.
7. McCabe JC, Roser SM: Evaluation and management of the cardiac patient for surgery. Oral Maxillofac Surg Clin North Am 10:429–443, 1998.
8. Muzyka BC, Glick M: The hypertensive dental patient. J Am Dent Assoc 128:1109–1120, 1997.

17. RESPIRATORY DISORDERS

Robert E. Doriot, D.D.S., and Kenneth J. Benson, D.D.S.

1. What is the normal adult oxyhemoglobin dissociation curve for blood at 37%, pH of 7.4, PCO₂ of 40 mmHg?

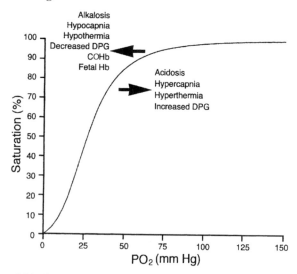

Normal oxyhemoglobin dissociation curve. (From Hess D: Arterial blood gases. In Parsons PE, Heffner JE (eds): Pulmonary/Respiratory Therapy Secrets. Philadelphia, Hanley & Belfus, 1997, pp 31–40, with permission.)

2. Which way would this curve shift if the pH was more acidic?
To the right.

3. What are the general rules concerning the dissociation curve shifts?
- A low pH or a high PCO₂ shifts the curve to the right.
- A high pH or a low PCO₂ shifts the curve to the left.
- Elevated body temperature shifts the curve to the right.
- Lower body temperature shifts the curve to left.

4. How does the interpretation of the curve change when the curve shifts to the left?
With a shift to the left, a lower PO₂ is required to bind a given amount of oxygen (O₂). The lower the oxygen half-saturation pressure (P-50), the higher the affinity of hemoglobin for O₂; the higher the P-50, the lower the affinity of hemoglobin for O₂. If the curve is shifted to the right, the P-50 increases, and if the curve is shifted to the left, the P-50 decreases.

5. Which way does carbon monoxide move the curve?
Small amounts of carbon monoxide in blood increase the affinity of remaining oxygen for hemoglobin and therefore cause a leftward shift of the curve.

6. What is 2,3-diphosphoglycerate (2,3-DPG)?
2,3-DPG is produced by erythrocytes and normally is present in fairly high concentrations in red blood cells (RBCs).

7. When is 2,3-DPG produced?

2,3-DPG is produced mainly during chronic hypoxic conditions. An increase in 2,3-DPG shifts the curve to the right and allows more O_2 to be released from hemoglobin at a particular O_2 level.

8. How does decreased 2,3-DPG affect the dissociation curve?

With a decrease in 2,3-DPG, the curve will shift to the left, indicating an increased affinity for O_2 by hemoglobin. Hemoglobin does not release O_2 in the tissues except at a very low PO_2.

9. How does 2,3-DPG affect blood supply in blood banks?

Blood stored for as little as 1 week will have depleted 2,3-DPG unless steps are taken to restore normal levels of 2,3-DPG.

10. How does the aging process affect $PaCO_2$?

$PaCO_2$ and alveolar ventilation are unchanged by the aging process.

11. How does the aging process affect PaO_2?

PaO_2 decreases with age. This decrease can be calculated according to the following formula:

$$PaO_2 = 100.1 - (0.323 \times \text{age in years})$$

Thus, the PaO_2 of a 30-year-old would be calculated $100.1 - (0.323 \times 30) = 90.41$.

12. How is the forced expiratory volume in one second (FEV_1) changed with age?

FEV_1 declines linearly with age increase.

13. What are the most significant changes of pulmonary function associated with aging?
- Loss of lung elasticity, which leads to increased mean alveolar diameter and volume and reduced FEV_1
- Decreased power of the respiratory musculature
- Increased rigidity of rib cage

All these changes start becoming apparent in third decade of life.

14. What does PEEP mean?

*P*ositive *e*nd-*e*xpiratory *p*ressure during mechanical ventilation. PEEP aids in preventing alveolar and small airway collapse and may help recruit lung units that were previously collapsed.

15. What are the beneficial effects of PEEP?
- Increased functional residual capacity
- Increased compliance
- Increased PaO_2
- Increased ventilation-perfusion (V/Q) ratio (when initially low)
- Decreased pulmonary shunt

16. What is the effect of PEEP on cardiac output?

Because of increased intrathoracic pressure and decreased venous return when using PEEP, cardiac output may be decreased secondarily.

17. What are the normal blood gas values?

pH	7.40 ± 0.05 units
(H^+)	40 ± 5 mEq/L
pCO_2	40 ± 5 mmHg

As a rule, each 0.1 increment of pH corresponds to 12 mmHg of pCO_2, which equals a base change of 6 mEq/L.

Golden rule #1: a pH of 0.08 = $PaCO_2$ of 10 mmHg.

Golden rule #2: a pH of 0.15 = base change of 10 mEq/L.

18. Define acidosis and alkalosis.

Acidosis is the metabolic state when only excessive quantities of metabolic acids are produced or when the buffering systems or renal function are abnormal. **Alkalosis** occurs when there is excessive ingestion of a base (e.g., bicarbonate) or a loss of excess acid (e.g., hypovolemia, vomiting).

19. How is the diagnosis of respiratory acidosis made?

Respiratory acidosis is usually evident from the clinical examination, especially if respiration is obviously depressed. Analysis of arterial blood gases (ABGs) will confirm the diagnosis: arterial pH will be < 7.35 and PCO_2 will be > 45 mmHg.

20. What are some causes of respiratory acidosis?

Any disease or condition that may affect the respiratory function can cause respiratory acidosis, including:

Chronic obstructive pulmonary disease (COPD)
Pulmonary edema
Cardiac arrest
Pneumonia
Chest wall or airway injury
Drug effects
Central nervous system (CNS) depression
Extreme obesity (e.g., pickwickian syndrome)

21. How is the diagnosis of respiratory alkalosis made?

Clinically, respiratory alkalosis usually manifests as hyperventilation. However, depending on its severity and acuteness, hyperventilation may not be evident, but an analysis of arterial blood gases will demonstrate an arterial pH of > 7.45 and a PCO_2 of < 35 mmHg.

22. What are some causes of respiratory alkalosis?

Hyperventilation
CNS injury
Fever
Pulmonary embolus
Excessive mechanical ventilation

23. With what is bronchial carcinoma most often associated?

Up to 50% of cases of carcinoma of the hypopharynx and upper part of the esophagus are associated with Plummer-Vinson syndrome.

24. Where is the respiratory center?

The respiratory center is a widely dispersed group of neurons located bilaterally in the reticular substance of the medulla oblongata and pons.

25. What influences the respiratory center?

Excess CO_2 and hydrogen ions (H^+) affect respiration mainly by direct excitatory effects on the respiratory center itself. Oxygen does *not* have a significant direct effect on the respiratory center. O_2 acts almost entirely peripherally on the carotid and aortic bodies.

26. How does metastatic bronchiogenic carcinoma usually reach the mandible?

The mandible is affected by metastatic tumors much more often than the maxilla is. Studies have shown that 82–85% of metastatic tumors involve the mandible. The molar area is predominantly involved because it contains a rich deposit of hematopoietic tissue. Also, because the mode of spread is usually hematogenous, tumor cells tend to be deposited in the vascular medullary tissue.

27. What is the normal rate of breathing?

The respiratory rate (RR) is 10–20 breaths per minute in normal adults and 44 breaths/min in infants. An RR > 20/min is considered tachypnea, and RR < 10/min is bradypnea.

28. What is Cheyne-Stokes breathing?

Periods of hyperpnea (deep breathing) alternating with periods of apnea. Children and the elderly normally show this pattern in sleep. In normal adults, causes of this pattern of breathing include heart failure, uremia, drug-induced respiratory depression, and brain damage.

29. What causes stridor?

Stridor, an airway emergency that demands immediate attention, is caused by partial obstruction of the airway at the level of larynx or trachea.

30. What is the definition of acute respiratory failure?

Respiratory failure is an inadequate exchange of O_2 and CO_2 secondary to failure of the ventilatory apparatus or gas exchange system. It results in hypoventilation and therefore hypercapnia and hypoxemia.

31. How is the diagnosis of respiratory failure made?

Respiratory failure is primarily based on arterial blood gases. Hemoglobin saturation of < 92% (which corresponds to a PaO_2 of < 60 mmHg, a $PaCO_2$ > 50 mmHg, and a pH of < 7.35 (respiratory acidosis).

32. How is respiratory failure treated?

Secure and maintain a patent airway in order to deliver appropriate O_2 therapy using mechanical or supportive ventilation. The airway may be in the form of oral and nasal endotracheal intubation, tracheostomy, or cricothyrotomy.

33. What are the indications for elective intubation and mechanical ventilation?

The indications for intubation and mechanical ventilation are based on clinical and laboratory values. These include:
- Respiratory rate > 30–40 breaths/min
- Negative inspiratory pressure < 25 cm H_2O
- Vital capacity < 10–15 ml/kg or a $PaCO_2$ > 50 mmHg with a pH < 7.3

34. What are the guidelines for withdrawing mechanical ventilatory support (weaning parameters)?

Mechanical ventilation can be withdrawn if one or more of the following parameters is met:
PaO_2 > 60 mmHg with an FiO_2 < 0.4
$PaCO_2$ (35–45) acceptable with normal pH
Tidal volume > 4–5 ml/kg
Vital capacity > 10–15 ml/kg
Minute ventilation < 10 L/min
Respiratory rate < 25/min
Negative inspiratory pressure > 20 cm H_2O

35. What is pleural effusion?

Pleural effusion occurs when fluid accumulates in the pleural space (i.e., volume overload, infection) and the air-filled lung separates from the chest wall.

36. What is atelectasis?

Atelectasis occurs when mucus or a foreign object obstructs airflow in a mainstem bronchus causing collapse of the affected lung tissue into an airless state. It typically occurs 36 hours postoperatively and presents with mild dyspnea, low-grade fever, and hypoxia.

37. How is postoperative atelectasis managed?

Treatment of postoperative atelectasis is aimed at expansion of the lung, and, for most patients, incentive spirometry is adequate. However, in patients with severe atelectasis, endotracheal suction and even bronchoscopy may be warranted.

38. What are the signs of pneumothorax?

Pneumothorax occurs when air leaks into the pleural space causing the lung to recoil from the chest wall. The signs of intraoperative pneumothorax include unexplained hypotension, ventilatory hypoxia with bulging diaphragm, jugular venous distention, tympanic thorax, and trachea deviated to one side. In an awake patient, a pneumothorax typically presents with dyspnea, chest pain, absence of breath sounds on the affected side, and evidence of pneumothorax on chest x-ray. Tracheal deviation may be present.

39. What is the appropriate treatment of pneumothorax?

Pneumothorax is definitively treated with placement of a thoracostomy tube and connected to closed suction of 20 cm H_2O. However, if tension pneumothorax is suspected, immediate needle decompression through the second intercostal space in the midclavicular line using a 14-gauge needle should be performed.

40. What is the mechanism of asthma?

Asthma is a chronic disorder characterized by inflammation and increased responsiveness of the tracheobronchial tree to diverse stimuli resulting in a varying degree of airway obstruction.

41. What is the clinical presentation of acute asthma?

Patients present with dyspnea or tachypnea, wheezing, hypoxemia, and, occasionally, hypercapnia.

42. What is the appropriate management of an acute asthma attack?

An acute asthmatic attack is best treated by administration of supplemental O_2 with inhaled beta-adrenergic agonistic (albuterol, 3.0 ml [2.5 mg], in 2 ml of normal saline every 4–6 hours, in a nebulizer). If the patient is resistant to beta agonists, theophylline should be considered. Therapy also may include parenteral steroids such as methylprednisolone (50–250 mg over 4–6 hours). In a severe asthmatic attack that is unresponsive to the above, administer 0.3 mg of 1:1000 epinephrine subcutaneously.

43. What drugs interfere (interact) with aminophylline?

The most commonly cited drug is erythromycin, which increases serum levels of aminophylline. Cimetidine also increases serum levels of aminophylline.

44. Why do chronic emphysema patients have a barrel-chest appearance?

In patients with emphysema, the distal air spaces become enlarged, and the lungs become hyperinflated.

45. What is adult respiratory distress syndrome (ARDS)?

ARDS is a C5a-induced neutrophil aggregation in the lung. This aggregation is one of the major mechanisms of pathology of ARDS. The damaged capillaries leak protein-rich fluid into interstitium, which leads to changes in pulmonary function.

46. What causes ARDS?

ARDS usually results from an injury to the alveolar-capillary membrane. It also can be caused by an existing underlying disease such as systemic sepsis, fat embolism, head injury, aspiration, pancreatitis, or inhalation injury. Patients typically show severe dyspnea and hypoxemia refractory to supplemental O_2 with diffuse pulmonary infiltrates on chest radiograph.

47. What is the appropriate management of ARDS?

Management of ARDS includes immediate transfer to an intensive care unit and placement of a pulmonary artery catheter with mechanical ventilation to maintain the pulse oximetry (SpO_2) > 90%, which corresponds to PO_2 > 60 mmHg. In addition, the pulmonary capillary pressure should be kept in the range of 12–15 mmHg, and the cardiac index should be maintained above 3 L/min/m². Treatment of ARDS is generally supportive to achieve O_2 saturation of ≥ 90% while minimizing barotrauma and oxygen toxicity.

48. Describe the features of ARDS.

- History of major insult
- Increased respiratory distress
- Diffuse infiltration on chest x ray
- Hypoxemia (PaO_2 < 60 mmHg with FiO_2 > 0.6)
- Respiratory alkalosis
- Normal pulmonary capillary wedge pressure (PCWP)
- Decreased pulmonary compliance
- Increased shunt function
- Increased dead space and ventilation

49. What is the appropriate management of aspiration of gastric contents?

Treatment of aspiration is generally supportive and should include administration of O_2, endotracheal intubation, and antibiotics. The patient should not be given anything orally (NPO) and may require total parenteral nutrition or enteral feedings. These patients generally will present with acute dyspnea and fever 2–3 hours after the event, secondary to chemical pneumonitis. Note that the chest radiograph in these patients may be normal initially but eventually will demonstrate diffuse interstitial infiltrates.

50. Name the possible complications of aspiration.

ARDS, pneumonia, and lung disease.

51. What are the signs and symptoms of pulmonary embolus (PE)?

Symptoms of PE	*Signs of PE*
Dyspnea	Tachypnea
Chest pain	Tachycardia
Cough	Possible syncope
Possible hemoptysis	

52. How is PE diagnosed?

PE should be considered in any postoperative patient with unexplained dyspnea, hypoxia, or tachypnea. Immediate SpO_2, electrocardiogram (ECG), and chest x-ray should be obtained. Desaturation will be evident, and nonspecific ST or T wave changes will be noted. Spiral computed tomography (CT) scans are helpful in diagnosis.

53. What is the appropriate management of postoperative PE?

Treatment should include the administration of O_2 to correct hypoxemia and intravenous fluids to maintain blood pressure. In addition, intravenous or subcutaneous heparin should be initiated immediately with a target partial thromboplastin time (PTT) of 1.5–2.4 times the control. Warfarin therapy should be started while the patient is on heparin until the patient's therapeutic prothrombin time (PT) is reached (within 5–7 days). The treatment is continued for 2–3 months. Finally, placement of an inferior vena cava (IVC) filter should be considered. Embolectomy may also be considered.

BIBLIOGRAPHY

1. Barash P, Cullen B, Stoelting R, et al (eds): Clinical Anesthesia, 2nd ed. Philadelphia, Lippincott-Raven, 1996.
2. Bates B, Bickley L, Hoekelman R: The thorax and lungs. In Bates B (ed): A Guide to Physical Examination and History Taking, 6th ed. Philadelphia, J.B. Lippincott, 1995.
3. Kollef M, Goodenberger D: Critical care and medical emergencies. In Ewald G, McKenzie C (eds): The Washington Manual of Medical Therapeutics. Boston, Little, Brown, 1995.
4. Miller R, Stoelting R: Acid-base and blood gas analysis. In Miller R (ed): Basics of Anesthesia, 3rd ed. New York, Churchill Livingstone, 1994.
5. Pettit TW, Cobb JP: Critical care. In Doherty G, et al (eds): The Washington Manual of Surgery. Boston, Little, Brown, 1997.
6. Roser SM: Management of the medically compromised patient. In Kwon P, Laskin D (eds): Clinician's Manual of Oral and Maxillofacial Surgery, 2nd ed. Chicago, Quintessence Publishing, 1997.

18. HEMATOLOGY

James A. Giglio, D.D.S., M.Ed., and Robert E. Doriot, D.D.S.

1. Which blood clotting factors are dependent on vitamin K for their synthesis?
Factors II, VII, IX, and X.

2. Which blood test is used to monitor the effect of warfarin?
Prothrombin time (PT) test.

3. What is the International Normalized Ratio (INR)?
The INR is a calculated value developed to normalize the reporting of PT.

$$INR = \left(\frac{patient\ protime}{mean\ of\ the\ normal\ range} \right)^{ISI}$$

The ISI is the International Sensitivity Index value assigned by the manufacturer to each lot of thromboplastin calibrated to the World Health Organization reference material. The INR standardizes reporting of anticoagulation activity and monitors patients on stabilized oral anticoagulant therapy only. The therapeutic INR range is 2.0–3.0 for most clinical situations. Patients with mechanical prosthetic heart valves are maintained at 2.5–3.5.

4. What are the three phases of hemostasis?
Vascular, platelet, and coagulation phases.

5. What effect can long-term antibiotic therapy have on hemostasis?
Long-term antibiotic therapy can suppress the normal flora in the gastrointestinal tract that are necessary for the synthesis of vitamin K. Clotting factors II, VII, IX, and X require vitamin K for their synthesis.

6. What disease is a factor IX deficiency?
Hemophilia B or Christmas disease.

7. If warfarin (Coumadin) is to be discontinued prior to oral surgery, how soon should this occur before the planned procedure?
Although dose dependent, in general, the duration of action for warfarin is 3–5 days with an onset in 12–24 hours. The half-life is 1.5–2.5 days. Warfarin should be discontinued at least 3 days prior to the procedure and a PT test should be done within 24 hours of the surgery.

8. How does administering vitamin K affect warfarin?
Vitamin K reverses the action of warfarin. Once vitamin K is administered, the patient may be resistant to further anticoagulation with warfarin for a few days. In addition, certain patients may have an underlying thrombotic tendency that puts them at risk for thrombosis and embolic complications should the effects of the anticoagulant be stopped abruptly. Therefore, administering vitamin K or abruptly stopping warfarin medication can be harmful to some patients.

9. How does heparin affect blood clotting?
Heparin is a naturally occurring conjugated polysaccharide formed by many cells including mast cells located in connective tissue, especially in the lung. Heparin calcium is commercially prepared from porcine intestinal connective tissue whereas the sodium form is prepared from either porcine intestinal connective tissue or bovine lung. Heparin affects the

intrinsic and common pathways of blood coagulation. It prevents the formation of prothrombin activator and inhibits the action of thrombin on fibrinogen. Heparin increases the normal clotting time (4–6 minutes) to 6–30 minutes. Its duration of action is 3–4 hours.

10. How can the effects of heparin be reversed?

Protamine sulfate is used to reverse the effects of heparin. Protamine, which itself is an anticoagulant, must be administered with caution. When protamine is given with heparin, the anticoagulant effect of both drugs is lost. Careful control of the protamine dosing is necessary to prevent bleeding from an overdose. Too rapid administration of protamine can result in hypertensive and anaphylactoid reactions.

11. How does aspirin affect blood coagulation?

Aspirin (acetylsalicylic acid [ASA]) and other nonsteroidal anti-inflammatory drugs (NSAIDs) affect the platelet phase of coagulation. These drugs alter cyclooxygenase activity within platelets. Cyclooxygenase controls the release of the adhesive proteins from platelets that are necessary for them to aggregate and "stick together" in response to trauma. Inhibition of cyclooxygenase activity by either aspirin or another NSAID will cause the development of an ineffective platelet plug resulting in prolonged bleeding. This side effect of ASA has led to its accepted controlled use as a prophylactic measure against coronary and cerebral vessel thrombosis.

12. What are the components of the extrinsic, intrinsic, and common pathways of the coagulation cascade?

The components of the intrinsic pathway are factors XII, XI, IX, and VIII. The components of the extrinsic pathways include tissue factors and factor VII. The common pathway involves factors X and XIII, prothrombin, thrombin, fibrinogen, and fibrin.

13. What factors are measured by PT and which ones are measured by partial thromboplastin time (PTT)?

PT measures factors II, VII, IX, X, and fibrinogen. PTT measures the integrity of the intrinsic pathways prior to the activation of factor X and the activity of factors I, II, V, VIII, IX, X, XI, and XII, and fibrinogen.

14. What are the indications for transfusion of fresh frozen plasma (FFP)?

Fresh frozen platelets are used for replacement of deficiencies of factors II, V, VII, IX, and XI when specific component therapy is not available or desirable. In an average size adult, each unit of FFP increases the level of all clotting factors by 2–3%, and most bleeding can be controlled by transfusion of FFP at a dose of 10 ml/kg of body weight.

15. What is anemia?

A decrease in the oxygen carrying capacity of the blood. General symptoms include weakness, fatigue, palpitations, tingling and numbness of the fingers and toes, a burning tongue, bone pain, and shortness of breath. Clinical signs of anemia include pallor, spooning and brittle nails, and a smooth, red tongue caused by loss of filiform papillae.

16. What causes iron deficiency anemia?

Iron deficiency anemia is caused by low serum ferritin and blood loss. A diagnosis of iron deficiency anemia is based on a low hemoglobin, a low white blood cell count and microcytic, hypochromic erythrocytes. Iron supplement and correction of any underlying cause of blood loss is the treatment for this anemia. Plummer-Vinson syndrome is a clinical triad of esophageal webbing, dysphagia, and oral symptoms of glossitis and xerostomia in a patient with iron deficiency anemia.

17. What is pernicious anemia?
Red blood cells (RBCs) require vitamin B_{12} and folic acid for their maturation and development. Vitamin B_{12} requires intrinsic factor, which is secreted by the parietal cells in the stomach, for its absorption. Pernicious anemia will develop if there is a deficiency of intrinsic factor, folic acid, or vitamin B_{12}.

18. What causes sickle cell anemia?
Sickle cell anemia is caused by a defect in the beta chain of hemoglobin causing the RBCs to become sickle shaped when exposed to low oxygen tension or increased pH. The inherent defect causing sickle cell anemia is the substitution of valine for glutamic acid on the beta chain of the hemoglobin molecule.

19. What is the perioperative management of a patient with sickle cell disease?
Perioperative management of a sickle cell anemia patient involves avoiding all possible precipitating factors, which include hypoxia, dehydration, stress, and infection. This can be done with intravenous fluids, sedation, oxygen supplementation, and all measures that prevent infection including antibiotic coverage. In patients with severe sickle cell disease who are undergoing major surgical procedures, exchange transfusions may be used to dilute the defective RBCs by 50% keeping the hematocrit under 35%. Treatment of sickle cell crisis involves maintenance of hydration, administration of oxygen, and analgesics.

20. What is the result of a deficiency of glucose-6 phosphate dehydrogenase (G-6-PD)?
Red blood cell glucose is metabolized by either the glycolytic or the hexose monophosphate shunt pathways. Reduced nicotinamide adenine dinucleotide phosphate (NADPH) formed by the hexose monophosphate shunt is necessary to rid the cell of oxidants. G-6-PD is a necessary enzyme for the hexose monophosphate shunt pathway to function properly. A deficiency of G-6-PD results in an accumulation of cell oxidants and ultimately a hemolysis of RBCs. ASA medications should not be prescribed to patients with G-6-PD deficiency because it can cause hemolysis.

21. What is the normal white blood cell count?
Between 4,500 and 11,000/mm³. An increase in white blood cells is termed *leukocytosis*, and a decrease is *leukopenia*.

22. What are the forms of leukemia?
Leukemia can be either acute or chronic. There are two types of acute leukemia: acute lymphocytic and acute myelogenous leukemia. Chronic leukemia is classified as chronic lymphocytic or chronic myelogenous leukemia.

23. Which form of leukemia is most often associated with the Philadelphia chromosome?
Chronic myelogenous leukemia. This marker can be found in the metaphase and is associated with a poorer prognosis.

24. What is the primary difference between Hodgkin's disease and non-Hodgkin's lymphoma?
Both diseases are lymphoproliferative diseases. Hodgkin's disease usually begins as a single tumor focus whereas non-Hodgkin's lymphoma is usually multifocal.

25. What is Plummer-Vinson syndrome?
Plummer-Vinson syndrome occurs with iron deficiency anemia and is a predisposing factor to oral carcinoma. It is found primarily in women in the 4th and 5th decades of life. Clinical signs include cracking at the lip commissure, lemon-tinted pallor, smooth red painful tongue with atrophy of the filiform, and later fungiform papillae. A characteristic esophageal

webbing or stricture is also identified. Iron deficiency anemia responds well to iron replacement therapy.

26. What is von Willebrand's disease? How is it managed in a patient who is about to undergo surgery?

Von Willebrand's disease is an inherited disorder (autosomal dominant) in which von Willebrand's factor, required for platelet adhesion, is either deficient or defective. Management of von Willebrand's disease depends on the severity of the disease, because bleeding is variable from patient to patient. In mild cases, one of the following routes can be followed: preoperative administration of 50–100 gm/kg of intravenous aminocaproic acid (Amicar); oral Amicar 3 hours after surgery and then every 6 hours for 7 days; or intravenous infusion of 0.3 mg/kg of desmopressin (DDAVP) diluted in 50 ml of normal saline over 15–30 minutes, which will produce maximum levels of factor VIIIc in 90–120 minutes and will last for 6 hours. In severe cases, a transfusion of cryoprecipitate (20 bags) is warranted in order to achieve factor VIIIc, VIII vw levels of 1 U/ml immediately before surgery. In addition, Amicar should be initiated 12–24 hours preoperatively and continued for 12 days.

27. Differentiate hemophilia A and B.

Hemophilia A is an X-linked recessive disorder in which factor VIII is deficient, while the affected serine protease in type B is factor IX. Initially, the two coagulation disorders will present similarly with elevated PTT and normal PT and bleeding time, but they are managed differently.

28. Name some other causes of bleeding disorders.

Liver disease, anticoagulant therapy, aspirin therapy, disseminated intravascular coagulation (DIC), vitamin K deficiency, malabsorption syndrome, thrombocytopenia, polycythemia vera, iron deficiency, B_{12} deficiency, and thalassemia major can also cause bleeding disorders.

29. What is DIC?

Disseminated intravascular coagulation is the consequence of intravascular activation of both the coagulation and fibrinolytic systems. DIC varies greatly in its clinical presentation because it can show up as either bleeding or thrombosis. Generally treatment involves correction of the underlying process, which can be neoplasm, infection, liver disease, snake bites, spider bites, obstetric complications, trauma, shock, extensive burns, connective tissue diseases, or acute leukemia.

30. How should a patient with hemophilia A who is about to undergo a surgical procedure be managed?

Patients with hemophilia A are managed according to the severity of their disorder and anticipated blood loss. Patients with severe hemophilia should receive replacement of factor VIII with factor VIII concentrate. The minimal level of factor VIII required for hemostasis is 30%, and the half-life of factor VIII in the circulation is 10 hours. A loading dose of 30 U/kg immediately before surgery is followed by continuous infusion of 3 U/kg for 5 days and then a single dose of 30 U/kg for an additional 5 days. Patients with less severe disease can be managed with cryoprecipitate or DDAVP, 0.3 mg/kg every 24 hours, and/or Amicar, 4 gm by mouth every 4 hours for 5–7 days.

31. What is the replacement therapy for hemophilia B?

Replacement therapy for hemophilia type B is similar to factor VIII deficiency, but the dosing interval differs because the half-life of factor IX is 24 hours. Factor IX concentrate should be given every 18–24 hours.

BIBLIOGRAPHY

1. Beirne O, Koehler J: Surgical management of patients on warfarin sodium. J Oral Maxillofac Surg 54:1115–1118, 1996.
2. Herman W, Konzelman J, Sutley S: Current perspectives on dental patients receiving Coumadin anti-coagulant therapy. J Am Dent Assoc 128:327–335, 1997.
3. Lew D: Blood and blood products. In Kwon PH, Laskin DM (eds): Clinician's Manual of Oral and Maxillofacial Surgery, 2nd ed. Carol Stream, IL, Quintessence, 1997, pp 105–116.
4. Little J, Falace D, Miller C, Rhodes N: Dental Management of the Medically Compromised Patient, 5th ed. St. Louis, Mosby, 1997.

19. LIVER DISEASES

Mark A. Oghalai, D.D.S.

1. What are the risk factors for liver disease?
Intravenous drug abuse
Cocaine use
Contact with blood
Blood transfusion before 1989
Alcohol abuse
Multiple sexual contacts
Diabetes
Family history of liver disease
Intake of certain medications and food supplements

2. Which liver function tests are useful for assessing hepatocellular damage?
Alanine aminotransferase (ALT) and aspartate aminotransferase (AST). These enzymes are released from damaged hepatocytes. ALT is a more sensitive indicator of liver damage because it is found only in hepatic cells while AST is also found in heart, skeletal muscle, pancreas, kidney, and red blood cells. Increased bilirubin, decreased albumin, decreased cholesterol, and abnormal prothrombin time (PT) are other laboratory abnormalities in liver disease.

3. How is drug metabolism affected by liver cirrhosis?
Fibrosis leads to decreases in blood flow from the hepatic artery to the most distal areas. These areas are concentrated with the cytochrome P450 system, which is important in metabolizing many drugs. Prolonged plasma half-life of these drugs is a consequence of cirrhosis.

4. What are the signs of liver failure?
• Jaundice
• Portal hypertension (dilated chest, abdominal or rectal veins, liver and spleen enlargement)
• Hepatic encephalopathy
• Asterixis
• Palmar erythema
• Testicular atrophy
• Ascites
• Dupuytren's contracture
• Gynecomastia
• Spider telangiectasia

5. What laboratory test is used to assess hepatic dysfunction secondary to biliary obstruction?
Alkaline phosphatase (ALP). ALP is present in bile duct cells; even slight degrees of bile duct obstruction result in large increases in plasma concentration.

6. How is drug protein binding affected by liver disease?
Decreased albumin production by the liver results in a decreased number of protein-binding sites. The amount of unbound, pharmacologically active drug is, in turn, increased.

7. What is the effect of inhaled anesthetics on hepatic blood flow?
A 20–30% decrease in hepatic blood flow results from decreased perfusion pressure.

8. Describe the effect of positive pressure ventilation on hepatic blood flow.

Decreased hepatic blood flow secondary to increased central venous pressure decreases hepatic perfusion pressure.

9. What class of drugs can cause spasm of the choledochoduodenal sphincter?

Opioids.

10. Which inhaled anesthetic is best for maintaining hepatic blood flow and hepatocyte oxygenation?

Isoflurane.

11. Which muscle relaxant is the best choice to use in a patient with liver dysfunction?

Cis-atracurium, because it is eliminated by Hofmann elimination and therefore is independent of liver function.

12. How does liver dysfunction affect metabolism of procaine?

The liver is responsible for the production of pseudocholinesterase, which metabolizes procaine (and other ester anesthetics). Decreased production can result in prolonged half-life of these drugs.

13. What mechanism is responsible for metabolism of amide anesthetics?

Hepatic microsomal enzymes have the major role in metabolism of amide local anesthetics. A decrease in liver function can, therefore, prolong the plasma half-life of amide anesthetics.

14. What is the most accurate test for evaluation of liver disease?

The liver biopsy. The biopsy can detect cirrhosis, fibrosis, fat deposition, iron overload, and inflammatory processes as well as determine the prognosis.

15. How can liver disease affect the bleeding time?

The bleeding time may be increased in patients with portal hypertension by splenic sequestration of platelets leading to thrombocytopenia.

16. Which clotting factors does the liver produce?

Factors II, V, VII, IX, and X. Factors II, VII, IX, and X are vitamin K–dependent clotting factors.

17. What laboratory values will be affected by a deficiency in the factors produced by the liver?

PT and partial thromboplastin time (PTT).

18. What is the treatment of bleeding diathesis from liver disease?

Fresh frozen plasma. If the patient is thrombocytopenic, he or she may need platelet transfusion as well. Vitamin K–dependent clotting factors alone are not sufficient because they do not include factor V, which is also produced in the liver.

19. What is Gilbert syndrome?

Gilbert syndrome, the most common cause of idiopathic hyperbilirubinemia, is an autosomal dominant trait with variable penetrance. Decreased bilirubin uptake by hepatocytes results in increased plasma concentration of unconjugated bilirubin.

20. What are the most common drugs used in the dental office that are metabolized primarily by the liver?

Local anesthetics including lidocaine (Xylocaine), mepivacaine (Carbocaine), prilocaine (Citanest), and bupivacaine (Marcaine) are metabolized by the liver. Analgesics that are metabolized in the liver include aspirin, acetaminophen (Tylenol), codeine, meperidine (Demerol), and ibuprofen (Motrin). The most commonly used sedation drug that is metabolized in the liver is diazepam (Valium). Antibiotics that are metabolized in the liver include ampicillin and tetracycline.

21. What are the different types of viral hepatitis?

To date, five distinct types of hepatitis have been designated according to the etiologic viruses: types A, B, C, D (delta), and E. Each of these viruses belongs to a different family of virus with distinct autogenic properties.

22. What are the differences among the various viral hepatides?

Hepatitis A virus (HAV) is a 28-nm RNA virus whose mode of transmission is primarily fecal-oral. The diagnostic marker for hepatitis A is anti-HAV. Infected patients are treated with immune globulin and will develop lifetime immunity to HAV. A vaccine is available for HAV.

Hepatitis B virus (HBV) is a 42-nm DNA virus whose mode of transmission is predominately parenteral or through sexual contact. **Hepatitis D** occurs only as a coinfection or superinfection with hepatitis B. Diagnostic markers for HBV include IgM anti-HBc (acute), HbsAg (acute/chronic/infective), HbeAg (infectious), anti-HBs (recovery/immunity), and anti-HBcIg (ongoing or past infection). Infected patients are treated with hepatitis B immunoglobulin, and infected patients will develop lifetime immunity. A vaccine is available for HBV.

Hepatitis C virus (HCV) is a 38–50-nm RNA virus whose mode of transmission is predominantly parenteral. Diagnostic markers include anti-HCV (recovery/immunity) and HCV RNA (infectivity). Effectiveness of treatment modalities for infected patients has not yet been established. Immunity following infection is weak and ineffective, and no vaccine currently exists.

Hepatitis E virus (HEV) is a 32-nm RNA virus whose mode of transmission is predominately fecal-oral. The diagnostic marker used is anti-HEV (recovery). No treatment is currently used for infected patients. Infected patients will develop lifetime immunity, but no vaccine is currently available for HEV.

23. List the orofacial features of patients with chronic alcoholism.

Poor oral hygiene	Jaundice of the oral mucosa
Glossitis	Parotid gland enlargement
Angular cheilosis	Impaired healing
Candidiasis	Bruxism
Petechiae	Xerostomia

24. What precautions should be taken before oral and maxillofacial surgery in a patient with viral hepatitis?

The patient's liver function status should be determined by means of liver function enzymes (AST, ALT, ALP). Drug choice and dosage should be determined with these laboratory values in mind. The patient's bleeding tendency should also be assessed by PT, PTT, international normalized ratio (INR), and bleeding time. For patients undergoing major surgical procedures, if the PT or PTT more than $1\frac{1}{2}$ times greater than control values or if the INR is $\geq$ 3.0, transfusion of fresh frozen plasma should be considered. This supplies the patient with factors II, VII, IX, X, XI, XII, and XIII and heat-labile factors V and VII. In patients with a platelet count of $< 50,000/mm^3$, platelet administration to a level above $50,000$ mm^3 is indicated. Universal precautions should also be taken to prevent hepatitis exposure to the surgeon and assistants.

25. Describe the preoperative therapy for patients with liver disease.

Preoperative maximization of liver function in patients with liver disease should include evaluating and optimizing the nutritional status and correcting electrolytes and coagulation abnormalities. The patient should stop alcohol intake and increase protein intake. If the patient has active hepatitis, all elective surgeries should be postponed until the hepatitis has resolved completely. Defects in coagulation should be corrected with fresh frozen plasma. If the patient is taking steroids, intravenous corticosteroids should be given. Finally, preoperative or operative sedation should be done to a degree that is compatible with the patient's decreased ability to metabolize drugs by the liver, especially benzodiazepines, barbiturates, and other sedatives.

26. What are the intraoperative considerations in patients with liver disease?

It is important to maintain adequate liver perfusion during surgery by maintaining adequate blood pressure. This can be done by infusing saline, fresh frozen plasma, and platelets if there is thrombocytopenia. If the patient swallowed blood, the stomach should be evacuated to prevent protein loading and false-positive blood in the stool. If the patient is taking corticosteroids, supplemental steroids should be given.

27. What are the surgical considerations in post-liver transplant patient?

During the first 3 months of the postoperative period, and in patients with chronic rejection of the graft, only emergency oral surgical procedures should be rendered. Such procedures should be performed only after consultation with the patient's transplant service, and whenever possible antibiotic prophylaxis should be given to prevent bacterial endarteritis. After the first 3 months, the patient is usually on immunosuppressants. If the patient has a stable functional graft, good liver function is established. However, there is still the risk of acquired infection including influenza, fungal infections, and post-transplant viral infections. In these patients, prevention and treatment of any possible infection is important and consideration must be given to the patient's immunosuppressant doses, supplementation of steroid (if necessary), and use of effective infection control measures.

BIBLIOGRAPHY

1. Cerulli MA: Management of the patient with liver diseases. Oral Maxillofac Surg Clin North Am 10:465–470, 1998.
2. Douglas LR, Douglas JB, Sieck JO, Smith PJ: Oral management of the patient with end-stage liver disease and the liver transplant patient. Oral Surg Oral Med Oral Pathol Oral Radiol Endod 86:55–64, 1998.
3. Duke J: Renal function and anesthesia. In Duke J (ed): Anesthesia Secrets, 2nd ed. Philadelphia, Hanley & Belfus, 2000, pp 237–248.
4. Little JW, Falace DA: Liver disease. In Little JW, Falace DA (eds): Dental Management of the Medically Compromised Patient. St Louis, Mosby, 1997, pp 274–293.
5. Stoelting RK, Dierdorf SF: Diseases of the liver and biliary tract. In Stoelting RK, Dierdorf SF (eds): Anesthesia and Co-existing Disease, 3rd ed. New York, Churchill Livingstone, 1993, pp 251–275.
6. Stoelting RK, Miller RD: Liver and biliary tract disease. In Stoelting RK, Miller RD (eds): Basics of Anesthesia, 3rd ed. Philadelphia, Churchill Livingstone, 1994, pp 301–314.
7. Ziccardi VB, Abubaker AO, Sotereanos GC, Patterson GT: Maxillofacial considerations in orthotopic liver transplant patient. Oral Surg Oral Med Oral Pathol 71:21–26, 1991.

20. RENAL DISEASES

Mark A. Oghalai, D.D.S., and William A. Carvajal, D.D.S.

1. What are five main functions of the kidney?
1. Elimination of metabolic waste
2. Maintenance of fluid balance
3. Maintenance of electrolyte balance
4. Maintenance of acid and base balance
5. Endocrine and metabolic functions, including erythropoietin secretion and vitamin D conversion

2. Which compound is used as a sensitive, indirect measurement of glomerular filtration rate (GFR)?
Creatinine is used because it is filtered by the glomeruli but minimally secreted or reabsorbed.

3. Define renal failure.
Renal failure is defined as impairment in renal function, as measured by the GFR. It is classified as either acute or chronic.

4. Describe acute renal failure (ARF).
This syndrome is characterized by sudden decline in renal function, resulting in retention of nitrogenous waste with corresponding elevations of serum creatinine and blood urea nitrogen (BUN). It is usually reversible if treated early.

5. What are the major classes of ARF?
1. **Prerenal.** This class is the most common type and is associated with insufficient renal perfusion. Examples include hypovolemia, impaired cardiac function, and sepsis.
2. **Renal.** Glomerular diseases, acute tubular necrosis, and acute interstitial nephritis fall under this classification.
3. **Postrenal.** This type of renal failure includes bilateral urethral obstruction and bladder neck obstruction.

6. Describe chronic renal failure (CRF).
CRF is an irreversible, advanced, and progressive renal insufficiency.

7. What are the major causes of CRF?
1. Diabetic nephropathy
2. Hypertension

8. What are the clinical manifestations of CRF and end-stage renal disease (ESRD)?
The clinical manifestations of CRF and ESRD depend on the stage of the disease, but include:

Fluid and electrolyte disturbances	Peripheral neuropathy
Hypertension and pericarditis	Anemia and thrombocytopenia
Uremia and uremic osteodystrophy	Nausea and vomiting
Tiredness and insomnia	Pruritus and hyperpigmentation

9. What are the main treatment options for ESRD?
1. Peritoneal dialysis
2. Hemodialysis
3. Renal transplant

10. What endocrine abnormality is often associated with CRF?

Secondary hyperparathyroidism. As the kidneys lose their ability to convert vitamin D, intestinal absorption of calcium decreases, causing hyperparathyroidism.

11. List the oral manifestations of renal disease.

Patients with renal disease or CRF often demonstrate orofacial signs and symptoms that are not necessarily specific for ESRD but are related to the systemic manifestations of the disease. The most common of these manifestations are:

- Enamel hypoplasia and staining of teeth
- Halitosis and metallic taste
- Stomatitis and xerostomia secondary to fluid intake restriction
- Gingival bleeding, ecchymosis, petechiae, and pale and inflamed gingiva
- Osteolytic bone defects in the mandible, mandibular condyles, and maxilla; loss of lamina dura; and decreased trabeculation of bone
- Skeletal facial deformities secondary to altered growth
- Accelerated dental calculus accumulation

12. What are the laboratory findings in patients with CRF?

- Elevated BUN and creatinine resulting from decreased glomerular filtration
- Metabolic acidosis secondary to impaired tubular function, causing an accumulation of ammonia
- Multiple electrolyte abnormalities including hyperkalemia, hypocalcemia, and hypermagnesemia
- Anemia from decreased renal production of erythropoietin

13. How does renal disease affect the pharmacodynamics of administered drugs?

The effects of drugs may be potentiated by increased volume of distribution, decreased protein binding, and decreased glomerular filtration and renal tubular secretion. Renal failure may modify drug bioavailability, distribution, pharmacologic action, or elimination when the kidney excretes the drug or its metabolites. For the ESRD patient, most drugs are administered in an initial loading dose to provide therapeutic blood concentrations. Sustained effects are controlled by dosage adjustments and time-interval alterations and are based on serum drug levels.

14. How do nonsteroidal anti-inflammatory drugs (NSAIDs) affect renal function?

NSAIDs inhibit prostaglandin synthesis and, therefore, decrease prostaglandin-associated intrinsic renal vasodilatation.

15. What classes of drugs should be avoided in patients with renal disease?

1. Nephrotoxic drugs including NSAIDs, aminoglycosides, and IV dyes
2. Drugs that are converted to toxic metabolites, including meperidine and propoxyphene
3. Drugs that contain excessive electrolytes, including penicillin G and magnesium citrate

16. What analgesics should be avoided in patients with renal disease?

- Aspirin
- Acetaminophen
- NSAIDs
- Meperidine—accumulation of meperidine can result in seizures
- Morphine—dose decreased secondary to accumulation of morphine-6-glucuronide

17. What antibiotics should be avoided in patients with renal disease?

Cephalosporins	Tetracycline
Erythromycin	Aminoglycosides

18. In severe renal dysfunction patients, are metabolic end products from local anesthetics contraindicated?

No. Local anesthetics are metabolized in the liver and plasma, then excreted. Therefore, anesthetics can accumulate and not be a factor in patients with renal disease.

19. What effect might general anesthetics have on renal blood flow and GFR?

General anesthetics that can cause myocardial depression also can cause decreased renal blood flow and glomerular filtration rate that is proportional to the depth of anesthesia. Methoxyflurane is no longer in use because of fluoride-induced nephrotoxicity. Halothane, enflurane, and isoflurane produce much lower fluoride levels and are safer to use with regard to nephrotoxicity. Therefore, it is important to choose the type of agent and the appropriate level of anesthesia in renal failure patients in order to minimize further injury and likelihood of renal failure.

20. Which metabolites from halogenated general anesthetics can lead to nephrotoxic renal failure?

Inorganic fluoride from the metabolism of methoxyflurane. Sevoflurane also increases inorganic fluoride, and its use is controversial in patients with renal disease.

21. Which halogenated general anesthetics do not significantly increase plasma inorganic fluoride concentrations?

Isoflurane, halothane, and desflurane.

22. What length of time prior to and after surgery should dialysis be performed?

One day prior to surgery and 1–2 days after surgery in order to correct potassium and fluid balance while minimizing bleeding complications.

23. What laboratory tests should be performed for renal failure patients prior to surgery?

CRF patients should have bleeding time, prothrombin time (PT), partial thromboplastin time (PTT), platelet count, complete blood cell count (CBC), and serum potassium and protein levels. Bleeding time is the most sensitive test for a bleeding tendency in CRF patients. If the bleeding time is elevated, the patient should receive vigorous dialysis and, if necessary, deamino-D-arginine vasopressin (DDAVP) intravenously or nasally, at a dose of 0.3 µg/kg, 30 minutes before surgery. Hyperkalemia can also be corrected with preoperative dialysis. If surgery is emergent and dialysis cannot be performed preoperatively, hyperkalemia should be treated aggressively to decrease the arrhythmogenic effect of hyperkalemia. This can be done by intravenous infusion of calcium chloride, glucose, and insulin to drive extracellular potassium into cells.

24. What is the cause of CRF-induced anemia?

Decreased erythropoietin production from the kidneys.

25. What is the treatment of CRF-induced anemia prior to surgery?

Anemia in CRF patients should be treated with administration of recombinant human erythropoietin until the patient's hematocrit is raised to at least 30–33%.

26. What is the difference between peritoneal dialysis and hemodialysis?

In peritoneal dialysis, a hypertonic solution is placed into the peritoneal cavity and removed a short time later. During the removal process, dissolved solutes such as urea are drawn out. Peritoneal dialysis does not require anticoagulation and is less expensive than hemodialysis. However, peritoneal dialysis requires more frequent sessions than hemodialysis, is less effective, and has a higher incidence of complications such as infection, hypoglycemia, and protein loss. The most common use for peritoneal dialysis is the treatment of patients with ARF.

Hemodialysis is the most commonly used method of dialysis for CRF and is performed at 2–3-day intervals. Surgical placement of a permanent arteriovenous (AV) fistula for large-bore cannulation is required; the patient's blood is filtered through a dialysis machine and returned to the patient via the AV fistula. Administering heparin prevents clotting. Patients receiving hemodialysis are at risk for contracting hepatitis B, hepatitis C, and HIV because of multiple blood exposures. In addition, these patients are at risk for infection of their AV shunts, which predisposes them to septic emboli, septicemia, infective endarteritis, and infective endocarditis.

27. Outline the steps that should be taken prior to oral surgical procedures on ESRD patients.

- Review laboratory values to detect possible bleeding diathesis (bleeding time, platelet count, PT, PTT).
- Monitor blood pressure.
- Avoid nephrotoxic drugs such as acyclovir, aspirin, NSAIDs, and high-dose acetaminophen.
- Decrease dosage of drugs metabolized by the kidney.
- Aggressively manage orofacial infections.
- Ensure that patients receiving hemodialysis do not undergo surgery for at least 4 hours after hemodialysis to avoid heparin-induced bleeding.

28. What preoperative adjustments need to be made in drug dosing or interval in patients with CRF?

DRUG	PRESURGERY ADJUSTMENT
Aspirin	Increase interval between doses and avoid it completely if GFR is low
Acetaminophen	Increase interval between doses and avoid it completely in cases of severe failure
Penicillin V, cephalexin, tetracycline	Increase interval between doses in severe failure
Ketoconazole	Reduce dose
Lidocaine, codeine, erythromycin, clindamycin, metronidazole	No adjustment necessary

29. What medical considerations should be given to patients receiving dialysis prior to oral surgical procedures?

No adjustments are required for patients receiving peritoneal dialysis, but there are several concerns for patients receiving hemodialysis. Surgically created bacteremia can cause infection of the AV fistula. Because graft endothelialization takes up to 3–6 months after placement, standard American Heart Association antibiotic prophylaxis is strongly recommended for the first 6 months following fistula placement and may be beneficial for all graft patients undergoing oral surgery. The arm that contains the AV shunt should not be used for blood pressure recording because the shunt could collapse. Likewise, intravenous administration of medications should be avoided in the arm because clot formation could jeopardize the shunt. The quality of the AV thrill should be assessed initially and then periodically during surgery. During long surgeries, the use of a circulating heating pack over the arm is advocated.

Patients should be screened for bleeding tendencies because hemodialysis destroys platelets. Surgery should be delayed for at least 4 hours after hemodialysis to prevent heparin-induced bleeding. Patients should be screened periodically for hepatitis B, hepatitis C, and HIV. Universal precautions should be followed by the surgical team when treating any patient undergoing hemodialysis. The positioning of the containing access site must be observed during surgery to avoid pressure on the site.

30. How are bleeding problems prevented and managed in patients with renal failure?

Bleeding encountered in patients with renal failure is best managed initially with local hemostatic procedures, such as good surgical technique, primary wound closure whenever possible, hemostatic agents and topical thrombin, and electrocautery. Preoperative IV (0.3 µg/kg) or intranasal (3.0 µg/kg) DDAVP temporarily corrects the increase in bleeding time in uremic patients for up to 4 hours. It also may be useful as a therapeutic modality in acute postsurgical hemorrhage. Cryoprecipitate has a peak effect in 4–12 hours and duration of 24–36 hours but generally is reserved for acute bleeding that is not easily managed. Conjugated estrogen, which has duration of up to 30 days and peak effects in approximately 2–5 days, also may be used.

BIBLIOGRAPHY

 1. Bennett WM, Muther RS, Parker RA, et al: Drug therapy in renal failure: Dosing guidelines for adults. Part I: Antimicrobial agents, analgesics. Ann Intern Med 93:62–89, 1980.
 2. Carl W, Wood RH: The dental patient with chronic renal failure. Quintessence Int 7:9–15, 1976.
 3. Duke J: Renal function and anesthesia. In Duke J (ed): Anesthesia Secrets, 2nd ed. Philadelphia, Hanley & Belfus, 2000, pp 287–298.
 4. Little JW, Falace DA: Chronic renal failure and dialysis. In Little JW, Falace DA (eds): Dental Management of the Medically Compromised Patient. St. Louis, Mosby, 1997, pp 260–273.
 5. Silverstein KE, Adams MC, Fonseca RJ: Evaluation and management of the renal failure and dialysis patient. Oral Maxillofac Surg Clin North Am 10:417–427, 1998.
 6. Stoelting RK, Dierdorf SF: Renal disease. In Stoelting RK, Dierdorf SF (eds): Anesthesia and Co-existing Disease, 3rd ed. London, Churchill Livingstone, 1993, pp 289–310.
 7. Stoelting RK, Miller RD: Renal disease. In Stoelting RK, Miller RD (eds): Basics of Anesthesia, 3rd ed. Philadelphia, Churchill Livingstone, 1994, pp 301–314.
 8. Swell SB: Dental care for patients with renal failure and renal transplants. J Am Dental Assoc 104:171–177, 1982.
 9. Westbrook DS: Dental management in patients receiving hemodialysis and kidney transplants. J Am Dental Assoc 96:464–468, 1978.
10. Ziccardi VB, Saini J, Demas PN, Braun TW: Management of the oral and maxillofacial surgery patient with end-stage renal disease. J Oral Maxillofac Surg 50:1207–1212, 1992.

21. ENDOCRINE DISEASES

Maria Iuorno, M.D.

1. What is calcitonin?
Calcitonin, a 32–amino acid polypeptide, is a hormone produced by the parafollicular cells or C cells of the parathyroid glands.

2. What are the signs and symptoms associated with adrenal insufficiency?

Chronic Signs and Symptoms	Associated Mineralocorticoid Deficiency Symptoms
Anorexia	Acute (adrenal crises) mental status changes
Bronzing of the skin	Confusion
Dehydration	Hyperkalemia
Dizziness	Hyponatremia
Fatigue	Hypotension
Hypertension	Lethargy
Hypoglycemia	
Nausea	
Vomiting	
Weakness	
Weight loss	

3. Where is aldosterone produced?
Aldosterone, a mineralocorticoid, is produced within the zona glomerulosa of the adrenal cortex.

4. What influence does aldosterone have on sodium (Na) and potassium (K)?
Major influence on sodium balance by increasing renal tubular reabsorption of sodium in distal tubular segment (mostly collecting tubules). The net result is Na resorption and K excretion.

5. Which hormone is also known as vasopressin?
Antidiuretic hormone (ADH).

6. Where is ADH produced and released?
Posterior pituitary.

7. What effect will an increased release of ADH have on urine concentration?
Because ADH affects the renal collecting tubule's permeability, water will be reabsorbed, resulting in a more concentrated urine.

8. What causes ADH release?
ADH is released in response to changes in the serum osmolality detected by the hypothalamus. Osmolality that decreases to about 295 mOsm/kg initiates release.

9. Where are angiotensin I and II produced?
In the kidney.

10. How does angiotensin II cause an increase in blood pressure?
Angiotensin II actively increases vascular tone, stimulates catecholamine release, and increases sodium reabsorption (at distal tubule). It also stimulates release of aldosterone from zona glomerulosa of the adrenal cortex.

11. What are the diagnostic criteria for differentiating among acute tubular necrosis, prerenal azotemia, and postrenal obstruction?

	PRERENAL AZOTEMIA (OBSTRUCTION)	ATN (TUBULAR INJURY)	POSTRENAL OBSTRUCTION
Urine osmolality	> 500	< 350	Varies
U/P osmolality	> 1.25	< 1.1	Varies
U/P urea	> 8	< 3	Varies
U/P creatinine	> 40	< 20	< 20
Urine sodium	< 20	> 40	> 40
FENa	< 1	> 3	> 3

ATN = acute tubular necrosis; U/P = urea/plasma ratio; FENa = fractional excretion of sodium

12. What is azotemia?
Nitrogen retention resulting from factors other than primary renal disease.

13. What is the syndrome of inappropriate secretion of ADH (SIADH)?
SIADH is the nonphysiologic secretion of ADH from sites other than the pituitary gland. It is the most common cause of hospital-acquired hyponatremia. Several conditions can cause SIADH:
- Some tumors, such as oat cell lung carcinoma (small cell), secrete biologically active ADH.
- Central nervous system (CNS) disorders, such as meningitis and encephalitis, may affect osmoreceptors that regulate pituitary ADH secretion.
- Pulmonary infections cause decreased serum sodium concentration by an unknown mechanism.
- Pharmacologic agents such as clofibrate, cyclophosphamide, and the oral hypoglycemic chlorpropamide enhance secretion of ADH or duplicate the kidney's response to ADH.
- Mechanical ventilation, narcotics, hypercarbia, and pain may trigger ADH.

14. How is SIADH diagnosed?
Clinical examination may reveal weakness, lethargy, seizure, confusion, and coma.
Laboratory findings usually show persistent hyponatremia, serum hypo-osmolarity greater than plasma, and an inappropriately concentrated urine and abnormally high sodium. Dehydration must be ruled out before diagnosis of SIADH can be made.

15. Describe the treatment for SIADH.
Treatment of SIADH depends on the symptoms. Mild to moderate symptoms are treated with fluid restriction (500–1000 ml/24 hours). Severe water intoxication requires hypertonic saline (5%, 200 ml) in addition to free water restriction. Water restriction is effective in most cases of chronic SIADH. Demeclocycline, which inhibits ADH action at the renal tubular cell, can also be used.

16. What is diabetes insipidus (DI)?
DI is a disease of ADH deficiency. It is less common than SIADH and occurs primarily after head trauma, cranial surgery, anoxic encephalopathy, metastatic neoplasms to the pituitary (e.g., breast cancer), and granulomatous destruction (e.g., sarcoid) of the posterior pituitary. Drugs that inhibit ADH release (phenytoin and ethanol) can stimulate a mild form of DI. Idiopathic central DI causes polyuria, polydipsia, and astounding urine volumes (5–10 L/day).

17. How is DI diagnosed?
DI is characterized by dilute urine with increased serum osmolality. The diagnosis is made by fluid restriction for 6–10 hours. A patient with an intact neurohypophyseal axis will

increase urine osmolality up to 500–1400 mEq/L while keeping serum osmolality < 295 mEq/L. A patient with full-blown DI cannot protect his or her serum osmolality. As a result, levels of serum osmolality > 320 with a urine osmolality < 200 may be seen. When this patient is given parenteral ADH, the urine osmolality rises significantly.

18. How is central DI treated?

Treatment of central DI depends on etiology. DI due to trauma or surgery is often transient and self-limited. DDAVP (1-deamino-8-D-arginine vasopressin), an ADH analogue with an antidiuretic pressor activity ratio of 2000:1, is the treatment of choice for DI from other etiologies. Duration of action is 6–20 hours when taken intranasally or subcutaneously. It requires once- or twice-daily dosing.

19. What is nephrogenic DI and how does it differ from central DI?

In nephrogenic DI, the renal distal tubular cells are unable to respond to ADH. Causes of nephrogenic DI include lithium use and pregnancy. Nephrogenic DI is differentiated from central DI by evidence that ADH administration will not increase urine osmolality. Nephrogenic DI should be treated with thiazide diuretics and strict salt restriction. Psychogenic polydipsia (compulsive water drinking) may mimic DI.

20. What is the result of resection of the parathyroid gland?

Hypoparathyroidism is characterized by decreased excretion of calcium. Blood chemistry shows low serum calcium and high serum phosphorus. If calcium falls to 7–8 mg/dl, neuromuscular symptoms will develop. If serum levels fall to 5–6 mg/dl, tetany and the characteristic carpopedal spasms are apparent. Chronic calcinosis sometimes precedes idiopathic hypoparathyroidism, possibly inducing an immune response.

21. Describe the three types of multiple endocrine neoplasia syndrome (MENS).

TYPE	CHARACTERISTICS
MEN I	Hyperplasia of pituitary, parathyroid, adrenal cortex, pancreatic islet cells, and peptic ulcer
MEN II MEN IIa MEN IIb	Parathyroid tumor: adenoma, pheochromocytoma, and medullary carcinoma of thyroid
MEN III	Mucocutaneous neuroma, pheochromocytoma, and medullary carcinoma of thyroid and a marfanoid appearance

22. What are MEN IIa and MEN IIb associated with?

MEN IIa is associated with hyperparathyroidism, and MEN IIb is associated with marfanoid habitus and hyperplastic joints.

23. How is adrenal crisis recognized? How is it treated?

Adrenal crisis is characterized by acute-onset fatigue, mental status changes, and hypotension. Electrolyte abnormalities are also present in the form of hyponatremia, hyperkalemia, and non–anion gap acidosis. Appropriate therapy includes 0.9% normal saline infusion and corticosteroid replacement with hydrocortisone, 100-mg IV every 6–8 hours. If adrenocorticotropic hormone (ACTH; cosyntropin) stimulation test is needed, dexamethasone (2–4 mg every 8 hours) should be used for replacement instead; this drug, unlike hydrocortisone, is not measured as serum cortisol in the blood. Mineralocorticoid replacement with Flourinef is not indicated in the acute management of adrenal crisis.

24. How does one test for primary adrenal insufficiency?

The gold standard test for primary adrenal failure is the ACTH (cosyntropin) stimulation test. Cosyntropin (Cortrosyn) is an ACTH analogue that stimulates the adrenal gland and its

ACTH receptor. The test is performed by drawing a serum cortisol between 7 o'clock and 8 o'clock in the morning, administering cosyntropin (125 mg IM or IV), and drawing the serum cortisol again at 30 minutes and 60 minutes after the cosyntropin administration. The serum cortisol level should rise to > 20 µg/dl if there is adequate adrenal function.

25. How long can high-dose exogenous corticosteroids produce potential significant adrenal insufficiency?
Exogenous steroids in excess of 10–20 mg of prednisone daily can produce significant endogenous adrenal axis suppression after ≥ 2 weeks in chronic therapy for such conditions as asthma, chronic obstructive pulmonary disease (COPD), and rheumatoid arthritis. Preoperatively, these patients should be treated with high-dose (100 mg of hydrocortisone) stress-level steroids for at least 24 hours before surgery and every 8 hours thereafter to avoid adrenal crisis.

26. What are some clinical signs and symptoms of anterior pituitary tumors?
The many functional types of anterior pituitary tumors are based on the predominate pituitary hormone that the tumor secretes. They also produce functional deficiencies of the anterior pituitary. Common tumors include:

HORMONE-ASSOCIATED TUMORS	SIGNS AND SYMPTOMS
Prolactin	Amenorrhea or galactorrhea in women
Nonsecreting chromophobe adenoma	Often none, unless large
Luteinizing hormone and follicle-stimulating hormone secretory (gonadotropin-secretory) tumor	Impotence in men
Asymptomatic, TSH-secreting, ACTH-secreting tumors	Cushing's disease
Growth hormone-secreting tumors	Acromegaly

TSH = thyroid-stimulating hormone

Typical signs such as impotence, amenorrhea, headaches, bitemporal hemianopia, and visual field disturbance worsen as the tumor increases in size.

27. Name the preferred medical agents used to treat hypertension in hyperaldosteronism.
The usual agents are K^+-sparing diuretics. Hyperaldosteronism is characterized by potassium-wasting hypertension. Spironolactone is the drug of choice because it is a direct aldosterone antagonist at the level of the kidney. Aldactone is an alternative.

28. What are the characteristic electrolyte abnormalities of hyperaldosteronism?
Hyperaldosteronism is usually characterized by extreme hypokalemia (< 3.1) and possible signs of insufficiency such as increased serum creatinine and blood urea nitrogen (BUN). The hypokalemia may be exacerbated by the use of loop diuretics such as furosemide and thiazide drugs.

29. What is appropriate therapy for the treatment of symptomatic hypercalcemia?
Symptomatic hypercalcemia can be life-threatening and needs to be treated on an emergency basis. Usually, therapy includes aggressive IV hydration with normal saline (not lactated Ringer's solution, which contains calcium). After 6–12 hours of hydration, furosemide (Lasix) therapy may be initiated to help with aggressive diuresis of calcium. IV pamidronate, a biphosphonate, may be given (60 mg IV over 4–6 hours) to help sequester serum calcium back into bony sites. A one-time dose will deliver adequate therapy for up to 2 weeks.

30. What is the proper management of a palpable solitary nodule within the thyroid gland?

An isolated palpable nodule needs to be evaluated for thyroid cancer. Thyroid cancer is usually occult and slow growing, which permits time for evaluation. Masses > 1 cm are more suspicious for malignancy. Palpable nodules may be evaluated first by fine-needle aspiration biopsy. The results of the biopsy can be read quickly by a pathologist; if the preliminary results come back consistent with malignancy, the patient should be referred for surgery. If the results are benign, the nodule may be followed every 6 months to evaluate for an increase in size. Lesions that are undetermined can undergo thyroid iodine I^{123} scanning. "Cold" nodules with low uptake are suspicious for malignancy and should be referred to surgery. Also, at the initial visit, a TSH may be drawn. If TSH is low or suppressed, the patient should be referred for thyroid scan to rule out a benign "hot" nodule.

31. What laboratory thyroid function test and findings characterize sick euthyroid syndrome?

Sick euthyroid syndrome is a euthyroid condition common in the critically ill patient. It is due to excessive conversion of thyroxine (T_4) to reverse triiodothyronine (rT_3) instead of its more potent isomer T_3 and possibly hypothalamic suppression of TSH. These patients are clinically euthyroid. Laboratory findings include a normal to low TSH, low to normal T_4, and low free T_4 index. Direct free T_4 by equilibrium dialysis, however, is normal. Reverse T_3 is high, and T_3 is low.

32. Does empiric therapy benefit critically ill patients with euthyroid sick syndrome?

Studies of critically ill patients 24–72 hours after coronary artery bypass grafting failed to demonstrate that patient survival and morbidity improved following therapy with exogenous T_3 (Cytomel).

33. What common postoperative complication is associated with subclinical hypothyroidism?

Significant respiratory suppression with inability to wean from a respirator can be seen in patients who have even mild untreated hypothyroidism that is otherwise asymptomatic. Thyroid function tests alone may be needed to make this diagnosis. Preoperative TSH is the best screening test. This test should be elevated even in mild hypothyroidism.

34. What is the most common cardiac arrhythmia present in the elderly with hyperthyroidism?

Hyperthyroidism in the elderly may be of the **clinical** form or the **apathetic** form. In the latter, patients rarely present with classic signs and symptoms such as anxiety, sweat, weight loss, or palpitations. Rather, they may present with depressed mood or somnolence, cognitive impairment, or poor appetite. A TSH that is suppressed is the most sensitive indicator of hyperthyroidism. Even patients who are elderly and symptomatic are at significantly increased risk for cardiac arrhythmia, most commonly atrial fibrillation.

35. What are the contraindications to the use of metformin (glucophage) in type 2 diabetes?

Metformin therapy is strictly contraindicated in alcoholics, patients with significant renal insufficiency or failure (serum creatinine > 1.5), and patients with liver disease. These conditions considerably increase the risk of the fatal side effect, lactic acidosis. Patients who are older than 70 years and those with cardiac ejection fractions less than 50% are also not candidates for metformin therapy. Patients about to receive iodine contrast for cardiac catheterization or who are to undergo major surgery should discontinue metformin therapy 48–72 hours prior to the procedure.

BIBLIOGRAPHY

1. Arnaud CN: The calcitropic hormones and metabolic bone disease. In Greenspan FS, Baxter JD (eds): Basic and Clinical Endocrinology, 4th ed. Stamford, CT, Appleton & Lange, 1994, pp 227–306.
2. Deftos LJ, Catherwood BD: Syndromes involving multiple endocrine glands. In Greenspan FS, Baxter JD (eds): Basic and Clinical Endocrinology, 4th ed. Stamford, CT, Appleton & Lange, 1994, pp 713–728.
3. Favus JJ (ed): Primer on the Metabolic Bone Diseases and Disorders of Mineral Metabolism, 3rd ed. New York, Lippincott-Raven, 1996.
4. Greenspan FS: The thyroid gland. In Greenspan FS, Baxter JD (eds): Basic and Clinical Endocrinology, 4th ed. Stamford, CT, Appleton & Lange, 1994, pp 160–226.
5. Halpern LR, Chase DC: Perioperative management of patients with endocrine dysfunction: Physiology, presurgical, and postsurgical treatment protocols. Oral Maxillofac Surg Clin North Am 10:491, 1998.
6. Karam JH, Forsham PH: Diabetes mellitus. In Greenspan FS, Baxter JD (eds): Basic and Clinical Endocrinology, 4th ed. Stamford, CT, Appleton & Lange, 1994, pp 571–631.
7. McDermott MT (ed): Endocrine Secrets, 2nd ed. Philadelphia, Hanley & Belfus, 1998.
8. Orth DN, Kovacs WJ: Adrenal cortex. In Wilson JD, Daniel F, Kronenberg HM, Larsen PR (eds): Williams Textbook of Endocrinology, 9th ed. Philadelphia, Wilson & Foster, 1998, pp 517–664.
9. Reeves FG, Bichel CB, Andreoli TE: Posterior pituitary and water metabolism. In Wilson JD, Daniel F, Kronenberg HM, Larsen PR (eds): Williams Textbook of Endocrinology, 9th ed. Philadelphia, Wilson & Foster, 1998, pp 341–388.

22. MANAGEMENT OF THE DIABETIC PATIENT

Bradley A. Gregory, D.M.D.

1. What is diabetes?

Diabetes is a chronic disorder of carbohydrates, fat, and protein metabolism whereby a defective or deficient insulin secretory response leads to impaired glucose use. Diabetes creates a physiologic predisposition for developing generalized microvascular, macrovascular, and neuropathic complications.

2. How is glucose normally metabolized?

Blood glucose level is normally maintained between 60 and 130 mg/dl. Excess glucose is converted to glycogen, which is stored mostly in liver and muscle. Triglycerides (omega-3 fatty acids attached to glycerol) are used during periods of energy deprivation through lipolysis, and various amino acids can be converted to glucose in the liver through gluconeogenesis.

3. How does insulin facilitate uptake of glucose into cells?

Insulin is released in a rapid surge during the first 10–30 minutes after a meal. This is followed by a second phase of a slower, sustained release of insulin. Insulin receptors in the cell membrane have alpha and beta subunits. Insulin binds to subunit alpha, which causes the aforementioned change in subunit beta. Subunit beta promotes the activity of the enzyme tyrosine kinase. Tyrosine kinase is essential because it phosphorylates intracellular insulin receptors that bring glucose into the cell.

4. Where is insulin secreted?

Insulin is secreted from the beta cells of the endocrine pancreas.

5. How does insulin lower the plasma glucose?

Insulin promotes glucose uptake into most tissues *except* brain, kidney tubules, intestinal mucosa, and red blood cells. Insulin promotes glycogenesis, the formation of glycogen from glucose. At the same time, it will inhibit glycogenolysis. Insulin also inhibits gluconeogenesis, especially in the liver and kidney.

6. How does insulin lower blood levels of amino acids?

Insulin promotes the uptake of amino acids into muscles. This facilitates protein synthesis. At the same time, insulin inhibits proteolysis.

7. What is the effect of insulin on free fatty acids (FFAs)?

Insulin lowers the blood levels of FFAs by promoting their uptake into adipose tissue. In addition, insulin promotes the formation of triglycerides (lipogenesis). Also, insulin inhibits hormone-sensitive lipase, which is the enzyme necessary for the breakdown of triglycerides to FFAs.

8. Where is glucagon secreted?

Glucagon is secreted by alpha cells of the endocrine pancreas. It is also found in the gastrointestinal mucosa.

9. What metabolic effects does glucagon regulate?

The metabolic effects exerted on liver, muscle, and adipose tissue are opposite those of insulin. Glucagon mobilizes stored energy by promoting glycogenolysis (especially at the liver), gluconeogenesis, and lipolysis by activating hormone-sensitive lipase. Other effects of glucagon include stimulating the secretion of insulin by increasing plasma glucose and stimulating the secretion of growth hormone.

10. How is cortisol secreted and regulated?

Corticotropin releasing hormone (CRH) is released from the hypothalamus. CRH stimulates the release of adrenocorticotropic hormone (ACTH) from the anterior pituitary. ACTH stimulates cortisol release from the zona fasciculata of the adrenal glands, causing negative feedback to CRH and ACTH.

11. What metabolic role does cortisol play in glucose metabolism?

Cortisol protects plasma glucose and stores glucose as glycogen by promoting the breakdown of protein from muscle, stimulating hepatic gluconeogenesis and glycogenesis, and facilitating lipolysis by growth hormone and epinephrine. Cortisol also has an anti-insulin effect on muscle and adipose tissue.

12. How does epinephrine exert its metabolic controls?

Effects are mediated through beta receptors located on the exterior of cells. The inhibition of insulin secretion at the beta cell of the pancreas is through alpha receptors. Epinephrine stimulates gluconeogenesis at the liver through alpha receptors.

13. What is the role of epinephrine in glucose regulation?

The overall goal of epinephrine is to protect plasma glucose. In the muscle and liver, it promotes glycogenolysis. Epinephrine promotes gluconeogenesis as well. In addition, it will inhibit insulin release and stimulate glucagon release through alpha receptors in the pancreas. In the bloodstream, it will inhibit glucose uptake. Finally, epinephrine stimulates hormone-sensitive lipase to facilitate lipolysis in muscle and adipose tissue.

14. What is the role of growth hormone in glucose regulation?

Growth hormone is secreted by stimuli such as exercise-induced hypoglycemia, fasting, and stress from trauma, fever, and surgery. Growth hormone release is inhibited by glucose and FFAs. Growth hormone increases plasma glucose, mobilizes FFAs and protein stores by promoting lipolysis, increases glycogenolysis, and inhibits glucose uptake by muscle and adipose tissue.

15. What are the four different types of diabetes mellitus?

1. **Type 1 diabetes.** This form is usually associated with young people. These patients require insulin to maintain glucose homeostasis secondary to beta cell destruction in the pancreas.

2. **Type 2 diabetes.** These patients' cells have lost their sensitivity to insulin secondary to environmental and genetic factors. Therefore, their muscle and adipose cells cannot transport glucose.

3. **Gestational diabetes.** This usually develops secondary to pregnancy. Up to 40% of women with gestational diabetes will develop type 2 diabetes within 10 years of developing gestational diabetes.

4. **Secondary diabetes.** This is related to a specific cause such as removal of the pancreas.

16. What is the pathogenesis of type 1 diabetes?

- A **genetic susceptibility** predisposes some people to autoimmunity against beta cells of the pancreas.
- **Autoimmunity** develops spontaneously or, more commonly, is stimulated by an environmental agent.
- **Environmental injury** can damage beta cells, which are then recognized as foreign by the immune defenses.

17. What is the pathogenesis of type 2 diabetes?
- Genetics plays a significant, but not well understood, part.
- It is a combination of insulin resistance and an insulin secretory defect.
- Environmental factors play a very important role. This includes obesity, which will not cause diabetes but can unmask it. Also in this group are inactivity, pregnancy, and stress. Stress releases cortisol and catecholamines, which oppose insulin and raise the blood sugar level.

18. What metabolic abnormalities are associated with type 1 diabetes?
Abnormalities are classified into those of carbohydrate, protein, and lipid metabolism.
1. Type 1 patients generally have a combination of glucose underutilization and excessive glucose production resembling the fasting state. Glucose is unable to get into certain tissues, which causes the renal threshold to be surpassed resulting in polyuria. Polyuria leads to dehydration, which triggers polydipsia. In addition, because cells are not getting nourishment, patients experience polyphagia.
2. These patients breakdown protein from muscle to make glucose. Proteins are required for antibody production, white blood cell production, and healing of wounds. This leads to susceptibility of infections and poor wound healing.
3. Insulin deficiency leads to lipolysis of triglycerides into FFAs, which yields acetyl coenzyme A (CoA). Ultimately, ketone bodies are formed, which can lead to metabolic acidosis.

19. What metabolic abnormalities are associated with type 2 diabetes?
The metabolic abnormalities are classified into those of insulin resistance, loss of sensitivity of cells to insulin, and insulin secretion. Insulin is unable to get into cells because either a post receptor defect prevents uptake or there is a problem of insulin binding to target cells in the liver, muscle, and adipose tissue. In addition, type 2 diabetics may have a gradual decrease in basal levels of insulin secretion because the pancreas loses sensitivity to glucose level changes.

20. Which acute complication is most often associated with type 1 diabetes?
Diabetic ketoacidosis (DKA) almost exclusively occurs in type 1 diabetics. DKA is the result of severe insulin deficiency coupled with an absolute or relative increase of glucagon. Patients with DKA usually have blood glucose levels > 250 mg/dl, ketones in the urine and serum, pH < 7.2, and plasma bicarbonate < 15 mEq/L. Clinical manifestations include nausea and vomiting to compensate for the metabolic acidosis and Kussmaul respirations to reduce carbon dioxide levels in blood. The goals of treatment are to correct dehydration by starting 0.9% normal saline IV, using regular insulin, reversing the acidosis, and treating the potassium deficiency.

21. What is the acute complication most associated with type 2 diabetes?
Hyperosmolar nonketotic coma usually occurs in patients who are 65 years or older. The symptoms may go unrecognized for weeks. These patients have enough insulin to prevent a ketotic state, but they are severely hyperglycemic (usually above 600). Left untreated, they become severely dehydrated and progress into a comatose state. The treatment includes increased insulin and slow fluid replacement to prevent cerebral edema because of the sorbitol accumulation in the brain.

22. What tissues do not require insulin for glucose transport?
Nervous tissue
Lens of the eye
Kidney tubules
Brain
Blood vessels

23. What pathophysiologic mechanisms cause major chronic complications of diabetes?
Neuropathy
Macroangiopathy
Microangiopathy
Retinopathy
Nephropathy

24. What biochemical pathways are suspected of contributing to diabetic complications?
The pathways suspected are enzymatic glycosylation and the buildup of sorbitol. Enzymatic glycosylation is the process by which glucose attaches to proteins throughout the body at a rate proportional to the plasma glucose concentration. The proteins glycosylated include serum albumin, collagen, basic myelin protein, and low-density lipoproteins (LDLs). The function of the proteins is altered.

Hyperglycemia leads to buildup of glucose in tissues that do not require insulin for uptake. Excess glucose is metabolized to sorbitol, which creates an osmotic gradient favoring water diffusing into the cell.

25. Name the enzyme that is responsible for the breakdown of glucose into sorbitol.
Aldose reductase.

26. How do advanced glycosylation end-products (AGEs) contribute to diabetic complications?
AGEs are the result of enzymatic glycosylation. They get incorporated into the collagen that comprises the basement membranes of capillaries located in the eye, kidney, nerves, and skin. This results in thickening of basement membranes and a reduction in production of relaxing factors by the endothelium, causing vasoconstriction and ultimately hypertension. In addition, AGEs irreversibly attach to collagen walls in larger vessels. This impedes the normal efflux of LDLs entering the vessel wall and promotes cholesterol deposition.

27. How does sorbitol accumulation lead to diabetic complications?
Cells of the tissues that do not require insulin for glucose transport (see question 22) become hypertonic. In Schwann cells, the hypertonicity causes loss of feeling in extremities and a decrease in sensation. In the lens of the eye, water accumulation leads to cataracts, macular edema, and glaucoma. Damage to endothelial cells leads to thickening of basement membranes, resulting in microangiopathies of the retina, arterioles of the kidneys, and small vessels of the skin.

28. What is the importance of nonenzymatic glycosylation of hemoglobin?
The degree of nonenzymatic glycosylation is dependent on the amount of plasma glucose levels. Therefore, high levels result in more glycosylation of hemoglobin. The normal hemoglobin A1c is 4–6%. In diabetics, levels may reach 16–20%. Because the life span of a red blood cell is about 120 days, and the glycosylation occurs continuously over that span, hemoglobin A1c concentrations provide an index of the average blood glucose over the preceding 60–90 days.

29. How does glycosylation of platelets affect microvascular disease?
Glycosylation of platelets increases platelet adhesiveness. This allows platelets to produce excessive thromboxane, which makes the platelets hypercoagulable. This hypercoagulable state predisposes a diabetic to microvascular disease.

30. What are the criteria for the diagnosis of diabetes mellitus?
The diagnosis is made based on one or more of the following criteria:
1. Signs and symptoms plus a random plasma glucose concentration $\geq$ 200 mg/dl

2. A fasting plasma glucose ≥ 126 mg/dl at least two times
3. Oral glucose tolerance test with a 2-hour postload glucose concentration ≥ 200 mg/dl and a time 0 serum glucose level > 126 mg/dl

31. What test is accepted by the American Diabetes Association for diagnosing diabetes?
The **fasting plasma glucose test** is a diagnostic marker for diabetes. The patient fasts overnight for at least 8 hours, and the test is performed the next morning. This test is performed only on nonpregnant adults who are not taking any medications or have any other metabolic conditions that would lead to abnormal results. A normal fasting plasma glucose is usually 65–110 mg/dl.

32. What is the oral glucose tolerance test and how is it performed?
This test measures a person's ability to handle a glucose load over a period of time. The patient fasts overnight. In the morning, the fasting blood glucose is determined. The patient then ingests a 75-gm glucose load. In children and nonpregnant adults, the blood glucose is tested every 30 minutes for 2 hours. The test is considered normal if the fasting blood glucose is < 110 mg/dl and the 2-hour postload blood glucose is < 140 mg/dl.

33. Describe the different categories of hypoglycemia.
Categories of hypoglycemia can be broken down depending on the level of plasma glucose and associated signs and symptoms.

Categories of Hypoglycemia

	PLASMA GLUCOSE LEVEL	SIGNS/SYMPTOMS
Mild	60–70 mg/dl	Tachycardia; palpitations; pallor; shakiness; irritability
Moderate	50–60 mg/dl	Impaired central nervous system function: confusion, inability to concentrate, slurred speech, blurred vision
Severe	≤ 40–50 mg/dl	Loss of consciousness; difficulty awakening; seizures

34. How do you treat mild to moderate hypoglycemia?
Initially, treat with 10–15 gm of carbohydrates. Give the patient ½ cup of orange juice or a *regular* soda, 3–5 hard candies, 1 cup of milk, 3 glucose tablets, *or* 2 tablespoonfuls of raisins. Evaluate plasma glucose levels as soon as possible. If symptoms do not improve in 15 minutes, treat with an additional 10–15 gm of a carbohydrate source.

35. How do you treat severe hypoglycemia?
If a glucagon kit is available, the patient should be given an injection of glucagon. The adult dose is 1 mg; children < 5 years, 0.5 mg; and infants < 1 year, 0.25 mg. If no kit is available and the patient can swallow without risk of aspiration, 15–50 gm of a carbohydrate source can be given on the inside of the cheek. Sources include glucose gel, 1–4 teaspoonfuls of honey (except in infants), syrup, *or* jelly. When the patient is more alert, follow with a liquid such as orange juice.

36. What is the best route to administer agents to stimulate insulin release?
Oral glucose and amino acids have a greater stimulatory effect on insulin than IV-administered solutions because of stimulation of intestinal hormones by ingested substances. These hormones include gastric inhibitory peptide, cholecystokinin (CCK), glucagon, and gastrin. All are stimulators of insulin secretion.

37. Describe the different insulin preparations.

	TYPE OF INSULIN	ONSET	PEAK	DURATION
Short-acting	Regular	0.5–1 hr	2–4 hrs	5–7 hrs
Intermediate-acting	Isophane (NPH)	1–2 hrs	6–14 hrs	18–24 hrs
	Lente	1–2 hrs	6–14 hrs	18–24 hrs
Long-acting	Ultralente	6 hrs	18–26 hrs	36+ hrs

38. How do you manage the postsurgical patient with diabetes that is controlled by diet only?

If plasma glucose levels exceed and remain above 250 mg/dl as a consequence of surgical stress or infection, sliding scale insulin therapy should be instituted.

39. How do you manage a surgical patient who controls her diabetes with oral hypoglycemic agents?

Use of oral agents other than chlorpropamide should be discontinued on the day of the procedure. Chlorpropamide, which has a longer half-life than other oral hypoglycemics, should be discontinued the day before surgery. These patients often require insulin perioperatively during major surgical procedures. Postoperatively, follow the same regimen that is adhered to for diabetes controlled by diet.

40. What is the management of a patient with insulin-controlled diabetes who is undergoing major surgery?

Most diabetic patients who receive insulin use a combination of intermediate acting (NPH) and regular insulin. In these patients, total insulin dosage is usually given in the morning or divided between morning and afternoon. Usually, two-thirds of the total dose is NPH, and one-third is regular insulin. Management of these patients in the perioperative period includes:

1. Half of the normal daily insulin is given as NPH in the morning. An IV line is placed and lactated Ringer's solution started. A preoperative blood sugar is obtained.

2. During surgery, plasma glucose, serum electrolytes, and arterial blood gases (ABGs) should be monitored. Additional regular insulin is provided as needed by titrating an insulin infusion of 5–10 units an hour either subcutaneously or in the IV fluids.

3. Postoperatively, blood glucose is checked every 4–6 hours. Regular insulin should be administered to maintain plasma glucose between 150 and 200 mg/dl.

4. Once the patient has resumed oral intake, NPH insulin is started. The patient's plasma glucose is monitored, and the insulin dosage is adjusted with regular insulin as needed.

41. How do you manage a patient with insulin-controlled diabetes who is undergoing ambulatory surgery?

One-half of the daily NPH insulin dose is given on the morning of surgery, and the regular insulin is withheld if the patient is expected to be able to resume oral intake shortly after surgery. The remaining one-half of NPH is given in the afternoon but not too late in the afternoon. If given too late in the afternoon, the peak effect of the NPH will occur while the patient is sleeping.

42. What oral hypoglycemic is categorized as a biguanide?

Metformin (Glucophage) reduces hepatic glucose production and enhances glucose utilization by muscle. It is normally used by type 2 diabetics.

43. What is the pharmacology of the sulfonylureas?

These type 2 diabetic agents acutely increase insulin secretion from the beta cells and potentiate insulin action on several extrahepatic tissues. Long-term sulfonylureas increase peripheral utilization of glucose, suppress hepatic gluconeogenesis, and possibly increase the sensitivity or number of peripheral insulin receptors.

44. What drugs make up the sulfonylureas?

Sulfonylureas

DRUG	TRADE NAME	DOSE	DURATION
Tolbutamide	Orinase	2 gm	6–12 hrs
Tolazamide	Tolinase	250 mg	10–18 hrs
Glipizide	Glucotrol	10–15 mg	12 hrs
Glyburide	Micronase	5–10 mg	16 hrs
Acetohexamide	Dymelor	1 gm	8–12 hrs
Chlorpropamide	Diabinese	250 mg	1–3 days

45. What are the contraindications to the use of metformin in type 2 diabetes?
Metformin therapy is strictly contraindicated in alcoholics, patients with significant renal insufficiency or failure (serum creatinine > 1.7), and patients with liver disease. These conditions considerably increase the risk of lactic acidosis, a fatal side effect. Patients who are older than 70 years and those with cardiac ejection fractions < 79% are also not candidates for metformin therapy. Patients who are about to receive iodine contrast dye, such as prior to cardiac catheterization, or who are to undergo major surgery should discontinue metformin 48–72 hours prior to the procedure.

46. What is the physiologic effect of a decrease in plasma glucose?
A decrease protects plasma glucose levels. Therefore, there would be an increase production of glucagon, epinephrine, growth hormone, and cortisol to increase plasma glucose.

47. What are the laboratory findings in type 2 diabetes?
High plasma glucose, glucose in the urine, and a high urine volume.

48. What is the response of insulin and glucagon to dietary protein?
An increase in both hormones.

49. Which hormones are considered ketogenic? Why?
Epinephrine, glucocorticoids, glucagon, and growth hormone because they promote lipolysis.

50. What is the response by insulin to parasympathetic stimulation?
Insulin release will be increased.

51. How will epinephrine released from the adrenal medulla affect plasma glucose?
Epinephrine decreases glycogen synthesis in the liver. In addition, its release is increased in response to hypoglycemia.

52. Where is the major site of action for glucagon?
The breakdown of hepatic glycogen to glucose.

53. What hormones antagonize the action of insulin on blood sugar?
Growth hormone, cortisol, glucagon, and epinephrine.

54. What are the effects of infection and surgical stress on blood sugar in diabetic patients?
Surgical stress can be related to trauma to the tissues during the procedure, pain that the patient experiences after the procedure, and anxiety before and after the surgery. Infections

cause stress on tissues and can cause trauma to tissues. Stress leads to surges of epinephrine. As discussed earlier, epinephrine will antagonize insulin and cause an increase in plasma glucose. In addition, stress from surgery and infections may override negative feedback mechanisms to result in cortisol surge. Cortisol will contribute to the effects of epinephrine on glucose.

55. What are the most common types of infections in diabetics and why?

Diabetic patients have enhanced susceptibility to infections of the skin, tuberculosis, pneumonia, and pyelonephritis. Together, these infections cause the death of about 5% of diabetics. In addition, diabetics are very susceptible to fungal infections. The susceptibility to infections is a combination of impaired leukocyte function, inability to make antibodies against the bacteria, and vascular insufficiency.

BIBLIOGRAPHY

1. Cada DJ, Covington TR, Hebel SK (eds): Facts and Comparisons. St. Louis, Wolters Kluwer, 1998.
2. Kumar V, Cotran RS, Robbins SL: Basic Pathology, 5th ed. Philadelphia, W.B. Saunders, 1991.
3. Roser M: Management of the medically compromised patient. In Kwon PH, Laskin DM (eds): Clinician's Manual of Oral and Maxillofacial Surgery. Carol Stream, IL, Quintessence, 1997, pp 194–196.
4. Steil CF: Diabetes: An Overview. In CVS Pharmacy Pharmaceutical Care Module—Diabetes. Woonsocket, RI, CVS Pharmacy, 1998.

23. THE IMMUNOCOMPROMISED SURGICAL PATIENT

A. Omar Abubaker, D.M.D., Ph.D., and Noah Sandler, D.M.D., M.D.

1. What are the types of immunodeficiency?

Immunodeficiency can be either **primary** or **acquired** (secondary). Primary immunodeficiency is usually caused by a defect in a specific aspect of the immune system, such as a specific immunoglobulin. Acquired immunodeficiency can be secondary to disease or iatrogenic causes, such as the result of chemotherapy, and may involve more than one aspect of the immune system.

2. What are the common causes of immunosuppression and immunodeficiency?

Immunodeficiency can be caused by any of several factors including advancing age, malnutrition, trauma, burns, surgery, diabetes mellitus, radiation, and organ failure. Causes of immunosuppression also include malignancy, acquired or congenital immunodeficiency, and iatrogenic causes such as post-transplant drug immunosuppression (see Table).

Common Causes of Immunosuppression

Acquired/congenital immunodeficiency	Malnutrition
Advanced age	Organ failure
Burns	Radiation
Diabetes	Surgery
Drugs/iatrogenic	Trauma
Malignancy	

Adapted from Sandler NA, Braun TW: Current surgical management of the immunocompromised patient. Oral Maxillofac Surg Clin North Am 10:445–455, 1998.

3. What are the different classes of systemic immunity?

Systemic immunity can be classified into an **antigen-specific** or **nonspecific immunity**. Antigen-specific can be either humoral or cell-mediated immunity. Parts of the nonspecific immunity system are the phagocytes and complement cascade.

4. What is the effect of deficiency in cell-mediated immunity and what are the appropriate methods of testing for such deficiency?

Deficiencies in cell-mediated immunity predispose the patient to infection from gram-negative organisms, mycobacteria, viruses, *Pneumocystis carinii*, and *Toxoplasma*. The best test for cell-mediated immunity is delayed-type hypersensitivity (DTH) skin testing in which patients' reactions to intradermal injections of *Candida*, tuberculin, *Trichophyton*, and other antigens are observed. Direct measurement of T-cell function by the use of monoclonal antibodies is, however, a more specific test. The ratio of helper T-cells (CD4) to suppressor T-cells (CD8) (normally 1.8:2.2) is often used as a measure of this immune type function.

5. How is deficiency in humoral immunity manifested and what are the appropriate methods of testing for humoral immunity?

Deficiency in humoral immunity predisposes patients to infection from pyogenic bacteria, hepatitis viruses, *Cytomegalovirus*, parasites, and *Pneumocystis carinii*. Measuring serum immunoglobulin levels tests humoral immunity. Testing for the presence of antibodies to previous vaccination or infections can also indicate the status of the patient's humoral immunity. Other tests for humoral immunity such as circulating B-cell count and in vitro B-cell testing can also be performed.

6. What infections are caused by deficiency in polymorphonuclear neutrophils (PMNs)?

Deficiencies of neutrophilic leukocytes predispose patients to infections from staphylococci, *Serratia*, *Escherichia coli*, *Pseudomonas*, *Proteus*, *Enterobacter*, *Salmonella*, *Candida*, and *Aspergillus*. Neutrophil absolute count and most functions of polymorphonuclear leukocytes can be tested.

7. What is the effect of deficiency in complement and how can complement functions be tested?

Deficiency in complement predisposes patients to infections from *Neisseria* and viruses. The status of complement cascade can be measured by the $C'H_{50}$ (50% hemolyzing dose of complement) assay and by individual assay or C3 and C4 levels.

8. What are the possible complications of immunosuppressive drugs in transplant patients?

Although newer immunosuppressive medications have reduced the amount and severity of acute transplant rejection, these new regimens are not without consequences. An increased risk of infection is seen in these patients secondary to decreased host resistance, with an increased risk for graft rejection in patients with severe infection. Infection is also the leading cause of death in transplant patients. Therefore, any transplant patients with active infections should be treated aggressively. Another risk for transplant patients is the increased incidence of de novo cancer. There may be a 100-fold increased incidence of cancer in the transplant patient. The most prevalent neoplasms are lymphoma and squamous cell carcinoma of the lips and skin. The incidence of tumors such as non-Hodgkin's lymphoma is approximately 2%, and this risk increases with the duration of immunosuppressive therapy. Most of these lesions occur in the head and neck, gastrointestinal tract, and transplanted allograft. These lesions are seen primarily with the use of cyclosporine and tacrolimus and are believed to be related to the inhibition of Epstein-Barr virus (EBV) cytotoxic T cells. Transplant patients on immunosuppressive therapy, therefore, should be examined carefully for lip and skin lesions, nonhealing ulcers, and lymphadenopathy, and questionable lesions should undergo biopsy.

9. What are the most common types of orofacial infection seen in immunocompromised patients?

T-cell deficiency is commonly found in post-transplant patients on immunosuppressive therapy, in AIDS patients, in some patients with certain forms of carcinoma, and in patients on cancer therapy. Viral and fungal infections are more common in these patients. Viral infections are most often produced by the Herpesviridae family (i.e., herpes simplex, varicella zoster virus, and cytomegalovirus). The clinical presentation of these infections is typically an acute, vesiculobullous lesion with a lack of inflammatory response in leukopenic patients. If not treated aggressively with antiviral agents such as acyclovir or ganciclovir, these infections can lead to significant local and possible systemic morbidity.

Among fungal infections, *Candida albicans* is the most common fungal pathogen, but others such as *Aspergillus* and *Cryptococcus* are commonly encountered. The more aggressive fungi show an invasive behavior that often involves deeper tissues. Patients should be monitored carefully for signs of local tissue trauma that may predispose the patient to viral or fungal colonization.

10. Describe the characteristics of bacterial oral infections in immunocompromised patients.

Oral infections in immunocompromised patients typically occur with significant local symptoms and may spread to involve adjacent or distant anatomic sites. These infections tend to progress more rapidly and may produce systemic symptoms or local osteomyelitis. Infections may be caused by gram-negative enteric flora secondary to colonization of these organisms in the oral cavity. These bacteria are often resistant to penicillin and cephalosporins. Broad-spectrum antibiotic prophylaxis should be used empirically before definitive identification of the causative microorganism in immunocompromised patients with evidence of infection.

11. Explain the general principles of the preoperative evaluation of immunocompromised patients.

Immunosuppression is not in itself a contraindication to well-planned surgery. The general approach to the care of these patients when they are to undergo surgery is to increase host resistance to infection and to maximize wound healing. The patient's immune status should be evaluated by means of a history, physical examination, and laboratory studies. The history should include questions about the patient's underlying disease, previous infections, use of medications and other therapy, previous anesthesia, and trauma. The physical examination should also determine the patient's nutritional status and include a search for signs of existing infection and lymphadenopathy.

High-risk patients should have elective procedures scheduled at the beginning of the day. The possibility of reducing the dosages of immunosuppressive drugs must be weighed against the effect this might have on the reason why the patient is being treated with these agents. Other considerations include the removal of any infected foreign bodies; assessment of the need of invasive devices; restoration of cardiac and renal function, including tissue perfusion; correction of nutritional deficiencies, if present; assessment of the patient's need for vaccinations; and the administration of prophylactic antibiotics. Also, regardless of the etiology, hemostasis should be achieved with pressure, packing, or suturing, and if the platelet count is below 50,000/mm^3, platelet transfusion should be considered. In the case of dental extractions, alveolectomy and primary closure are recommended. If platelet counts are less than 40,000/mm^3, platelets should be transfused 30 minutes before surgery to achieve platelet levels of more than 40,000/mm^3. One unit (pack) of platelets typically raises the platelet count by 10,000/mm^3. Although correcting the patient's immunodeficiency is usually difficult or impossible, defects in B-cell function may be partially treated by administering immunoglobulin.

12. What preoperative laboratory studies should be included in evaluation of immunocompromised patients?

- Chest radiograph
- Urinalysis
- Serum albumin determination
- Liver and kidney function tests
- Culture of material from any infected sites

Because some of these patients may present with neutropenia as well as thrombocytopenia, other tests include:

- Complete blood count with platelet count
- Prothrombin time (PT)
- Partial thromboplastin time (PTT)
- Specific testing of the patient's T cells, B cells, PMNs, and complement should be checked before surgery

13. What are the effects of chemotherapeutic and immunosuppressant drugs on the immune system?

The effects of these drugs vary from agent to agent. For example, chemotherapeutic agents depress the number and activity of the neutrophilic leukocytes. The nadir of white cell counts varies with the agents used, but generally occurs 10–20 days after administration. The patient is susceptible to infection when the absolute neutrophil count (ANC) falls below 1500/mm^3. The susceptibility increases significantly when the count falls below 500/mm^3. Corticosteroids, on the other hand, decrease the leukocyte response to inflamed tissue and also depress T-cell function. Wound healing is slowed, and the ability to localize infection is reduced. Cyclosporine has almost no effect on the local inflammatory reaction but causes the initiation of interleukin-2 production and the suppression of T-helper and cytotoxic cells. Antilymphocyte antibodies appear to work by lysing target cells. With all of these agents, increased dosage is associated with increased predisposition to infection. These patients should receive prophylactic antibiotics before most surgical procedures.

14. When should prophylactic antibiotics be used in chemotherapy patient?

Prophylactic antibiotics should be considered if the granulocyte count is less than 2000/mm^3. Surgery generally should be performed at least 3 days before chemotherapy is initiated in cancer patients because granulocyte levels may fall below 500/mm^3 1 week after the initiation of many types of chemotherapeutic agents. When surgery needs to be performed during severe neutropenia (granulocyte counts < 500/mm^3), it is recommended that the procedure be performed in a hospital setting with broad-spectrum antibiotic prophylaxis administered during the perioperative period.

15. What type of virus is HIV and what is its cell target?

Human immunodeficiency viruses (HIV) are a group of retroviruses that can be acquired by the transmission of body fluids, including transfusions, and through the infection of infants by infected mothers. The specific target of the virus is the CD4 T-cell lymphocytes. The virus multiplies in the cell and eventually destroys it. Cell-mediated immunity is thereby severely affected.

16. What are the general categories of HIV-infected patients?

1. Asymptomatic patients with evidence of HIV infection demonstrated by the presence of HIV antibodies in the serum or in the secretions of these patients.

2. Patients with AIDS-related complex (ARC), manifested by presence of symptoms including lymphadenopathy, unexplained fever, weight loss, and hematologic and neurologic abnormalities.

3. Patients with AIDS as defined by the Centers for Disease Control and Prevention (CDC) (i.e., HIV infection and CD4 lymphocyte count < 200).

17. What are the laboratory tests to determine the status of the HIV patient?

Diagnosis of HIV infection is made by detection of antibodies to HIV. Antibodies to HIV are determined by the enzyme-linked immunosorbent assay (ELISA) method or by the Western blot method; both tests require the patient's consent in many states.

The status of patient with HIV infection and potential risk of surgery is evaluated by assessing the viral load (as determined by the HIV RNA), and the CD4+ lymphocyte count. Information regarding the overall physical status of the patient and the patient's symptomatic and physical manifestation of HIV-related diseases are also helpful in assessing the HIV patient risk for surgery.

Viral load measurements give an indication of the amount of current viral activity and have been shown to correlate with disease progression. Studies have demonstrated that viral loads of more than 30,000–50,000 HIV RNA copies per milliliter of plasma correlate with poor prognosis, whereas viral loads of less than 5000 copies per milliliter correlate with better short-term prognosis.

The CD4+ lymphocyte gives an indication of the degree of immunologic destruction. Laboratory findings in patients with AIDS include low lymphocyte counts and depressed CD4 T-cells, with the CD4-to-CD8 ratio of 1:0 or less (normally 1.8:2.2).

18. What are the clinical manifestations of AIDS?

Signs and symptoms
Lymphadenopathy
Weight loss
Diarrhea
Thrombocytopenia
Anemia
Leukopenia

Opportunistic infections
Pneumocystis carinii (pulmonary)
Toxoplasmosis (cerebral)
Cryptosporidiosis (diarrhea)
Candidiasis (esophageal)
Cryptococcus (meningitis)
Herpes
Varicella viruses (skin)
Histoplasmosis
Tuberculosis

Neurologic abnormalities
Dementia
Encephalopathy
CNS toxoplasmosis
Lymphoma

Neoplasms
Kaposi's sarcoma
Lymphoma

19. What are the principles of drug therapy of AIDS patients?

The major goal of therapy of patients with AIDS is treatment of the opportunistic infections including antiviral therapy. Prophylaxis is essential for all persons with symptomatic HIV disease, AIDS, or CD4+ counts less than 200/µl. Survival has also been prolonged in HIV-positive patients by prophylaxis against the opportunistic infections such as *Pneumocystis carinii* pneumonia (PCP), the mycobacterium avium complex (MAC), and other fungal infections. PCP prophylaxis commonly is with trimethoprim-sulfamethoxazole, although dapsone-trimethoprim or clindamycin-primaquine may be used alternately. Prophylaxis for MAC usually consists of a macrolide antibiotic, clarithromycin, or azithromycin and is recommended when the CD4+ cell count falls below 75 or 50/µl. Prophylaxis against *Candida* or other fungal diseases is currently not recommended, although many immunocompromised patients may be taking an antifungal medication such as fluconazole or another azole when they have manifestations of fungal infection. Current antiretroviral therapies have been shown to reduce viral counts and slow disease progression, and they can be effective in raising the CD4+ lymphocyte counts considerably. The most effective antiretroviral treatment strategies are multiple drug therapies that combine nucleoside analog drugs with protease inhibitors and, when patients are able to tolerate these regimens, triple drug therapy with two nucleoside analog drugs plus a protease inhibitor.

20. What are the considerations in the surgical treatment of an HIV-infected person?

Patients with early HIV infection and with no immunologic impairment generally tolerate elective oral surgical procedures well, and recent studies have demonstrated no increased incidence in infection, bleeding, or dry socket in extractions. In fact, routine prophylactic antibiotics are not indicated for these patients and may even further predispose them to candidiasis or drug reactions. In contrast, patients with AIDS and ARC are not good surgical candidates because of their hematologic abnormalities and predisposition to AIDS infection. Patients with mandibular fractures who have AIDS infection have an increased incidence of postoperative infections compared to asymptomatic HIV-positive patients. Accordingly, it is recommended that patients with AIDS (as defined by CD4+ count of < 200 cells/µl or history of AIDS-defining illness such as lymphoma, tuberculosis, or *P. carinii*) should not undergo elective surgery. When urgent and emergency surgery is necessary, these patients should receive broad-spectrum prophylactic antibiotics before undergoing any surgical procedure and proper attention to the prevention of wound infection, care must be taken to prevent transmission of the virus to personnel caring for the patient.

21. What are the potential drug interactions in HIV-infected patients?

Potential Interactions of Drugs Used by HIV-Infected Patients

DRUG	DRUG USED TO TREAT HIV	MECHANISM OF INTERACTION	EFFECT	RECOMMENDATION
Benzodia-zepines	Ritonavir, indinavir (protease inhibitors)	Inhibition of hepatic metabolism	↑ Concentration of benzodiaze-pines	Adjust benzodiaze-pines dosage, use alternate agent, or monitor closely for toxicity
Cisapride	Azole antifungals, clarithromycin, ritonavir, indinavir	Inhibition of hepatic metabolism	Cardiotoxic ef-fects (incl. fatal arrhythmias)	Avoid concomitant use
Clarithro-mycin	Ritonavir, indinavir	Inhibition of hepatic metabolism	↑ concentration of clarithromycin	Dosage reduction not required for patients with normal renal function
Didanosine (nucleoside analog)	Oral ganciclovir	Unknown	↑ didanosine	Monitor for didano-sine toxicity, dosage reduction may be required
Ganciclovir	Zidovudine (thymi-dine analog)	Pharmacody-namic inter-action	Enhanced bone marrow toxicity	May require decreased dose of zidovudine or concomitant G-CSF
Ketocona-zole	Saquinavir (protease inhibitor)	Inhibition of hepatic metabolism	↑ saquinavir concentration	Under investigation to maximize saquinavir exposure
Metronida-zole	Ritonavir (liquid only)	Alcohol in liquid formulation	Disulfiram-like reaction	Monitor for toxicity, change form of ritonavir
Opiate anal-gesics (especial-ly meperi-dine, pro-poxyphene, fentanyl)	Ritonavir	Inhibition of hepatic metabolism	↑ opiate concen-tration	Use alternate pain medication; monitor for toxicity
Terfenadine, astemizole (H_1 anti-histamines)	Azole antifungals, clarithromycin, ritonavir	Inhibition of hepatic metabolism	Accumulation of cardiotoxic un-metabolized antihistamine	Avoid concomitant use

Adapted from Sandler NA, Braun TW: Current surgical management of the immunocompromised pa-tient. Oral Maxillofac Surg Clin North Am 10:445–455, 1998.

22. What is the management of health care workers exposed to HIV-infected blood or body fluids?

The rate of seroconversion of health care workers exposed to HIV-infected blood or body fluid has been reported to be 0.42%. The management of occupational exposures of contami-nated or suspected contaminated fluids is controversial. Currently, the CDC recommends that, after informed consent is obtained, the patient should be tested for HIV. If the patient is HIV positive, the exposed health care worker should then undergo HIV testing immediately and then at 6 weeks, 12 weeks, and 6 months. Initiation of zidovudine prophylaxis after exposure remains controversial because of its yet unproven efficacy.

23. Describe the mechanism of action of immunosuppressant agents used in transplant patients.

Several new immunosuppressive agents are available for clinical use or are undergoing clinical trials in this country. These new drugs suppress the immune system at sites complementary to traditional immunosuppressive medications (see Figure). Many transplant patients currently are on two or more of these drugs in an attempt to prevent rejection. This may predispose the patient to overimmunosuppression or potential drug interactions.

Antigen						
↓						
Antigen Presenting Cell	IL-1 →	CD-4 T-helper Cell	IL-2 →	B-cells T-cells	→ →	Plasma cells Activated T-cells
Corticosteroids		Cyclosporine Tacrolimus Monoclonal antibodies	Sirolimus	Azathioprine Mycophenolate mofetil	Gusperimus	

Sites of action of immunosuppressive drugs used in transplant patients. (From Sandler NA, Braun TW: Current surgical management of the immunocompromised patient. Oral Maxillofac Surg Clin North Am 10:445–455, 1998, with permission.)

24. What are the side effects of immunosuppressant drugs in transplant patients?

Side Effects of Immunosuppressant Drugs Used in Transplant Patients

MEDICATION	POTENTIAL SIDE EFFECTS
Corticosteroids	Cushing's syndrome, adrenal insufficiency
Azathioprine	Myelodepression (leukopenia, thrombocytopenia)
Cyclosporine	Nephrotoxicity, neurotoxicity, hypertension, hepatotoxicity
Tacrolimus	Nephrotoxicity, neurotoxicity, diabetogenic effects
Mycophenolate mofetil	Myelodepression (leukopenia, anemia), gastrointestinal (diarrhea, emesis)
Sirilimus	Myelodepression (leukopenia, thrombocytopenia), potential nephrotoxicity
Gusperimus	Myelodepression (leukopenia, anemia, thrombocytopenia)
Monocloncal antibodies	CNS (seizure, encephalopathy, psychosis)*

* Increased risk of encephalopathy and psychosis reported with indomethacin use.
Adapted from Sandler NA, Braun TW: Current surgical management of the immunocompromised patient. Oral Maxillofac Surg Clin North Am 10:445–455, 1998.

25. What are the oral manifestations of cyclosporine use?

Cyclosporine is associated with gingival hyperplasia in the dental papillae of the anterior teeth, which typically occurs after 3–6 months of immunosuppressant therapy. Studies suggest that approximately 30% of patients medicated with cyclosporine alone experience significant gingival changes. Calcium channel blocking agents that may be prescribed to counter the hypertension caused by cyclosporine may also induce gingival hyperplasia with an additive effect to that of cyclosporine. When the two drugs are used simultaneously, they can result in nearly a 40% incidence of gingival hyperplasia. Other significant risk factors that influence gingival overgrowth include age and sex (with younger men having an increased susceptibility), duration of therapy, serum creatinine levels, and the HLA-B37 haplotype. Decreases in the dosage of the drug or discontinuing the drug early may result in reversal of this side effect. However, surgical intervention that consists of gingivectomy and tissue recontouring is often necessary to improve aesthetics and function.

26. What are the different drug interactions of cyclosporine/tacrolimus?

Drug Interactions of Cyclosporine and Tacrolimus

DRUG	CLASS	MECHANISM
Increased cyclosporine		
Metoclopramide	Prokinetic	↑ cyclosporine absorption
Cisapride	Prokinetic	↑ cyclosporine absorption
Erythromycin	Macrolide antibiotic	Mechanism unclear
Increased cyclosporin/tacrolimus		
Clotrimazole	Imidazole	Inhibit cytochrome P450
Fluconazole	Antifungal	Inhibit cytochrome P450
Corticosterone	Corticosteroid	Inhibit cytochrome P450
Dexamethasone	Corticosteroid	Inhibit cytochrome P450
Bromocriptine	Dopamine agonist	Inhibit cytochrome P450
Cyclosporine/tacrolimus	Immunosuppressant	Inhibit cytochrome P450
Ergotamine	Alpha blocker	Inhibit cytochrome P450
Nifedipine	Ca channel blocker	Inhibit cytochrome P450
Diltiazem	Ca channel blocker	Inhibit cytochrome P450
Verapamil	Ca channel blocker	Inhibit cytochrome P450
Cimetidine	H_2 blocker	Inhibit cytochrome P450
Omeprazole	H/K ATPase blocker	Inhibit cytochrome P450
Increased tacrolimus		
Danazole	Androgen	?? renal impairment
Grapefruit juice		Inhibit intestinal cytochrome P450
Decreased cyclosporine/tacrolimus		
Rifampin	Antibiotic	↑ cytochrome P450 activity
Phenytoin	Anticonvulsant	↑ cytochrome P450 activity
Phenobarbital	Anticonvulsant	↑ cytochrome P450 activity
Decreased cyclosporine		
Sulfadimidine	Antibiotic	↑ cytochrome P450 activity
Trimethoprim	Antibiotic	↑ cytochrome P450 activity
Decreased tacrolimus		
Carbamazepine	Anticonvulsant	↑ cytochrome P450 activity
Primidone	Anticonvulsant	↑ cytochrome P450 activity

Adapted from Sandler NA, Braun TW: Current surgical management of the immunocompromised patient. Oral Maxillofac Surg Clin North Am 10:445–455, 1998.

27. What is tacrolimus and what are its major side effects?

Tacrolimus (FK-506) is a macrolide immunosuppressant isolated from *Streptomyces tsukubaensis* in 1984. This drug is 50–100 times more potent than cyclosporine. Initially used during episodes of severe graft rejection, it is now used for baseline immunosuppression.

The principal adverse effects associated with tacrolimus are similar to cyclosporine and include nephrotoxicity and neurotoxicity. In addition, diabetogenic effects are seen. The mechanism by which tacrolimus causes nephrotoxicity is related to an alteration of prostaglandin metabolism, by inducing vasoconstriction, and reduction in renal blood flow and a resultant decreased glomerular filtration rate. With the addition of a nonsteroidal anti-inflammatory drug (NSAID), the renal blood flow can become even more impaired. Therefore, the routine prescription of NSAIDs to patients on tacrolimus should be avoided.

Drugs that may induce nephrotoxicity and contribute to renal impairment such as aminogly-cosides, trimethoprim-sulfamethoxazole, amphotericin B, and acyclovir also should be avoided in patients who are taking tacrolimus.

28. Does tacrolimus interact with any drugs that are routinely used in oral and maxillo-facial surgery patients?
Yes. Tacrolimus is eliminated in the liver by cytochrome P450 isoenzymes and, therefore, may show a rise in concentration with the concomitant use of macrolide antibiotics such as erythromycin or clarithromycin, azole antifungal agents, or corticosteroids. Also, the antihist-amines terfenadine (Seldane) and astemizole (Hismanal) have been associated with cardiac arrhythmias after coadministration of tacrolimus or cyclosporine. Concurrent use of NSAIDs or nephrotoxic antibiotics and tacrolimus also increases the potential for nephrotoxicity.

29. What are the oral manifestations of graft versus host disease in the transplant patient.
Graft-versus-host disease results from the action of T cells in the transplanted organ against histocompatibility antigens of the host tissue. The oral cavity can be affected along with the liver, skin, and gastrointestinal tract. More than 80% of patients with graft-versus-host disease have oral lesions, which in many cases may be the first symptom. The clinical presentation of oral graft-versus-host disease resembles other collagen vascular diseases such as systemic lupus erythematosus or lichen planus. The oral mucosa may show erythema, ul-ceration, white striations, atrophy, or a pseudomembranous covering. Symptoms may range from mild discomfort to burning and severe pain and salivary dysfunction. Graft-versus-host disease is treated by augmenting immunosuppressive therapy. Careful monitoring of the pa-tient for signs of overimmunosuppression should also be performed during this period.

30. What are the preparative considerations of postsplenectomy patients?
Postsplenectomy patients have the potential to develop overwhelming sepsis with shock and disseminated intravascular coagulation (DIC). The most common organisms causing such infections are pneumococcus, meningococcus, and *Haemophilus*. Therefore, prior to splenec-tomy, patients should receive vaccination with pneumococcal polysaccharide. Prophylactic antibiotics should be given prior to surgical procedures in contaminated sites such as the oral cavity. Early aggressive treatment of infections in these patients is recommended.

BIBLIOGRAPHY

1. Carpenter CC, Fischl MA, Hammer SM, et al: Antiretroviral therapy for HIV infection in 1996: Recommendations of an international panel. International AIDS Society-USA. JAMA 276:146–164, 1996.
2. Centers for Disease Control and Prevention: USPHA/IDSA guidelines for the prevention of oppor-tunistic infections in persons infected with human immunodeficiency virus: A summary. MMWR Morb Mortal Wkly Rep 44:1–34, 1995.
3. Deeks SG, Smith M, Holodniy M, et al: HIV-1 protease inhibitors: A review for clinicians. JAMA 277:145–153, 1997.
4. Dodson TB, Parrott DH, Nguyen T, et al: HIV status and the risk of postoperative complications. J Oral Maxillofac Surg 49(suppl 1):81–82, 1991.
5. Grant D, Wall W, Duff J, et al: Adverse effects of cyclosporine therapy following liver transplanta-tion. Transplant Proc 19:3463–3465, 1987.
6. Ho M, Dummer JS: Risk factors and approach to infections in transplant recipients. In Mandell GL, Douglas RG, Bennett JE (eds): Principles and Practices of Infectious Diseases, 4th ed. New York, Churchill Livingstone, 1995, pp 2709–2716.
7. Lockhart PB, Sonis ST: Relationship of oral complications to peripheral blood leukocyte and platelet counts in patients receiving cancer chemotherapy. Oral Surg Oral Med Oral Pathol 48:21–28, 1979.
8. Martinez-Gimeno C, Acero-Sanz J, Martin-Sastra R, et al: Maxillofacial trauma: Influence of HIV infection. J Craniomaxillofac Surg 20:297–302, 1992.
9. Matsuda H, Iwasaki K, Shiriga T, et al: Interactions of FK506 (tacrolimus) with clinically important drugs. Res Commun Mol Pathol Pharmacol 91:57–64, 1996.

10. Maxymiw WG, Wood RE: The role of dentistry in patients undergoing bone marrow transplantation. Br Dent J 167:229–234, 1989.
11. Mignat C: Clinically significant drug interactions with new immunosuppressive agents. Drug Safety 16:267–278, 1997.
12. Pernu HE, Pernu LM, Huttunen K, et al: Gingival overgrowth among renal transplant recipients and uremic patients. Nephrol Dial Transplant 8:1254–1258, 1993.
13. Peterson DE, Sonis ST: Oral complications of cancer chemotherapy: Present status and future studies. Cancer Treat Rep 66:1251–1256, 1982.
14. Portery SR, Scully C, Luker J: Complications of dental surgery in persons with HIV disease. Oral Surg Oral Med Oral Pathol 75:165–167, 1993.
15. Reichart PA, Gelderblom HR, Becker J, et al: AIDS and the oral cavity. The HIV-infection virology, etiology, origin, immunology, precautions and clinical observation in 110 patients. Int J Oral Maxillofac Surg 16:129–153, 1987.
16. Robinson PG, Cooper H, Hatt J: Healing after dental extractions in men with HIV infections. Oral Surg Oral Med Oral Pathol 74:426–430, 1992.
17. Roser SM: Management of the medically compromised patient. In Kwon PH, Laskin DM (eds): Clinician Manual of Oral and Maxillofacial Surgery, 2nd ed. Chicago, Quintessence Books, 1996, pp 173–207.
18. Samaranayake LP: Oral mycoses in HIV infection. Oral Surg Oral Med Oral Pathol 73:171–180, 1992.
19. Schmidt B, Kearns G, Parrott D, et al: Infection following treatment of mandibular fractures in human immunodeficiency virus in seropositive patients. J Oral Maxillofac Surg 53:1134–1139, 1995.
20. Thomason JM, Seymour RA, Rice N: Determinants of gingival overgrowth severity in organ transplant patients. An examination of the role of HLA phenotype. J Clin Periodontol 23:628–634, 1996.
21. Thomason JM, Seymour RA, Rice N: The prevalence and severity of cyclosporine and nifedipine-induced gingival overgrowth. J Clin Periodontol 20:37–40, 1993.
22. Wysocki GP, Gretzinger HA, Laupacis A, et al: Fibrous hyperplasia of the gingiva: A side effect of cyclosporine A therapy. Oral Surg Oral Med Oral Pathol 55:274–278, 1983.
23. Yee J, Christou NV: Perioperative care of the immunocompromised patient. World J Surg 17:207–214, 1993.

24. MANAGEMENT CONSIDERATIONS IN THE JOINT REPLACEMENT PATIENT

Kathy A. Banks, D.M.D., and Jennifer Lamphier, D.M.D.

1. What are the two most common causes of prosthetic joint infections?

The majority of prosthetic joint infections are due to **wound contamination** occurring during placement of the prosthesis. Signs and symptoms of infection may occur immediately following joint placement or may arise weeks to months later. A smaller proportion of prosthetic joint infections are attributed to **hematogenous spread** of bacteria from distant sites of infection.

2. What major change in the surgical technique of prosthetic joint replacement is responsible for the low rate of postoperative infection?

Prophylactic antibiotic therapy is the single most important change in surgical technique and is mostly responsible for the low incidence (about 1%) of postoperative infections involving prosthetic joints. Prophylactic antibiotic therapy significantly decreases the risk of both early and late infections caused by wound contamination at the time of joint prosthesis placement. Antibiotic-impregnated cement used in the retention of the prosthesis and improvements in aseptic technique are contributing factors.

3. What bacteria are most commonly cultured from infected prosthetic joints?

Staphylococcus aureus and *Staphylococcus epidermidis* because the majority of infections involving prosthetic joints are caused by staphylococcal contamination during the placement of the prosthesis.

4. Which bacteria have been identified in cases of infected prosthetic joints arising via hematogenous spread of infection to the prosthesis from oral sites of infection?

Streptococcus viridans   *Streptococcus sanguis*

5. Which medical conditions place patients with prosthetic joints at high risk for developing hematogenous infection of the prosthetic joint?

- Active rheumatoid arthritis
- Systemic lupus erythematosus
- Severe type I insulin-dependent diabetes mellitus
- Steroid therapy
- Hemophilia
- Immunosuppressive disease
- First 2 years following joint placement

6. What conditions seem to predispose a prosthetic joint to development of infection?

- Loose prosthesis
- First 2 years following joint placement
- Second or third prosthesis in place
- Previous infection involving the joint
- Acute skin infections

7. Late infections involving prosthetic joints are associated with acute infections of which major organ systems?

Oral cavity   Respiratory system   Urogenital
Skin   Gastrointestinal

8. What bacteria most commonly cause infected prosthetic joints in the "high risk" group of patients?

Staphylococcus aureus and *Staphylococcus epidermidis*. The origin of the bacteria causing the joint infection is not different in this group.

9. What criteria are used to establish a diagnosis of hematogenous infection in prosthetic joint replacement?

The same strain of bacteria must be cultured from the following three sites:
1. Infected joint
2. Primary focus of infection
3. Blood

10. Describe the treatment options for a patient with an infected prosthetic joint.
- Remove the joint prosthesis
- Salvage the prosthesis with surgical debridement and antibiotic therapy
- Salvage the prosthesis with aspiration of pus and antibiotic therapy

11. When can transient oral bacteremias occur?
- During mastication
- During tooth brushing and flossing, and dental prophylaxis
- Sporadically in patients with moderate to severe periodontal disease
- Sporadically in patients with moderate to severe odontogenic infections
- During invasive dental and otolaryngology procedures

12. Which bacteria have been associated with transient oral bacteremias?
Streptococcus viridans and *Streptococcus sanguis*.

13. Which dental procedures have the highest incidence of bacteremia?
- Dental extractions
- All periodontal procedures
- Endodontic instrumentation
- Initial placement of orthodontic bands
- Intraligamentary injections of local anesthesia
- Dental prophylaxis of teeth or implants where bleeding is expected

14. Which dental procedures have the lowest incidence of bacteremia?
- Restorative dentistry:
  With or without retraction cord
  Placement of post and core buildup
  Placement of rubber dam
  Placement of removable appliances
- Injections of local anesthetic (except intraligamentary injections)
- Suture removal
- Taking oral impressions
- Fluoride treatments
- Taking oral radiographs
- Orthodontic bracket placement and adjustment

15. List the risks of antibiotic therapy.

Gastrointestinal upset	Anaphylaxis
Cross reactions with other drugs	Hearing loss
Emergence of resistant bacterium	Death
Allergic reactions	

16. What steps can be taken to minimize transient oral bacteremia in the prosthetic joint replacement patient?
- Elimination of active dental and periodontal disease prior to the joint replacement surgery
- Oral rinsing with chlorhexidine solution prior to dental, periodontal, and dental extraction procedures
- Aggressive treatment of acute dental and oral infections with antibiotics, surgery, and culture and sensitivity testing

17. What are the current recommendations of the American Dental Association and the American Academy of Orthopedic Surgeons regarding the use of antibiotic prophylaxis for routine dental procedures in patients with prosthetic joint replacements?
- Antibiotic prophylaxis is not indicated for dental patients with pins, plates, screws, nor is it routinely indicated for most dental patients with total joint replacements.
- Empiric prophylactic antibiotic therapy should be considered for patients who are considered to be at high risk for developing hematogenous prosthetic joint infection.
- The dentist is encouraged to consult with the orthopedic surgeon regarding the decision of whether to treat with antibiotic prophylaxis.

18. What are the current antibiotic prophylaxis guidelines recommended by the American Dental Association for dental patients with prosthetic joint replacements?

American Dental Association Antibiotic Prophylaxis Guidelines for Patients with Prosthetic Joint Replacements

PATIENT STATUS	ANTIBIOTIC	DOSE	ADMINISTRATION
Able to take oral penicillin	Cephalexin *or* Cephradine *or* Amoxicillin	2 gm 2 gm 2 gm	PO 1 hour prior to the dental procedure
Unable to take oral medications	Cefazolin *or* Ampicillin	1 gm 2 gm	IM or IV 1 hour prior to dental procedure
Allergic to penicillin	Clindamycin	600 mg	1 hour prior to dental procedure
Allergic to penicillin and unable to take oral medications	Clindamycin	600 mg	IV 1 hour prior to dental procedure

BIBLIOGRAPHY

1. Ainscow DA, Denham RA: The risk of haematogenous infection in total joint replacements. J Bone Joint Surg 66(B):580–582, 1984.
2. Bartzokas C, Johnson R, Jane M, et al: Relation between mouth and haematogenous infection in total joint replacements. BMJ 309:506–508, 1994.
3. Burton DS, Schurman DJ: Salvage of infected total joint replacements. Arch Surg 112:574–578, 1977.
4. Cozen L: Infection after knee replacement surgery. Orthopedics 1:222–223, 1978.
5. Little JW: Patients with prosthetic joints: Are they at risk when receiving invasive dental procedures? Spec Care Dentist 17:153–160, 1997.
6. Wahl M: Myths of dental-induced prosthetic joint infections. Clin Infect Dis 20:1420–1425, 1995.

VI. Management of the Oral and Maxillofacial Surgery Patient

25. APPLIED OROFACIAL ANATOMY

A. Omar Abubaker, D.M.D., Ph.D., and Kenneth J. Benson, D.D.S.

1. What are the sources for the blood and nerve supply to the sternocleidomastoid muscle (SCM)?

The blood supply to the SCM is provided from two sources. The **superior thyroid artery** supplies the middle third of the muscle, whereas the **occipital artery** branches, supplying the remainder of the muscle. The nerve supply is from the spinal accessory (cranial nerve [CN] XI) and from C2 and C3.

2. What are the sources of the blood and nerve supply to the temporomandibular joint (TMJ)?

The major arterial supply to the TMJ is derived from the superficial temporal artery and from the maxillary artery posteriorly, and from smaller masseteric, posterior deep temporal, and lateral pterygoid arteries anteriorly. The venous drainage is through a diffuse plexus around the capsule and rich venous channels that drain the retrodiscal tissue.

The nerve supply is from the auriculotemporal nerve, which provides the principal sensory innervation to the TMJ. The nerve gives off two or three branches, which enter the capsule inferiorly, medially, and laterally. The masseteric nerve also innervates the capsule from the frontal and medial sides of the joint. The posterior deep temporal nerve supplies the TMJ laterally and anteriorly.

3. How many origins and insertions does each masticatory muscle have?

For each muscle of mastication there are two insertions and two origins.

4. Discuss the insertions, origins, and functions of the lateral pterygoid muscle.

The lateral pterygoid muscle is triangular in shape and runs in a slightly inferior and posterior horizontal direction. The muscle has superior and inferior heads. The **superior head** arises from the infratemporal surface of the greater wing of the sphenoid and inserts into the articular capsule and disc. The function of the superior head is to stabilize the condyle and disc during closing movement.

The **inferior head** originates from the lateral surface of the lateral pterygoid plate and inserts into the pterygoid fovea of the neck of the condyle. The inferior head aids in translation of the condyle over the articular eminence during opening of the mouth.

5. Which muscles make up the pterygomandibular raphae?

The buccinator muscle anteriorly and the superior constrictor of the pharynx posteriorly make up the pterygomandibular raphae.

6. What embryologic structures form the external nose?

The **maxillary processes**, which originate from the dorsal ends of the first (mandibular) arch and the lateral nasal processes, grow toward the midline to merge with the downward-growing frontonasal process to form the external nose. The **frontonasal process** then continues to elongate, forming the median nasal process and fetal philtrum. The lateral nasal processes form the lateral portion of the adult nose (i.e., lower lateral cartilage and lobule). The **olfactory placode**, an ectodermal thickening, invaginates as a pit between the medial portion of the frontonasal process and the lateral nasal process. The olfactory placode finally comes to rest high in the nose as the analogue of the olfactory epithelium.

7. Discuss the nasal bones and cartilages that make up the external nasal skeleton.

Several bones and cartilages make up the external nose and give it its characteristic pyramidal shape. The nasal bones articulate with the nasal part of the frontal bone superiorly and the nasal process of the maxilla laterally. The nasal bones are attached at their inferior aspect to the upper lateral cartilages. The upper lateral cartilages in turn attach their inferior portion to the lower lateral cartilages and, medially, to the cartilaginous septum.

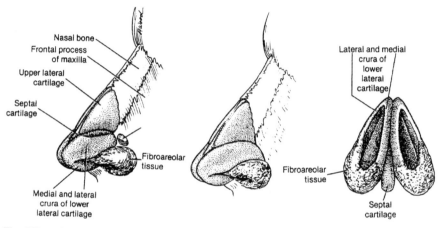

The different bones and cartilages that make up the nasal skeleton. (From Cummings CW, et al (eds): Otolaryngeology—Head and Neck Surgery. St. Louis, Mosby, 1986, p 514, with permission.)

Small rudimentary cartilages known as *sesamoid cartilages*, or *alar cartilages*, give additional support to the lateral nasal ala, where the lower lateral cartilage extends to meet the cheek. The fibrofatty tissue of the lower lateral cartilage, which contains the sesamoid cartilages, is known as the *lobule*.

The nasal septum is made up of quadrangle cartilage that continues with the lateral nasal cartilage toward the bridge of the nose, forming the cartilaginous portion of the septum. Posteriorly and above, the septal cartilage with the perpendicular plate of the ethmoid and the inferior edge of the septum fits into a groove on the vomer and the nasal crest.

8. Describe the vascular supply to the nose.

Branches from both the external and internal carotid arteries supply the nose. The external nose is supplied by the dorsal nasal of the ophthalmic artery superiorly, and the septal and lateral nasal of the angular artery inferiorly. The lower part of the dorsum of the nose is supplied by the external nasal, from the anterior ethmoidal artery.

The external carotid artery via the terminal branches of the internal maxillary artery, namely the sphenopalatine and greater palatine arteries, supplies the posterior inferior part of the internal nose. Branches from the anterior and posterior ethmoid arteries of the ophthalmic artery supply the anterior inferior nasal cavity, which is a branch of the internal carotid artery. Venous drainage of the nose corresponds to the arterial nomenclature, and occurs through the sphenopalatine, ophthalmic, and anterior facial veins.

9. Map out the sensory nerve supply to the nose.
- Olfactory fibers are located in the superior portion of the internal nose and serve the sensory function of smell.
- The sensory innervation of the skin of the root of the nose is derived from the supratrochlear and infratrochlear branches of the ophthalmic nerve.
- Branches of the infraorbital nerve supply the skin on the lower half of the nose's side.
- Nasociliary branches of the ophthalmic nerve supply the skin over the lower dorsum of the nose down to the tip.
- The trigeminal nerve supplies general sensory innervation to the anterior internal nose through the anterior ethmoidal, external, and internal nasal branches.
- The lateral posterior superior, pharyngeal, and lateral posterior inferior branches of the maxillary nerve supply the posterior portion.
- The terminal branches of the infraorbital nerve supply the lining of the nasal vestibule.
- The internal nasal (anterior ethmoidal) and medial posterior superior branches supply the septum anterior and posterior portions respectively.

10. Map out the motor nerve supply to the nose.
- The autonomic nerve supply of the nose controls the secretory function of the mucous glands.
- The preganglionic sympathetic innervation originates from the hypothalamus, passes through the thoracolumbar region of the spinal cord, and synapses in the superior cervical ganglion in the neck.
- Postganglionic sympathetic fibers then pass through the sphenopalatine ganglion to reach the nasal glands along the posterior nasal nerves.
- The parasympathetic nerve supply to the nose originates in the superior salvatory nucleus of the midbrain to reach the sphenopalatine ganglion through the greater petrosal nerve.
- The postganglionic fibers are carried out along the vidian nerve to finally reach the nose via the posterior nasal nerve.
- The motor nerve supply to all the muscles of the external nose are by the way of the facial nerve.

11. What are the most common vessels involved with anterior epistaxis?
Kiesselbach's plexus of septum arterioles is the source of 90% of nosebleeds. Four anastomosed arteries make up this plexus: the sphenopalatine, anterior ethmoidal, greater palatine, and superior labial arteries. The nasopalatine branch of the descending palatine artery anastomoses with septal branches of the sphenopalatine artery, the anterior ethmoidal artery, and superior lateral branches of the superior labial branch of the facial artery. Traumatic nasal bleeding can be caused by laceration of the nasal mucosa, and any of the nasal vessels can be the source of the bleeding (see figure, top of next page).

12. Describe the lymphatic drainage of the nose.
The lymphatics of the nose arise from the superficial portion of the mucous membrane and travel posteriorly to the retropharyngeal lymph nodes. Anteriorly, the lymphatics drain into the submandibular lymph nodes or the upper deep cervical nodes.

13. Where do the paranasal sinuses drain?
The sphenoid sinus drains into the sphenoethmoidal recess. The posterior ethmoid sinus drains into the superior nasal meatus, and the nasolacrimal duct drains into the inferior nasal meatus. All other sinuses (maxillary, frontal, and anterior and middle ethmoidal) drain into the middle nasal meatus.

14. What are Arnold's and Jacobsen's nerves? Which organ do they supply?
Both nerves provide sensory innervation to the ear. Arnold's nerve is a branch of the vagus nerve (CN X) and supplies the concha and auditory canal. Jacobsen's nerve is a branch of the glossopharyngeal nerve (CN IX) and supplies the concha, canal, and middle ear.

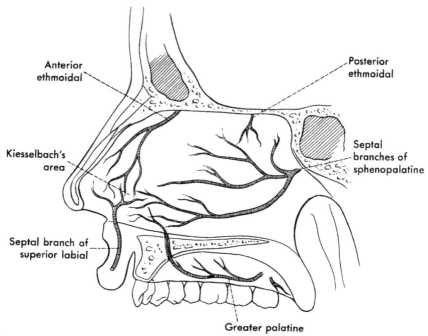

Anterior ethmoidal

Posterior ethmoidal

Kiesselbach's area

Septal branches of sphenopalatine

Septal branch of superior labial

Greater palatine

Vessels that make up Kiesselbach's plexus. (From Hollinstead H: Anatomy for Surgeons: The Head and Neck, 3rd ed. Philadelphia, Harper & Row, 1982, p 246, with permission.)

15. What other nerves supply the ear?

The auriculotemporal nerve (CN V_3) supplies the root helix, crus, tragus, and canal, whereas the auricular branch off the facial nerve (CN VII) supplies the concha and canal. Thus, in all, four cranial nerves (V, VII, IX, and X) provide sensory innervation for the ear.

16. What is the sensory innervation to the larynx?

The **vagus nerve** innervates the larynx via two laryngeal branches, the *internal laryngeal* and the *recurrent laryngeal*. The internal laryngeal branch provides sensory innervation to the mucous membrane above the vocal fold, while the recurrent laryngeal nerve provides sensory innervation to the mucous membrane below the vocal fold.

Motor function of the laryngeal muscles and vocal cords also is provided by the laryngeal branches of the vagus nerve (fibers of CN XI traveling with CN X). The *external laryngeal* branch innervates the cricothyroid muscle, and the recurrent laryngeal branch innervates all other intrinsic muscles.

17. What is the interval between open eyelids called?

The palpebral fissure (rima).

18. What is the average height of the inferior and superior tarsi?

The superior tarsus is 8–12 mm; the inferior tarsus is 5–7 mm.

19. Describe the autonomic innervation to the lacrimal gland.

Preganglionic parasympathetic fibers originate at the superior salivatory nucleus and are carried along the facial nerve to reach the sphenopalatine ganglion via the greater petrosal nerve. The postganglionic parasympathetic fibers travel via the zygomatic nerve to reach the lacrimal gland along the lacrimal nerve. Postganglionic sympathetic fibers from the superior cervical sympathetic ganglion travel through the deep petrosal nerve to reach the lacrimal gland in the same fashion as the parasympathetic fibers.

20. What are the components of the lacrimal drainage system?
Approximately a dozen small ducts under the outer corner of the upper eyelid drain tears onto the conjunctiva. From the superior and inferior punctae at the upper and lower eyelids at the medial canthus, the **lacrimal canaliculi** travel first vertically, then medially and downward (of superior canaliculi), and finally upward and medially (of inferior canaliculi) to converge at the **lacrimal sac**. The canaliculi length is approximately 8 mm. Often the canaliculi converge prior to the lacrimal sac and create a small dilation called the **sinus of Maier**. The lacrimal sac is 12 mm long and is found in the anterior aspect of the medial orbital wall. The **lacrimal crest** is covered by periosteum. The medial palpebral ligament lies anterior and superior to the sac. The lacrimal sac empties into the nasolacrimal duct, which drains into the inferior nasal meatus of the nose.

21. What is the relationship of the nasolacrimal duct to the nasal cavity and maxillary sinus?
The nasolacrimal duct lies within the thin, bony wall between the maxillary sinus and the nasal cavity. The duct ends at the inferior nasal meatus through the valve of Hasner. The position of the nasolacrimal duct beneath the inferior turbinate is 11–14 mm posterior to the piriform aperture and 11–17 mm above the nasal floor.

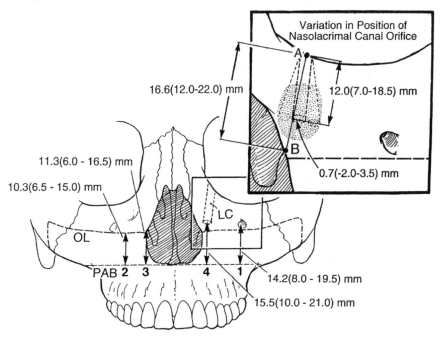

The relationship of the nasolacrimal duct to the nasal floor and turbinates. Heights (means and ranges) are from the piriform aperture base (*PAB*) to the infraorbital foramen (*1*), the simulated osteotomy (*2*), the anterior attachment of the inferior turbinate (*3*), and the inferior orifice of the nasolacrimal canal (*4*). The inset illustrates the variation in position of the nasolacrimal canal orifice relative to the x line drawn between the lacrimal fossa (*A*) and the anterior attachment of the inferior turbinate (*B*). LC = nasolacrimal canal, OL = simulated high-level Le Fort I osteotomy. (From You-ZH, Bell WH, Finn RA: Location of the nasolacrimal canal in relation to the high Le Forte I osteotomy. J Oral Maxillofac Surg 50:1075–1080, 1992, with permission.)

22. Which bones form the orbital cavity?

Lacrimal	Sphenoid
Ethmoid	Zygomatic
Palatine	Maxillary
Frontal	

23. What is Whitnall's orbital tubercle?

Whitnall's orbital tubercle is a bony protuberance present at the lateral orbital wall approximately 5 mm behind the lateral orbital rim. The tubercle is the area for attachment of the lateral horn of the levator aponeurosis, lateral palpebral ligament, and lateral check ligament. The attachment of these structures is in that order, from anterior to posterior.

24. Which orbital voluntary muscle does *not* originate at the orbital apex?

The inferior oblique muscle arises from the medial portion of the floor of the orbit just posterior to the orbital rim. The muscle then passes laterally and inserts on the posterolateral sclera.

25. Outline the anatomy, nerve supply, and function of the extraocular muscles.

Anatomy, Nerve Supply, and Function of the Extraoccular Muscles

MUSCLE	ORIGIN	INSERTION	NERVE SUPPLY	FUNCTION
Levator palpebrae superioris	Lesser wing of sphenoid	Anterior surface and upper border of superior tarsal plate		
• Voluntary portion			Oculomotor nerve	Raises upper eyelid
• Involuntary portion			Sympathetic nerves	
Superior rectus	Common tendinous ring	Sclera 6 mm behind corneal margin	Oculomotor nerve	Raises and medially rotates cornea
Inferior rectus	Common tendinous ring	Sclera 6 mm behind corneal margin	Oculomotor nerve	Depresses cornea medially rotates cornea
Lateral rectus	Common tendinous ring	Sclera 6 mm behind corneal margin	Abducent nerve	Moves cornea laterally
Medial rectus	Common tendinous ring	Sclera 6 mm behind corneal margin	Oculomotor nerve	Moves cornea medially
Superior oblique	Body of sphenoid	By way of pulley and attached to sclera behind coronal equator of eyeball; line of pull of tendon passes medial to vertical axis	Trochlear nerve	Moves cornea downward and laterally

(Table continued on next page.)

Anatomy, Nerve Supply, and Function of the Extraoccular Muscles (cont.)

MUSCLE	ORIGIN	INSERTION	NERVE SUPPLY	FUNCTION
Inferior oblique	Anterior part of floor of orbit	Attached to sclera behind coronal equator; line of pull of tendon passes medial to vertical axis	Oculomotor nerve	Moves cornea upward and laterally

Adapted from Snell RS: Clinical Anatomy for Medical Students, 5th ed. Boston, Little, Brown and Company, 1996, p 720.

26. What are the distance limits from the lateral, inferior, superior, and medial orbital rims for safe posterior dissection?

Although the distance from the orbital rim to the orbital apex is 4–4.5 cm, subperiosteal dissection along the orbital walls can be safely extended only up to 25 mm posteriorly from the inferior orbital rim and 25 mm from the lateral orbital rim. From the anterior lacrimal crest, dissection can be extended 25 mm posteriorly with minimal danger to the posterior orbital contents. From the superior orbital rim, dissection can be extended 30 mm. However, because most traumatic forces tend to displace all or part of these rims posteriorly, this displacement should be considered when carrying out posterior dissection in the orbit.

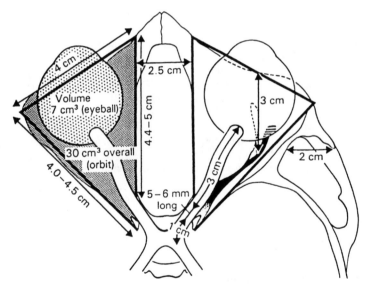

Major orbital dimensions and relationships. (From Ochs M, Buckley M: Anatomy of the orbit. Oral Maxillofac Surg Clin 5:420, 1993, with permission.)

27. Describe the autonomic nerve supply to the pupil.

Postganglionic sympathetic fibers have their cell bodies in the superior cervical ganglion. These nerves reach the dilator pupil muscles via the **short and long ciliary nerves**. Preganglionic parasympathetic fibers have their cell bodies in the Edinger-Westphal nucleus in the brain and travel to the ciliary ganglion in the orbit via the oculomotor nerve. The short ciliary nerves from the ciliary ganglion to the sphincter pupillary muscles carry the postganglionic fibers. Parasympathetic fibers contribute to pupillary constriction; the sympathetic supply activates pupillary dilator muscles.

28. What are the sebaceous and sweat glands of the eyelids called?

The sebaceous glands of the eyelid are called the *glands of Zeis*. The sweat glands of the eyelid are called the *glands of Moll*.

29. What are crocodile tears?

This condition results after injury to the fibers of the facial nerve carrying parasympathetic secretory fibers that normally innervate the salivary gland. The injury causes the fibers to heal in contact with fibers supplying the lacrimal gland, leading to "crying" when the patient eats.

30. What are the contents of the carotid sheath?

The carotid sheath contains the carotid artery, the jugular vein, and the vagus nerve. Within the carotid sheath, the vagus nerve (CN X) lies posterior to the common carotid artery and internal jugular vein.

31. How many branches does the external carotid artery give off? What are they?

The external carotid artery branches from the common carotid artery at the level of the upper border of the thyroid cartilage to be the principal artery supplying the anterior aspect of the neck, face, scalp, oral and nasal cavities, bones of the skull, and dura mater. Note that the orbit and its content are the only structures that are not supplied by the external carotid. There are eight branches (order of appearance from inferior to superior): (1) the superior thyroid, (2) the ascending pharyngeal, (3) the lingual, (4) the facial, (5) the occipital, (6) the posterior auricular, (7) the internal maxillary, and (8) the superficial temporal.

32. What is the course of the facial artery in the submandibular triangle?

The facial artery passes from behind and medial to the submandibular gland, up and over the gland, to emerge from the submandibular space laterally. It then proceeds into the face at the level of the anterior border of the masseter muscle. Thus, the facial artery may or may not be encountered in the incision and removal of the gland, and therefore may not require removal, but would have to be located during dissection by pinpointing the two lymph nodes, which overlie it at the level of the inferior border of the mandible.

Superior and deep to these lymph nodes is the marginal mandibular branch of the facial nerve. Posterior to the nodes is the facial vein. Because the vein is lateral to the gland, it is often necessary to ligate and cut this vessel during the dissection to remove the gland.

33. What is the relationship of the lingual nerve to Wharton's duct?

The submandibular gland, or Wharton's, duct is about 5 cm in length, and its lumen is 2–4 mm in diameter. It runs anteriorly above the mylohyoid muscle and on the lateral surface of the hyoglossus and genioglossus muscles. At first, the duct lies below the lingual nerve. Then, as the lingual nerve descends, it crosses lateral to the duct. As the duct and lingual nerve pass below the sublingual gland, the lingual nerve passes below the duct and crosses it medially. As the nerve continues toward the genioglossus, the duct continues anteriorly and medially. The duct loops from below upward beneath the lingual nerve at the level of the third molar, and then crosses above the lingual nerve at about the level of the second molar. Thus, the nerve loops almost completely around the duct (see figure, top of next page).

34. Describe the course and relationships of the hypoglossal nerves in the submandibular triangle.

The hypoglossal nerve emerges from hypoglossal canal and passes laterally between the internal jugular vein and the internal and external carotid arteries. It then descends steeply and crosses the stylohyoid and posterior belly of the digastric muscles on their medial surfaces. The hypoglossal nerve courses forward and upward on the lateral surface of the hyoglossus muscle and is accompanied by branches of the sublingual vein entering the oral cavity at the

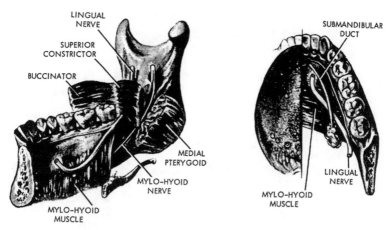

The course and relationships of the submandibular gland duct. (From Last J: Anatomy: Regional and Applied, 6th ed. New York, Churchill Livingstone, 1978, p 413, with permission.)

posterior border of the mylohyoid muscle, slightly above the digastric tendon. Here, beneath the tongue, the nerve curves forward and upward on the lateral surface of the genioglossus muscle, splitting into several branches that go into the substance of the tongue. These branches supply all extrinsic and intrinsic muscles of the tongue except the palatoglossus, which is supplied by CN XI via CN X.

35. What are the boundaries and significance of Lesser's triangle?

The triangle is made up by the angle between the tendon of the digastric muscle inferiorly, the hypoglossal nerve superiorly, and the posterior border of the mylohyoid muscle. The hyoglossal and mylohyoid muscles form the floor of this triangle. This triangle is useful in localization and ligation of the artery that lies at the inner surface of (beneath) the hyoglossus muscle deep to the floor of the triangle.

36. What is the superficial musculoaponeurotic system (SMAS)?

The SMAS is a layer of tissue that includes the platysma, risorius, triangularis, and auricularis muscles. Some authors also include the frontalis and the other muscles of facial expression in this tissue layer. The SMAS is connected to the dermis by a dense network of fibrous septae. These septae allow for movement of the overlying skin when the muscles in this tissue layer contract, giving rise to changes in facial expression. The skin can be dissected from the underlying SMAS by transection of these connecting fibrous septa, such as during rhytidectomy. The significance of the SMAS is related to its relationship to the nerves in the face: facial motor nerves deep to it, and sensory nerves more superficial to it (see figure, top of next page).

37. What are the layers of the scalp?

The scalp is made up of five tissue layers, the first three of which are intimately bound together and move as one unit called the *scalp proper*. The layers are:

Skin
Connective tissue layer
Aponeurosis
Loose areolar tissue occupying the subgaleal space
Periosteum or pericranium.

The aponeurosis is the tendinous sheet that connects the frontalis muscles to the occipitalis posteriorly and auricularis muscles and superficial temporal fascia laterally. Because the

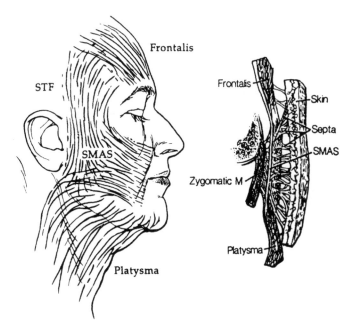

Anatomy of the SMAS. STF = superficial temporal fascia. (From Rees TD, Aston SJ, Thorne CHM: Blephroplasty and fascioplasty. In McCarthy JG (ed): Plastic Surgery. Philadelphia, W.B.Saunders, 1990, p 660, with permission.)

aponeurosis layer is the most distinct layer and covers the cranium like a helmet, it is also called the *galea*, which is Latin for "helmet."

38. Describe the blood supply and nerve supply to the scalp.

The scalp has a rich network of nerve and blood supply. Both the sensory nerves and the arteries of the scalp run in a radial fashion anterior to posterior, posterior to anterior, and laterally to the midline from both sides. All of these vessels and nerves meet at the vertex of the cranium, providing an even richer network of nerves and vessels in this region.

The **sensory nerves** supplying the cranium are a pair of supratrochlear and supraorbital nerves anteriorly (V1); the greater and third occipital nerves posteriorly (from the cervical); and the zygomaticotemporal (V2), auriculotemporal (V3), and lesser occipital nerves (C2–C3) laterally. The arterial supply consists of the supratrochlear and supraorbital arteries anteriorly (from the internal carotid); the occipital artery posteriorly; and the zygomaticotemporal, superficial temporal, and posterior auricular laterally (all from the external carotid) (see figure, top of next page).

The **motor nerves** to the muscles of the scalp (frontalis, occipitalis, and auricularis muscles) are supplied by the temporal and posterior auricular of the facial nerve.

39. What is the extension of the galea of the scalp into the temporal region?

The musculoaponeurotic layer covering the cranium is made of fascia (galea) in some locations and of muscles (frontalis, occipitals, and auricularis) in others. When this layer reaches the temporal region it is called the *superficial temporal fascia* or the *temporoparietal fascia*.

40. What is the extension of the temporoparietal fascia in the face?

The temporoparietal fascia in the temporal region of the face is confluent with the superficial musculoaponeurotic system (SMAS). This system consists of muscles of facial expression

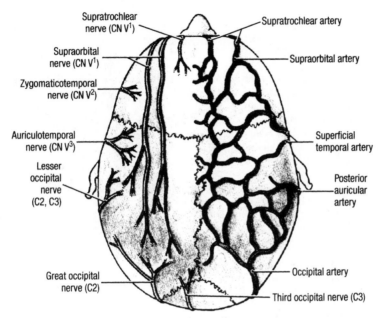

Supratrochlear nerve (CN V¹) — Supratrochlear artery

Supraorbital nerve (CN V¹) — Supraorbital artery

Zygomaticotemporal nerve (CN V²)

Auriculotemporal nerve (CN V³)

Lesser occipital nerve (C2, C3) — Superficial temporal artery

Posterior auricular artery

Great occipital nerve (C2) — Occipital artery

Third occipital nerve (C3)

The nerve and blood supply of the scalp. (From Snell RS: Head and neck anatomy. In Clinical Anatomy for Medical Students, 5th ed. Boston, Little Brown and Company, 1996, with permission.)

in some locations, and in other locations where there are no muscles it consists of a dense fascial layer.

41. List the other fascial layers of the temporal region.

In the temporal region, the temporalis fascia (the deep temporal fascia) becomes the extension of the pericranium, forming the periosteum covering the skull. In the preauricular region, roughly 2 cm superior to the zygomatic arch, the temporalis fascia splits into two layers (or leaflets): superficial and deep. These fascial layers form a pocket that contains the temporal fat pad. The two layers attach to the zygomatic arch and fuse with its periosteum.

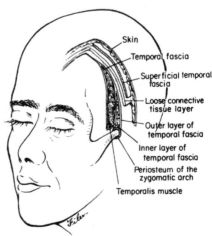

Skin

Temporal fascia

Superficial temporal fascia

Loose connective tissue layer

Outer layer of temporal fascia

Inner layer of temporal fascia

Periosteum of the zygomatic arch

Temporalis muscle

Anatomy of the different fascial layers of the temporal region. (From Abubaker AO, Sotereanos GC, Patterson GT: Coronal approach in treatment of craniofacial injuries. J Oral Maxillofac Surg 48: 579–586, 1990, with permission.)

42. What is the extension of the temporalis fascia below the level of the zygomatic arch?

The temporalis fascia extends below the zygomatic arch to invest muscles of mastication and adjacent structures, namely the masseter muscle and parotid gland. This layer is called *parotidomasseteric fascia.*

43. What are the extensions of the SMAS and parotidomasteric fascia in the neck?

In the neck, the extension of the SMAS is the superficial cervical fascia, which is similar to the SMAS in containing the muscle of facial expression of the neck, the *platysma.* This layer is loose in most areas, but is bound firmly to the underlying structures in a few places. The continuation of the parotidomasseteric fascia in the neck is the deep cervical fascia. This fascia also varies in thickness and splits in various sites to enclose the muscles of the neck, the submandibular gland, and the thyroid glands.

44. What is the blood supply to the temporalis muscle and the temporalis fascia?

The muscle is supplied primarily by the anterior and posterior deep temporal arteries (branches of the internal maxillary artery) and to a lesser extent by the superficial temporal artery.

The middle temporal artery, a branch of the superficial temporal artery, is the main supply to the fascia.

45. What is the blood supply to the temporal fat pad?

The blood supply to the temporal pad fat is from the middle temporal artery, which is a branch of the superficial temporal artery.

46. Describe the function and foramina of the twelve cranial nerves.

Cranial Nerves's Components, Function, and Foramen of Xxit from the Cranium

NERVE	COMPONENTS	FUNCTION	SKULL OPENING
I. Olfactor	Sensory	Smell	Opening in cribriform plate of ethmoid
II. Optic	Sensory	Vision	Optic canal
III. Oculomotor	Motor	Lifts upper eyelid, turns eyeball upward, downward, and medially; constricts pupil; accommodates eye	Superior orbital fissure
IV. Trochlear	Motor	Assists in turning eyeball downward and laterally	Superior orbital fissure
V. Trigeminal			
• Ophthalmic division	Sensory	Cornea, skin of forehead, scalp, eyelids, and nose; also mucous membrane of paranasal sinuses and nasal cavity	Superior orbital fissure
• Maxillary division	Sensory	Skin of face over maxilla and the upper lip; teeth of upper jaw; mucous membrane of nose, the maxillary air sinus, and palate	Foramen rotundum
• Mandibular division	Motor	Muscles of mastication, mylohyoid, anterior belly of digastric, tensor veli palatini, and tensor tympani	Foramen ovale
	Sensory	Skin of cheek, skin over mandible, lower lip, and side of head; teeth of lower jaw and temporomandibular joint; mucous membrane of mouth and anterior two-thirds of tongue	

(Table continued on next page.)

Cranial Nerves's Components, Function, and Foramen of Xxit from the

NERVE	COMPONENTS	FUNCTION	
VI. Abducent	Motor	Lateral rectus muscle; turns eye-ball laterally	
VII. Facial	Motor	Muscles of face, the cheek, and scalp; stapedius muscle of mid-dle ear; stylohyoid; and posterior belly of digastric	Internal acoustic meatus, facial canal, stylo-mastoid fora-men
	Sensory	Taste from anterior two-thirds of tongue; floor of mouth and palate	
	Secretomotor parasympa-thetic	Submandibular and sublingual salivary glands, the lacrimal gland, and glands of nose and palate	
VIII. Vestibulocochlear			
• Vestibular	Sensory	Position and movement of head	Internal acoustic meatus
• Cochlear	Sensory	Hearing	
IX. Glossopharyngeal	Motor	Stylopharyngeus muscle: assists swallowing	
	Secretomotor parasympa-thetic	Parotid salivary gland	Jugular foramen
	Sensory	General sensation and taste from posterior third of tongue and pharynx; carotid sinus and carotid body	
X. Vagus	Motor	Constrictor muscles of pharynx and intrinsic muscles of larynx; in-voluntary muscle of trachea and bronchi, heart, alimentary tract from pharynx to splenic flexure of colon; liver and pancreas	Jugular foramen
	Sensory	Taste from epiglottis and vallecula and afferent fibers from structures named above	
XI. Accessory			
• Cranial root	Motor	Muscles of soft palate, pharynx, and larynx	Jugular foramen
• Spinal root	Motor	Sternocleidomastoid and trapezius muscles	
XII. Hypoglossal	Motor	Muscles of tongue controlling its shape and movement (except palatoglossus)	Hypoglossal canal

Adapted from Snell RS: Clinical Anatomy for Medical Students, 5th ed. Boston, Little Brown and Company, 1996, p708.

47. At what distance from the stylomastoid foramen does the facial nerve bifurcate?

The nerve bifurcates into two main trunks (the zygomatico facial and the mandibular cer-vical) at variable distances after the nerve exits the skull, but on the average this distance is 1.3 cm.

,. **At what distance from the external auditory canal does the facial nerve bifurcate?**

The point of bifurcation of the facial nerve is located 1.5–2.8 cm inferior to the lowest concavity of the bony external auditory canal.

49. Define the "danger zone" for the frontal branch of the facial nerve as it crosses the zygomatic arch.

The frontal branch of the facial nerve crosses superficial to the zygomatic arch in an area that lies 0.8–3.5 cm anterior to the anterior concavity of the bony external auditory canal (an average of 2 cm anterior to the canal). A danger zone for injuring the frontal branch of the facial nerve during surgical procedures in the temporal and preauricular regions is located between two parallel lines drawn in the temporal region. The anterior line is drawn from the inferior attachment of the ear lobe to the most lateral extension of the eyebrow. The posterior line is drawn from a midpoint on the tragus of the ear to the most superior forehead crease of the forehead, or at least 2 cm from the first line or 2 cm above the supraorbital regions.

50. What is the "danger zone" for the marginal mandibular branch of the facial nerve?

The mandibular branch of the facial nerve courses in an area where incisions to approach the mandible and mandibular condyle are commonly placed. Accordingly, this area is considered a danger zone for injury to this branch. The zone is located between the inferior border of the mandible and a line in the retromandibular and submandibular region. This line extends from anterior to posterior and is 2 cm (1 thumb-breadth) behind the gonion and posterior border of the ascending ramus, 2 cm below the gonion, extending forward 2 cm below the inferior border of the mandible as far anteriorly as the level of the second premolar tooth. The anterior border of the zone is located at the intersection of two lines: a horizontal line 2 cm below and parallel to the inferior border of the body of the mandible, and another along the long axis of the lower second premolar.

51. How can the main trunk of the facial nerve be located during a parotidectomy?

As the facial nerve trunk travels from the stylomastoid foramen to the parotid gland, it passes anterior to the posterior belly of the digastric muscle, lateral to the styloid process and the external carotid artery, and posterior to the facial vein. Start a parotidectomy by mobilizing the tail of the parotid superiorly and retracting the anterior border of the sternocleidomastoid laterally, to identify the posterior belly of the digastric muscle. Follow this muscle superiorly toward its insertion at the mastoid tip. After bluntly separating the parotid from its attachment to the cartilage of the external auditory canal, the **tragal pointer** (outer surface of the external auditory cartilage) comes into view. The facial nerve trunk lies approximately 1 cm deep and slightly anteroinferior to the tragal pointer.

52. What are the branches of the facial nerve?

The facial nerve trunk has six major branches: temporal, zygomatic, buccal, mandibular, cervical, and auricular. The auricular branch comes off before the facial nerve turns into the parotid body, and innervates the superior auricular, posterior auricular, and occipitalis muscles, as well as provides sensation to the area behind the ear lobe. Within the parotid, the facial nerve divides into two main branches, the temporofacial and cervicofacial, which further divide into the temporal, zygomatic, buccal, mandibular, and cervical branches. The stylohyoid and posterior digastric are other minor branches of the nerve.

53. What is the relationship of the facial nerve to the parotidomasseteric fascia?

As the facial nerve branches leave the parotid gland, the parotidomasseteric fascia covers them. The SMAS is located superficial to this layer.

54. How do the facial muscles of expression receive their innervation?

All facial muscles except the mentalis, levator angularis superioris, and buccinator receive their innervation along their deep surfaces. However, because the above three muscles are located deep within the facial soft tissue and lie deep to the plane of the facial nerve, they receive their innervation along their superficial surfaces. All other facial muscles of expression are located superficial to the plane of the facial nerve and thus receive their innervation along their deep or posterior surfaces. For example, the platysma, orbicularis oculi, and zygomaticus major and minor are situated superficial to the level of the facial nerve.

55. What is the relationship of the frontal branch of the facial nerve to the SMAS and temporoparietal fascia?

Inferior to the zygomatic arch, the frontal branch of the facial nerve travels deep to the SMAS. As it crosses over the zygomatic arch it becomes very superficial. At this point it is sandwiched between the periosteum (extension of the temporal fascia) and the temporoparietal fascia (extension of the SMAS). Superior to the zygomatic arch, the frontal branch of the facial nerve travels within or on the under-surface of the temporoparietal fascia, but superficial to the outer layer of the temporal fascia.

56. How do the frontal and mandibular branches of the facial nerve differ from other facial branches?

Crossover communication between the frontal branch and adjacent branches and between the mandibular branch and adjacent branches is only about 15%. Crossover among the other branches is approximately 70%. Injury to either the frontal or mandibular branches leads to more marked deficit compared to the results of injury to the other branches.

57. Describe the relationship of the frontal and mandibular branch courses of the facial nerve.

The frontal branch of the facial nerve crosses the zygomatic arch deep to the SMAS and in the temporal region deep to the temporoparietal fascia (superficial temporal fascia). The nerve usually lies within 2 cm from the lateral border of the eyebrow and enters the frontalis muscle from its deep surface.

The mandibular branch courses within 2 cm of the inferior border of the mandible, posterior to the facial artery. The mandibular branch is at risk during an anterior dissection because in this area it becomes more superficial. It lies deep to the platysma and superficial to the facial artery.

58. How do I evaluate the five branches of the facial nerve during a physical examination?

Test each of the five branches of the nerve in the following manner:
- Cervical—contract the platysma muscles
- Marginal mandibular—whistle or pucker the lips
- Buccal—smile or show teeth
- Zygomatic—squeeze eyes shut tightly
- Temporal—raise eyebrows

59. List the most common causes of facial muscle paralysis.

Facial nerve paralysis, which may be unilateral or bilateral, can be a manifestation of any of several disease processes. These diseases can be idiopathic, neoplastic, traumatic, neoplastic, infectious, or congenital. The paralysis can also result from a systemic/metabolic process.

Idiopathic	Infection
Bell's palsy	Herpes zoster oticus (Ramsay-Hunt syndrome)
Recurrent facial palsy	Otitis media with effusion
Melkersson-Rosenthal syndrome	Acute suppurative otitis media
Neoplasia	Coalescent mastoiditis
Cholesteatoma	Chronic otitis media
Facial neuroma	Malignant otitis externa

Neoplasia (cont.)	Infection (cont.)
Glomus jugulareor tympanicum	(Pseudomonas osteomyelitis)
Carcinoma (primary or metastatic)	Tuberculosis
Schwannoma of lower cranial	Lyme disease*
nerves	AIDS
Meningioma	Infectious mononucleosis
Histiocytosis	**Congenital**
Rhabdomyosarcoma	Compression injury
Leukemia	Moebius syndrome*
Trauma	Lower lip paralysis
Temporal bone fractures*	**Metabolic and Systemic**
Birth trauma	Pregnancy
Facial contusions/lacerations	Diabetes mellitus
Penetrating wounds to face and	Sarcoidosis*
temporal bone	Guillain-Barré syndrome*
Iatrogenic injury	Autoimmune disorders

* May present as bilateral facial paralysis
Modified from Coker NJ: Acute paralysis of the facial nerve. In Bailey BJ, et al (eds): Head and Neck Surgery—Otolaryngology. Philadelphia, J.B. Lippincott, 1993.

60. Describe the retromandibular approach.

This approach is useful for procedures involving ramus and areas on or near the condylar neck/head. The incision begins 0.5 cm below the ear lobe and continues 3.0–3.5 cm inferiorly, approximately 2 cm posterior to the ramus. In some patients, this may limit the direct proximity of the skin incision to the mandible, which is one of the main advantages of this technique. Accordingly, some surgeons recommend placement of the incision more anteriorly at the posterior ramus, just below the earlobe. The deeper dissection of this approach is carried out bluntly through the parotid gland in an anteromedial direction (in the anticipated direction of the facial nerve) toward the posterior border of the mandible. The facial nerve, if identified, is avoided and deeper dissection is continued until the pterygomasseteric sling is identified and incised. The submasseteric dissection is continued to expose the ramus and condyle as needed.

61. Where should the skin incision be placed during a submandibular approach to avoid the mandibular branch of the facial nerve?

The submandibular approach is often referred to as the Risdon approach. It may be used to access the mandibular angle, ramus, condyle, inferior border of the mandibular body, and submandibular gland. The exact location of the skin incision differs mostly due to the disagreement over the course of the marginal mandibular branch of the facial nerve.

Dingman and Grabb showed in 192 patients that this branch is below the inferior border of the mandible, posterior to where the nerve crosses the facial artery. Anterior to that point, the facial nerve is above the inferior border in 100% of patients. In another study, Ziarah and Atkinson found that in 53% of patients, the marginal mandible of the facial nerve is below the inferior border of the mandible, posterior to the facial vessels, and in 6% this nerve continues to be below the inferior border anterior to the facial vessels.

Based on these findings, and to err well on the safe side, the recommended placement of the submandibular incision is **1.5–2.0 cm (a thumb-breadth) below the inferior border of the mandible**.

62. In a patient with a 3-cm vertical laceration of the anterior border of the masseter muscle, what findings are likely?

In such an injury there is a likelihood for paralysis of the frontalis, orbicularis occuli, nasalis muscles, and orbicularis oris. The paralysis of these muscles is due to severance of the frontal, zygomatic, and buccal branches of the facial nerve, respectively. The parotid duct and the parotid gland may also be involved.

63. What are the structures involved in resection of the mandible from mid ramus to the mental foramen?

Composite resection of the body of the mandible usually involves removal of bone, muscles, glands, lymph nodes, and vessels. The muscles involved are the masseter, medial pterygoid, platysma, mylohyoid, buccinator, depressor anguli oris, depressor labii inferioris, superior pharyngeal constrictor, and a small portion of the temporalis. The submandibular gland, sublingual glands, and the submandibular lymph nodes surrounding superficial and deep cervical nodes are also removed depending on the extent of the resection. The facial artery, anterior facial vein, and marginal mandibular branch of the facial nerve are also occasionally removed.

64. Describe the anatomy of taste sensory function.

Taste sensory function from the anterior part of the tongue is carried along corda tympani of the trigeminal nerve through the submandibular ganglion to reach the facial nerve. From the posterior or pharyngeal part of the tongue, taste sensation is carried along the glossopharyngeal nerve, through the pterygopalatine ganglion, to the major petrosal nerve and then the facial nerve. From the palatal region, the sensation is carried via the palatine nerves, which also pass through the pterygopalatine ganglion to ultimately reach the facial nerve.

Along with the facial nerve, taste fibers reach the tractus solitarius, which is concerned with visceral function including taste. Some textbooks state that taste fibers from the posterior part of the tongue reach the tractus solitarius directly via the glossopharyngeal nerve.

BIBLIOGRAPHY

1. Abbey SH: Facial nerve disorders. In Jafek BW, Stark AK (eds): ENT Secrets. Philadelphia, Hanley & Belfus, 1996, pp 123–131.
2. Abubaker AO, Sotereanos GC, Patterson GT: Use of bicoronal approach to treatment of craniofacial fractures. J Oral Maxillofacial Surg 48:579–586, 1990.
3. Anderson JE (ed): Grant's Atlas of Anatomy. Baltimore, Williams & Wilkins, 1983.
4. Coker NJ: Acute paralysis of the facial nerve. In Bailey BJ, et al (eds): Head and Neck Surgery—Otolaryngology. Philadelphia, J.B. Lippincott, 1993, p 1715.
5. Cummings CW, et al (eds): Otolaryngeology—Head abd Neck Surgery. St. Louis, Mosby, 1986.
6. Demas PN, Sotereanos GC: Incidence of nasolacrimal injury and turbinectomy-associated atrophic rhinitis with Le Fort I osteotomies: J Craniomaxillofac Surg 17:116–118, 1989.
7. Dingman RO, Grabbv WC: Surgical anatomy of the mandibular ramus of the facial nerve, based on the dissection of the facial halves. Plast Reconstruc Surg. 29:266–272, 1962.
8. Ellis E, Zide M: Surgical Approaches to the Facial Skeleton. Baltimore, Williams & Wilkins, 1984.
9. Frick H, Leanhardt H, Starck D: The Eye and the Orbit IN: Human Anatomy 2, 4th ed. Stuttgart, Germany, Thieme,. 1991.
10. Haller J: Trauma to the salivary glands. Otolaryngol Clin North Am. 32: 907–917, 1999.
11. Hollinstead H: Anatomy for Surgeons: The Head and Neck. 3rd ed. Philadelphia, Harper & Row, 1982.
12. Last J: Head and neck. In Last J: Anatomy: Regional and Applied, 6th ed. New York, Churchill Livingstone, 1978, pp 360–457.
13. Long CD, Granick MS: Head and neck ebryology and anatomy. In Weinzweig J (ed): Plastic Surgery Secrets. Philadelphia, Hanley & Belfus, 1996, pp 172–175.
14. Moore KL: Clinically Oriented Anatomy, 2nd ed. Baltimore, Williams & Wilkins, 1984.
15. Ochs M, Buckley M: Anatomy of the orbit. Oral Maxillofac Surg Clin 5:419–430, 1993.
16. Pansky B: The facial (VII) nerve. In Pansky B (ed): Review of Gross Anatomy. New York, Macmillan, 1984, pp 421–440.
17. Pitanguy I, Ramus A: The frontal branch of the facial nerve: The importance of its variation in face lifting. Plast Reconstruct Surg 38:352–356, 1966.
18. Rees TD, Aston SJ, Thorne CHM: Blepharoplasty and facioplasty. In McCarthy JG (ed): Plastic Surgery. Philadelphia, W.B.Saunders, 1990, pp 660–700.

19. Schow RS, Miloro M: Diagnosis and management of salivary gland disorders. In Peterson LJ, Ellis E 3rd, Hupp JR, Tucker MR (eds): Contemporary Oral and Maxillofacial Surgery, 3rd ed. St. Louis, Mosby, 1998, pp 488–509.
20. Schwember G, Rodriguez A: Anatomic dissection of the extraparaotid portion of the facial nerve. Plast Reconstruct Surg 81:183–188, 1988.
21. Sinha U, Ng M: Surgery of the salivary glands. Otolaryngol Clin North Am 32:888–905, 1999.
22. Snell RS: Head and neck anatomy. In Snell RS (ed): Clinical Anatomy for Medical Students, 5th ed. Boston, Little, Brown, 1995, pp 631–820.
23. Stuzin JM, Wagstrom L, Kawamoto HK, Wolfe SA: Anatomy of the frontal branch of the facial nerve: The significance of temporal fat pad. Plast Reconstr Surg 83:265–271, 1989.
24. You-ZH, Bell WH, Finn RA: Location of the nasolacrimal canal in relation to the high Le Fort osteotomy. J Oral Maxillofac Surg 50:1075–1080, 1992.
25. Ziarah HA, Atkinson ME: The surgical anatomy of the mandibular distribution of the facial nerve. Br J Oral Surg 19:159–170, 1981.

26. DENTOALVEOLAR SURGERY

James A. Giglio, D.D.S., M.Ed.

1. Why is it necessary to use a bite block when removing mandibular teeth?
To diminish pressure on the contralateral temporomandibular joint (TMJ).

2. Why isn't distilled water used for irrigation?
Distilled water is a hypotonic solution and will enter cells down the osmotic gradient causing cell lysis and rapid death of bone cells.

3. Why is buccal to lingual movement not efficient when removing mandibular posterior teeth?
Mandibular bone is too dense and does not expand in a similar fashion to that of the maxillary bone.

4. What anatomic structure can interfere with efficient removal of a maxillary first molar?
Root of the zygoma.

5. Which muscle is pierced by the needle when performing inferior alveolar nerve block anesthesia?
Buccinator muscle.

6. What muscles insert on the pterygomandibular raphe?
The buccinator muscle and the superior pharyngeal constrictor muscle.

7. What two structures form a V-shaped landmark for an inferior alveolar nerve block?
Deep tendon of the temporalis muscle and the superior pharyngeal constrictor.

8. What is the orthodontic indication for removal of an impacted third molar?
To facilitate distal movement of the second molar.

9. What is the "shift rule" as applied to impacted maxillary cuspids?
This radiographic technique determines the position of the impacted cuspid. A series of periapical radiographs are made. The film position is kept constant, but the head of the x-ray unit is moved either anteriorly or posteriorly after each exposure. If the impacted molar seems to move with the x-ray head, it is located on the palate. If it moves opposite to the unit head, it will be found on the buccal. This is also referred to as the SLOB rule: same lingual (palate), opposite buccal.

10. What is the advantage of an apically positioned mucoperiosteal flap for exposure of a buccally positioned impacted cuspid?
This flap design allows for the impacted tooth to erupt into attached mucosa and minimizes the possible development of periodontal defects and pocket formation.

11. Where is the inferior alveolar nerve most often located in relation to the roots of a mandibular third molar?

Buccal to the roots, and slightly apical.

12. The root of which tooth is most often dislodged into the maxillary sinus during an extraction procedure?

Palatal root of the maxillary first molar.

13. While trying to remove a root tip of a mandibular third molar, it disappears from view. Where might it be dislodged?

Inferior alveolar canal
Cancellous bone space
Submandibular space

14. What is the usually recommended sequence for extractions?

Maxillary teeth before mandibular teeth, and posterior teeth before anterior teeth.

15. What complications are associated with the removal of a freestanding, isolated maxillary molar?

Alveolar process fracture and fracture of the maxillary tuberosity.

16. How do you minimize the chance of dislodging an impacted maxillary third molar into the infratemporal fossa during its surgical removal?

Place a broad retractor distal to the molar while elevating it.

17. When performing a surgical removal, should you completely section through a mandibular molar?

No. The lingual plate is often thin, and complete sectioning may perforate the plate and injure the lingual nerve.

18. How is bleeding from pulsating nutrient blood vessels controlled following surgery on alveolar bone?

1. Burnish bone.
2. Crush with rongeurs.
3. Apply bone wax.

19. Name some common causes of postoperative bleeding following dental extractions.

• Failure to suture
• Failure to debride all granulation tissue
• Rebound blood vessel dilation following use of local anesthetic with a vasoconstrictor
• Torn tissue
• Torn surgical flaps

20. Why shouldn't a local anesthetic be used with a vasoconstrictor when treating postoperative hemorrhage?

The vasoconstrictor will mask the source of bleeding.

21. Why are mucoperiosteal flaps designed with a broad base?

To ensure an adequate blood supply to the flap margin.

22. Name the two basic flaps that are used in dentoalveolar surgery.

Full-thickness and split-thickness mucoperiosteal flaps.

23. What are the two basic types of full-thickness mucoperiosteal flaps?
1. Envelope flap
2. Envelope flap with a releasing component

24. Where are releasing incisions contraindicated?
Palate
Lingual surface mandible
Canine eminence
Through muscle attachments
In the region of the mental foramen

25. How do absorbable gelatin sponge (Gelfoam) and oxidized regenerated cellulose (Surgicel) assist with homeostasis?
They form a matrix or scaffold upon which a clot can form. Gelatin sponge does not become as readily incorporated into the clot as does the oxidized regenerated cellulose. Healing is delayed more often with cellulose than with the gelatin sponge, but oxidized regenerated cellulose is the more efficient homeostatic agent.

26. Why is a conventional dental handpiece that expels forced air contraindicated when performing dentoalveolar surgery?
Such an instrument can cause tissue emphysema or an air embolism. An air embolism can be fatal.

27. What are the cardinal signs of a localized osteitis (dry socket)?
Throbbing pain (often radiating)
Fetid odor
Bad taste
Poorly healed extraction site

28. Why is it contraindicated to curette a dry socket in order to stimulate bleeding?
Curetting a dry socket can cause the condition to worsen because healing will be further delayed, any natural healing already taking place will be destroyed, and there is a risk of causing the localized inflammatory process to be spread to the adjacent sound bone.

29. What is the treatment for a localized osteitis?
Conservative management is indicated. The wound should be irrigated gently with slightly warmed saline, and a sedative dressing should be placed. The dressing should be removed within 48 hours and replaced until the patient becomes asymptomatic. Systemic antibiotics are generally not indicated. Nonsteroidal anti-inflammatory analgesics should be prescribed if necessary.

30. What causes a dry socket?
The etiology of a dry socket is not absolutely clear but is thought to develop because of increased fibrinolytic activity causing accelerated lysis of the blood clot. Smoking, premature mouth rinsing, hot liquids, surgical trauma, and oral contraceptives have all been implicated in the development of a dry socket.

31. Why should flaps be repositioned and sutured over sound bone?
Unsupported flaps can collapse into bony defects, causing tension on the sutures. The sutures subsequently will pull through the tissue allowing the suture line to open and the wound to dehisce.

32. What percentage of dentoalveolar injuries include the primary maxillary central incisor?
70%

33. How are avulsed primary teeth treated?

No treatment is necessary; reimplantation is not indicated for primary teeth.

34. How is an extruded primary tooth treated?

If there is a gross interference with the opposing teeth, the tooth should be extracted. Otherwise, the teeth can be pressured and splinted in place.

35. What is the incidence of pulp necrosis after intrusion injuries of teeth?

With intrusion injuries, the risk of pulp necrosis for a tooth with a closed apex is 95% and for immature apex is 65%. Accordingly, any form of luxation should be followed with routine clinical and radiographic examinations.

36. How long should dentoalveolar fractures be splinted?

4–6 weeks.

37. What media can be used to transport avulsed teeth?

Saliva, fresh milk, balanced salt, or Hank balanced salt solution (HBSS). Water is harmful because, as a hypotonic fluid, it may cause periodontal ligament cell death when it enters cells down the osmotic gradient, causing cell lysis and death.

If the tooth is placed in an appropriate medium within 15–20 minutes, periodontal ligament cells can remain vital for 2 hours in saliva and 6 hours in fresh milk. Balanced salt solution can be used up to 24 hours if the initial dry storage was less than 30 minutes.

38. How long should extruded or avulsed teeth be splinted?

7–10 days.

39. What are the significant radiologic predictions of a close relationship between the inferior alveolar canal and the impacted mandibular third molar?

Signs of close proximity of the mandibular third molar to the inferior alveolar canal are mostly radiographic in nature and include:

Darkening and notching of the root
Deflected roots at the region of the canal
Narrowing of the root
Interruption of canal outlines
Diversion of canal from its normal course
Narrowing of canal outlines on the radiograph

40. What are the most important signs that may increase potential nerve injury with extraction of impacted mandibular third molars?

Of the above listed signs of close proximity of the canal to impacted third molar, diversion of canal, interruption of canal borders, and darkening of roots are the most reliable signs.

41. What are the possible complications of dentoalveolar surgery?

• Swallowing or aspiration of foreign objects
• Air emphysema
• TMJ pain
• Trismus
• Mandibular fracture
• Tuberosity fracture
• Root fracture
• Injuries to adjacent teeth
• Displacement of root and root fragments into the submandibular space, mandibular canal, or maxillary sinus

- Oral-antral communication, bleeding, infection, ecchymosis, and hematoma
- Localized osteitis (dry socket)
- Wound dehiscence
- Inferior alveolar and lingual injuries

Depending of the location and the nature of the surgery, these complications vary in severity and need for treatment.

42. How are roots or root tips displaced into the submandibular space managed?

Once displacement of a mandibular molar root into the submandibular space is suspected, manual lateral and upward pressure should be applied immediately on the lingual aspect of the floor of the mouth in an attempt to force the root back into the socket. If the root is visualized again in the socket, it may be retrieved from the socket with a root tip pick. If not, a mucoperiosteal soft tissue flap should be reflected on the lingual aspect of the mandible until the root tip is found; ensure that the mylohyoid muscle is sharply detached from its insertion in the mandible. Antibiotic coverage is indicated postoperatively. If the root is not visualized because of its location or uncontrollable bleeding, recovery is best performed as a secondary procedure when fibrosis occurs and stabilizes the tooth in a firm position, usually 4–6 weeks later. The patient should be placed on a short course of antibiotics.

43. How are roots or root tips that are displaced into the inferior alveolar canal managed?

When displacement of a root into the mandibular canal is suspected, periapical and occlusal radiographs should be taken for verification, because the root may be in a large marrow space or beneath the buccal mucosa. If the root is visualized, careful removal is indicated with a small hemostat after adequate alveolar bone removal. If the root is not visualized, delayed removal is recommended. Delayed removal is also indicated during persistent infection and nerve paresthesia. If the root fragment is small and does not become infected preoperatively, leaving the root in place is a viable and less invasive option.

44. How is a root or root fragment that is displaced into the maxillary sinus managed?

Once the root is suspected to be in the sinus, place the patient in an upright position to prevent posterior displacement and obtain a radiograph of the fractured tooth to determine its location and size. If the fragment is found to be in the sinus, local measures of retrieval should be attempted first, such as:

- Having the patient blow through the nose with the nostrils closed, and observing the perforation for the root to appear in the socket
- Using a fine suction tip to bring the root back into the defect
- Performing antral lavage with sterile isotonic saline in an effort to flush the root out through the defect
- Packing iodoform gauze into the antrum and removing it in one stroke; the root tip often adheres to the gauze

If local measures are unsuccessful, direct entry into the maxillary sinus via the Caldwell-Luc approach in the area of the canine fossa should be performed. Postoperative management includes a figure-of-eight suture over the socket, sinus precautions, antibiotics, and a nasal spray to keep the sinus ostium open and infection free.

45. How are oral-antral communications managed?

Probing, irrigation, and having the patient blow with the nostrils occluded are contraindicated because these maneuvers may enlarge an existing opening or create one that did not previously exist. For openings less than 2 mm, no surgical treatment is necessary providing adequate hemostasis is achieved. For openings of 2–6 mm, conservative treatment is indicated including placement of a figure-of-eight suture over the tooth socket and sinus precautions (avoid blowing the nose, violent sneezing, sucking on straws, and smoking). For openings greater than 6 mm, primary closure should be obtained with a buccal flap or a palatal flap procedure. Approximation of the gingiva can be facilitated by removal of a small amount of the buccal alveolar plate and scoring or incising the periosteum on the underside of the flap. Placement of a small piece of absorbable gelatin sponge into the occlusal third of the socket when the gingival margins cannot be coapted is not advisable because it introduces a foreign substance and could lead to subsequent breakdown of the clot. Antibiotics and nasal or oral decongestants are prescribed if there is evidence of acute or chronic sinusitis.

46. What steps should be taken for a tooth (maxillary third molar) that is displaced into the infratemporal fossa?

When a maxillary third molar is displaced into the infratemporal fossa, it is usually displaced through the periosteum and located lateral to the lateral pterygoid plate and inferior to the lateral pterygoid muscle with displacement. If there is good access and adequate light, a single cautious effort to retrieve the tooth with a hemostat can be made. If the effort is unsuccessful or if the tooth is not visualized, the incision should be closed, the patient should be informed, and prophylactic antibiotics should be prescribed. A secondary surgical procedure is performed 4–6 weeks later after lateral and posteroanterior radiographs are taken to locate the tooth in all three planes. After adequate anesthesia, a long needle—usually a spinal needle—is used to locate the tooth. Careful dissection is performed along the needle until the tooth is visualized and subsequently removed. If no functional problems exist after displacement, the patient may elect not to have the tooth removed. Proper documentation of this is critical.

47. How do you manage postoperative or secondary bleeding from extraction sites?

The first step in managing postoperative bleeding is to carefully examine and visualize the bleeding site to determine the precise source of bleeding. In the case of simple generalized oozing, a damp gauze is held over the site with firm manual pressure for 5 minutes. If unsuccessful, the area should be anesthetized and examined more closely. If sutures were placed, they should be removed and the existing clot should be curetted from the socket. Hemostatic agents such as an absorbable gelatin sponge, oxidized cellulose, and oxidized regenerated cellulose can be placed in the socket and sutured. If hemostasis is not achieved by local measures, laboratory screening tests should be performed to assist in diagnosis and treatment of the cause.

BIBLIOGRAPHY

1. Alling CC 3rd (ed): Dentoalveolar Surgery. Oral and Maxillofacial Surgery Clinics of North America, volume 5. Philadelphia, W.B. Saunders, 1993.
2. Lew D: Blood and blood products. In Kwon PH, Laskin DM (eds): Clinician's Manual of Oral and Maxillofacial Surgery, 2nd ed. Carol Stream, IL, Quintessence Publishing, 1997, pp 105–116.
3. Peterson L, Ellis E, Hupp J, Tucker M: Contemporary Oral and Maxillofacial Surgery, 3rd ed. St. Louis, Mosby, 1998.
4. Whitacre R: Removal of Teeth, 3rd ed. Seattle, Stoma Press, 1983.

27. DIAGNOSIS AND MANAGEMENT OF TRIGEMINAL NERVE INJURY

Kenneth J. Benson, D.D.S., and A. Omar Abubaker, D.M.D., Ph.D.

1. What are the two major classifications of nerve injury?
The Seddon and Sunderland classifications.

2. What is the pathophysiology of nerve injury?
Nerve injury is generally described as neuropraxia, axonotmesis, or neurotmesis.
- **Neurapraxia** is Seddon type I nerve injury resulting in conduction deficits without axonal or sheath degeneration. This type of injury is associated primarily with spontaneously reversing paresthesias.
- **Axonotmesis** is a traumatic nerve injury in which there is Wallerian degeneration distal to the point of injury, but the endoneural and perineural sheaths are intact. It is Seddon type 2 injury, expanded by Sunderland into second, third, and fourth degree injuries. There is potential for full recovery.
- **Neurotmesis** is a nerve injury with disruption of all axonal and sheath elements producing Wallerian degeneration and likely neuroma. This often requires microsurgical repair.

3. What is dysesthesia?
An unpleasant abnormal sensation produced by normal stimuli.

4. What is the difference between analgesia and anesthesia?
Analgesia is an absence of pain in response to stimulation that would normally be painful. Anesthesia is the absence of perception of stimulation by any noxious or non-noxious stimulation of skin or mucosa. It is divided into general (central), regional, and local types.

5. What is allodynia?
Allodynia is pain due to stimulus that does not normally provoke pain. Unlike hyperalgesia, hyperpathia, and hyperesthesia, allodynia may include emotionally induced sensations in the nerve-injured patient.

6. What is anesthesia dolorosa?
Anesthesia dolorosa is pain in an area or region that is anesthetic.

7. What is hyperalgesia?
Hyperalgesia is an increased response to a stimulus that is normally painful.

8. What is hyperesthesia?
Hyperesthesia is a increased sensitivity to any noxious or non-noxious stimulation of skin or mucosa, excluding the special senses; it includes allodynia and hyperalgesia.

9. What are the symptoms of hyperesthesia?
Patients describe a shooting, flashing, burning pain produced by normally nonpainful stimuli.

10. What is hyperpathia?
Hyperpathia is a painful syndrome characterized by increased reaction to a stimulus and increased threshold for response. It commonly is induced by repetitive mechanical pressures and characterized by faulty identification and localization of stimuli.

11. What is hypoalgesia?

Hypoalgesia is diminished pain response to normally painful stimulus.

12. Define paresthesia.

Paresthesia is an abnormal sensation, either evoked or spontaneous, that is not necessarily unpleasant or painful, as in dysesthesia.

13. What is sympathetically mediated pain (SMP)?

SMP is throbbing, diffuse, and hyperalgesic pain perpetuated by abnormal reflex activity in sympathetic pathways following peripheral nerve injury. The classic syndromes of causalgia and reflex sympathetic dystrophy are theorized to involve both peripheral and central mechanisms.

14. What are the symptoms of SMP?

The symptoms are often described as burning, hot, lancinating pain. Patients also complain of increased pain intensity during stressful periods.

15. What is Tinel's sign?

Tinel's sign is a provocative test of regenerating nerve sprouts in which light percussion over the nerve elicits a distal tingling sensation. It is used as a sign of small fiber recovery but is poorly correlated with functional recovery and easily confused with neuroma formation.

16. What is deafferentation pain?

Deafferentation pain is pain in body region of partial or complete traumatic peripheral nerve deficit in which retrograde central neuropathy has occurred. Deafferentation mechanisms have been implicated in phantom pain, hyperpathia, and allodynia.

17. How many axons are there in the inferior alveolar nerve?

Approximately 7000–12,000 axons and 10–24 fascicles.

18. What is the incidence of inferior alveolar and lingual nerve injury during removal of third molars?

The incidence of inferior alveolar, lingual, and, less frequently, long buccal nerve injury during mandibular third molar removal ranges between 0.6% and 5.0%. In general, the incidence of inferior alveolar nerve (IAN) injuries is higher than that of the lingual nerve; in one study, incidence was 1.2% for the IAN and 0.9% for the lingual nerve. Factors such as age, surgical technique, and proximity of the nerve to the tooth influence the incidence of these injuries. More than 96% of patients with lingual nerve injuries recover spontaneously.

19. What factors are associated with a higher incidence of lingual nerve injury during the course of third molar removal?

Lingually angled impactions are especially vulnerable to nerve injury during their removal because of the erosion or absence of the lingual cortical plate by infection or cyst exposing the nerve directly to damage during instrumentation to remove the tooth.

20. What is the average rate of an injured axons forward growth?

Approximately 1–2 mm/day.

21. List the potential clinical manifestations of a trigeminal nerve injury.

Nonpainful anesthesia and hypoesthesia
Painful anesthesia and hypoesthesia
Nonpainful hyperesthesia
Painful hyperesthesia

22. What is the recommended protocol for testing patients with decreased sensation without dysesthesia?

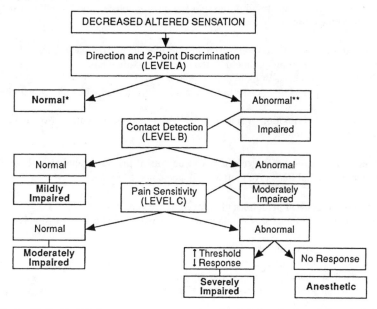

(From Zuniga JR, Essick GK: A contemporary approach to the clinical evaluation of trigeminal nerve injuries. Oral Maxillofac Surg Clin North Am 4:358–367, 1992, with permission.)

23. Outline the recommended nonsurgical treatment of chronic trigeminal dysfunction and dysesthesia.

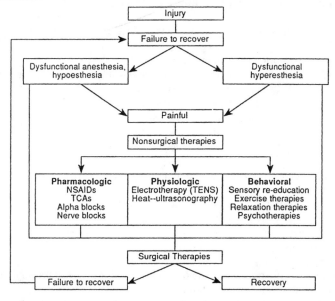

(From Allig CC, Schwartz E, Campbell RL, et al: Algorithm for diagnostic assessment and surgical treatment of traumatic trigeminal neuropathies and neuralgias. Oral Maxillofac Surg Clin North Am 4:555, 1992, with permission.)

24. How should open nerve injuries be managed?

If an open injury is observed, it is best managed with immediate primary repair. Delayed primary repair is performed within the first few postoperative days. A delayed secondary repair is performed more than 3 weeks after injury.

25. When should closed (unobserved) nerve injuries be addressed surgically?

Unobserved nerve injuries should be repaired if the patient has:

- Intolerable anesthesia of more than 3 months
- Painful symptoms that persist more than 4 months that may be relieved with proximal anesthetic block
- Intolerable deterioration of sensation beyond 4 months and no improvement of sensation beyond 4 months

26. What other method of nerve repair can be done if primary repair is not possible?

An interpositional free nerve graft and allogenic nerve guidance.

27. Explain the general principles of delayed nerve repair.

Repair must be completed without tension. First, extraneural decompression is performed to remove all irritative, foreign, or compressive forces from nerve contact. Next, the nerve must be inspected for continuity. If nerve continuity is seen, the nerve may be inspected with an epineural incision at the site of injury. Internal decompression (neurolysis) is performed and completed by closing the epineurium. If neuroma-in-continuity is too extensive, excision of neuroma along with part of the nerve is performed. A direct neurorrhaphy is performed in a tension-free manner.

28. What are the types of nerve repair?

Epineural, perineural, and group fascicular.

29. Which type of nerve repair is appropriate for the IAN?

Mixed motor and sensory nerves are best treated with the perineural and group fascicular suturing. The sensory IAN can be treated with the epineural suture technique.

30. What does coaptation refer to in nerve repair?

Bringing individual nerve fascicles into the best possible alignment. Direct neurorrhaphy can only be performed when the nerve is tension free.

31. If a defect is too large for a direct neurorrhaphy of the inferior alveolar nerve, which nerves may be considered as donors for free nerve graft?

The sural nerve, greater auricular, and median antebranchial nerves are considered.

32. What factors govern the choice of donor site for free nerve repair?

Accessibility

Diameter of donor nerve compared to the host nerve

Fascicular number and pattern

Length required

Patient preference

33. Which nerve is the best donor site for an interpositional graft for an inferior alveolar nerve defect of approximately 25 mm?

The sural nerve graft. The sural nerve can provide up to 30 mm of graft harvest. It provides sensation to the posterior and lateral aspect of the leg and foot. It also has up to 50% fewer axons and smaller axonal size than the inferior alveolar nerve.

34. Which free nerve may be used as a donor site for smaller defects (up to 15 mm long) of the IAN?

The greater auricular nerve can be used for short gaps (up to 15 mm). This nerve graft is a good match with the IAN in terms of axonal size and axonal numbers. However, compared to the host nerve, the greater auricular nerve is half the diameter and has half the fascicles. A cable graft (two parallel strands) may be used to provide a better size match.

35. How much nerve should be harvested for a nerve graft?

Because of primary contracture, the length of the harvested nerve should be at least 25% longer than the defect.

36. When is delayed nerve repair in the maxillofacial region indicated?

If a wound is grossly contaminated or if the mechanism of injury may cause scarring of the proximal and distal ends. Examples of such injuries are blunt, avulsive injuries such as gunshot wounds and injuries sustained in motor vehicle accidents.

37. How is the term *anastomose* applied to nerve injuries?

Trick question. Anastomose is not appropriate nomenclature when discussing nerve repair. Vessels are anastomosed, and nerves are repaired or reconstructed.

38. What type of sutures are most compatible for nerve repair?

Size 8.0 or 10.0 suture on a noncutting needle. Use the least tissue-reactive sutures (polyglycolic provokes less inflammation than nylon).

39. List potential alloplastic nerve conduits that may be used in nerve reconstruction.

For guided nerve growth up to 3 mm, the following nerve guides may be used for repair:
Collagen tubes
Polytetrafluoroethylene
Polyglycolic acid tubes

40. Describe a method for locating the great auricular nerve.

A line is drawn connecting the mastoid process and angle of mandible. A perpendicular line is then drawn to bisect the mastoid-mandible line. The great auricular nerve approximates this second line.

41. What is the success rate of microsurgical repairs of inferior alveolar and lingual nerve injuries?

	PATIENTS	SUCCESS*(%)	RANGE (%)	SEM
Hypoesthetic				
IAN	N = 192	85.4	66–94	3.68
Lingual nerve	N = 131	87.0	50–91	5.66
Hyperesthetic				
IAN	N = 124	55.6	25–80	7.01
Lingual nerve	N = 74	67.5	50–100	6.82

* Success defined as (1) minimum recovery of gross touch perception and (2) global pain reduction of > 30%. Overall success rate (N = 521) is 76.2%. SEM = standard error of the mean; IAN = inferior alveolar nerve.
Adapted from LaBanc JP, Gregg JM: Trigeminal nerve injuries: Basic problems, historical perspectives, early success, and remaining challenges. Oral Maxillofac Clin North Am 4:227–283, 1992.

BIBLIOGRAPHY

1. Allig CC, Schwartz E, Campbell RL, et al: Algorithm for diagnostic assessment and surgical treatment of traumatic trigeminal neuropathies and neuralgias. Oral Maxillofac Surg Clin North Am 4:555, 1992.

2. Donoff R: Surgical management of interior alveolar nerve injuries (part 1): Case for early repair. J Oral Maxillofac Surg 53:1327–1329, 1995.

3. Elusten K, Stevens M: Diagnosis and management of interior alveolar nerve injury. Compendium 16:1028–1038, 1995.

4. Greg J: Neurological complications of surgery for impacted teeth. In Alling CC, Helfric JF, Alling RD (eds): Impacted Teeth. Philadelphia, W.B. Saunders, 1993, pp 405–428.

5. Gregg J: Surgical management of inferior alveolar nerve injuries (part 2): Case for delayed management. J Oral Maxillofac Surg 53:1330–1335, 1995.

6. Gregg JM: Non-surgical management of traumatic trigeminal neuralgia and sensory neuropathies. Oral Maxillofac Surg Clin North Am 4:375–392, 1992.

7. LaBanc J: Reconstructive microneurosurgery of the trigeminal nerve. In Peterson LJ, et al (eds): Principles of Oral and Maxillofacial Surgery. Philadelphia, Lippincott, 1992, pp 1041–1087.

8. LaBanc JP, Van Bovan RW: Surgical management of inferior alveolar nerve injuries. Oral Maxillofac Surg Clin North Am 4:425–438, 1992.

9. LaBanc JP, Gregg JM: Glossary. Oral Maxillofac Surg Clin North Am 4:563, 1992.

10. Zuniga JR, Essick GK: A contemporary approach to the clinical evaluation of trigeminal nerve injuries. Oral Maxillofac Surg Clin North Am 4:353–367, 1992.

28. MAXILLOFACIAL TRAUMA

Ian McDonald, M.D., D.M.D., and Vincent B. Ziccardi, M.D., D.D.S.

1. What radiographs are included in a mandible series?

The mandible film series includes the right and left lateral oblique views, posteroanterior (PA) cephalogram, and reverse Towne's view. The lateral oblique views are useful to evaluate the body or ramus regions of the mandible. The PA view can assess the symphyseal region and evaluate the buccal-lingual displacement of body or angle fractures. The reverse Towne's view is helpful in assessing the mandibular condyles. Panoramic radiographs remain the gold standard for mandible fracture screening. Because these are seldom available in hospital radiology departments, an additional view that is oriented perpendicular to the lateral cortex can be substituted to accurately assess and diagnosis a fracture. A panoramic radiograph combined with a PA or reverse Towne's view is generally adequate for diagnosis.

2. What is a favorable fracture?

Favorability is determined by the forces exerted by the masticatory muscles on the fracture segments. A favorable fracture is one that is not displaced by masticatory muscle pull. Both horizontal and vertical components can be identified. The terms *horizontal* and *vertical* refer to the plane in which the fracture displacement is best visualized. Horizontal favorability is determined by cephalad-caudad stability while vertical favorability is evaluated in the buccal-lingual plane. An example of a horizontally favorable fracture is a body fracture where the inferior border is displaced above the superior border. In this instance, the pull of the pterygomasseteric sling would aid in stabilizing the reduction because of the fracture orientation.

3. What surgical techniques are available to treat mandible fractures?

The most frequently used treatment modalities available for the management of mandible fractures are:

- Closed reduction and maxillomandibular fixation with Ivy loops or arch bars
- Closed reduction and fixation with gunning splints secured to stable osseous structures (circummandibular or perialveolar wires)
- External pin fixation, used principally with comminuted and grossly contaminated fractures
- Open reduction with internal fixation using intra- or extraoral incisions and securing the segments with wires, plates, or lag screws with concomitant maxillomandibular fixation if rigid fracture fixation is not achieved

4. Name some of the common complications associated with mandibular fracture management.

Infection
Delayed union or nonunion usually resulting from infection or inadequate fixation
Malocclusion
Facial or trigeminal nerve injury
Damage to tooth roots
Hematoma
Wound dehiscence

5. What are the indications for removing a tooth in the line of fracture?

Because mandibular fractures commonly occur through the dental periodontal ligament space, much debate has been focused on whether or not to extract teeth in the line of fracture. By definition, a fracture that communicates with the oral cavity through the periodontal

ligament space is considered a compound fracture. The literature to date does not provide convincing evidence that infection is more likely to occur if a tooth is retained. Nonetheless, current recommendations for removal of teeth in the line of fracture include:
- Presence of obvious pathology such as caries or periodontal disease
- Gross mobility of involved teeth
- Teeth that prevent adequate reduction of fractures
- Teeth with fractured roots
- Teeth whose root surfaces or apices are exposed in the fracture site

6. What are the indications for open reduction and internal fixation of condylar fractures in adults?

Most fractures of the mandibular condyle are amenable to closed reduction with fixation and immobilization ranging from 7 to 21 days based on age of the patient, displacement of fracture, and number of other concomitant injuries. Intracapsular condylar fractures are generally treated with a short period of maxillomandibular fixation (10–14 days) followed by post-fixation physiotherapy to prevent ankylosis of the joint. The mandible will deviate clinically to the side of injury on opening because of unopposed pull of the contralateral lateral pterygoid.

Indications for open reduction of condylar fractures in adults were well described by Zide and Kent and divided into absolute and relative indications.

Absolute Indications
- Inability to obtain adequate occlusion using closed reduction techniques
- Displacement of the condyle into the middle cranial fossa
- Lateral extracapsular displacement of the condyle
- Foreign body in the joint capsule

Relative Indications
- Bilateral condylar fractures with concomitant comminuted midfacial fractures
- Bilateral fractures in an edentulous patient when splints are unavailable or impossible because of severe ridge atrophy
- Displaced condyle fracture in a medically compromised patient (e.g., seizure disorder, psychiatric problems, or alcoholism) with evidence of open bite or retrusion

7. What physical and radiologic findings are associated with zygomaticomaxillary orbital complex (ZMC) fractures?

Zygomatic fractures are commonly encountered in facial trauma because of their prominent position on the facial skeleton. They are second only to nasal fractures in frequency of involvement. Physical signs and symptoms associated with ZMC fractures include:
- Periorbital ecchymosis and edema.
- Subconjunctival hemorrhage that remains bright red for a prolonged period due to continued oxygen saturation of the blood through the oxygen-permeable conjunctiva.
- Flattening of the malar prominence or zygomatic arch.
- Step deformity and tenderness to palpation at the inferior orbital rim, zygomatic arch, frontozygomatic suture, or zygomatic buttress regions.
- Pain, especially in mobile fractures.
- Epistaxis on the side of fracture due to blood draining from the involved maxillary sinus. Direct nasal injury also must be ruled out.
- Diplopia (double vision), which results from displacement of the globe secondary to entrapment of extraocular muscles, edema, hematoma, neurologic injury, or increased orbital volume due to orbital floor defect or displacement of the lateral orbital wall.
- Infraorbital nerve paresthesia due to either direct trauma or impingement from the fractured segments of bone.
- Ecchymosis in the maxillary buccal vestibule (Guerin's sign).
- Trismus due to muscle spasm or the physical impingement of the coronoid process by the collapsed zygomatic arch.

Radiologic findings of ZMC fractures include:
- Waters' view or PA oblique demonstrates separation of frontozygomatic suture, possible distortion of orbital shape, steps in the orbital rim, or opacification of the ipsilateral maxillary sinus.
- Submental vertex view shows fractures of the zygomatic arch, which frequently presents with an M configuration. Rotation of the body of the zygoma around a vertical axis can also be assessed with this view.
- Computed tomography (CT) is the gold standard for assessing fracture location and displacement. Orbital defects as well as soft tissue injury can be evaluated accurately using both axial and coronal views.

8. Bilateral mandibular parasymphyseal fractures can predispose a patient to what potentially fatal outcome?

Bilateral parasymphyseal fractures result in a free-floating anterior mandibular segment. The genial tubercles are located on the lingual surface of the mandible to which the genioglossus muscle is attached. Lack of stability in this area allows for posterior displacement of the tongue with resultant airway embarrassment and inferior displacement by the suprahyoid musculature. This is known clinically as "gag bite" and can lead to death.

9. What management considerations are required in repairing an ear laceration?

A complete physical examination evaluating the pinna, external auditory canal, tympanic membrane, and hearing is essential prior to treatment of external ear injuries. The pinna is the most frequently lacerated component of the ear, consisting of a relatively avascular cartilage layer covered by a thin, but richly vascular, skin layer. Management includes local anesthesia without vasoconstrictor, conservative debridement, and placement of 6.0 nylon skin sutures aligning known landmarks and reapproximating the soft tissue envelope. Suturing the cartilaginous framework is seldom required; however, fine, permanent tacking sutures may be used. Hematoma formation requires drainage either through fine needle aspiration or a small incision to prevent future fibrosis and the aberrant cartilage formation known as "cauliflower ear deformity." Some type of pressure dressing is required to prevent reaccumulation of blood; this can be most easily accomplished using a transcartilaginous horizontal mattress suture and bolster dressing.

10. What anatomic structures need to be evaluated in a patient with a large through-and-through laceration of the cheek?

Cheek lacerations may involve several underlying vital structures including the parotid gland and duct, facial nerve branches, facial artery and its branches, and the buccal fat pad. Careful examination of the wound to identify these structures is warranted. Laceration of the parotid duct requires the placement of a stent and careful suturing of the cut ends with 6.0 nylon suture under magnification. Overlying tissues are then closed in layers. Gland injuries without duct involvement should be closed routinely and followed for sialocele or parotid fistula formation, which may be treated using pressure dressings or antisialogogues. Facial nerve lacerations proximal to a vertical perpendicular line through the lateral canthus are amenable to surgical repair. The buccal fat should be preserved and replaced if possible to prevent cosmetic deformity or cheek hollowing.

11. What is the significance of a nasal septal hematoma?

A nasal septal hematoma usually presents as a boggy, blue elevation of the septal mucosa. This finding is significant because it requires drainage to prevent secondary infection and necrosis of the septal cartilage leading to perforation and possible saddle nose deformity. Drainage can be accomplished by either needle aspiration or small mucosal incision. Transseptal resorbable sutures and nasal packing can be placed to prevent reaccumulation of blood.

12. What percentage of tissue can be lost without a significant cosmetic defect after primary closure in an avulsive injury of the upper and lower lips?

Avulsive injuries to the upper lip can involve 20–25% of lip structure and still be closed primarily without significant functional or cosmetic deformity. The lower lip is even more forgiving, allowing primary closure of defects involving 30–35% of lip structure. In all lip repairs, attention must be given to proper alignment of the vermilion border and orbicularis oris muscles. Significant avulsive injuries may be amenable to repair via Abbe or local rotational flaps.

13. What are the classical clinical findings in a patient with a naso-orbital-ethmoid (NOE) fracture?

The NOE fracture usually results from a direct blow to the bridge of the nose by a blunt object such as a steering wheel or dashboard during a motor vehicle accident. Patients classically present with a widened nasal bridge, periorbital edema and ecchymosis, epistaxis, cerebrospinal fluid (CSF) rhinorrhea (42%), and traumatic telecanthus (12–20%). Epiphora as an early or late finding indicates injury or outflow obstruction to the nasolacrimal apparatus. Treatment goals include restoration of normal intercanthal distance, fixation of the nasal bones, and careful evaluation and possible repair of the bony orbit and nasolacrimal apparatus.

14. What is difference between telecanthus and hypertelorism?

Telecanthus refers to a widening of the distance between the medial canthi, usually as a result of trauma such as NOE fractures. The normal caucasian adult intercanthal distance is approximately 33 mm. Hypertelorism is a widening of the orbits themselves and is measured as the interpupillary distance, normally 60 mm. Hypertelorism resulting from trauma is rare because tremendous force is required to fracture and displace the bony orbits. It is more commonly seen in congenital craniofacial deformities such as craniosynostosis.

15. Describe the etiologies of monocular and binocular diplopia.

Causes of monocular diplopia (double vision) include retinal detachment, dislocated lens, foreign body, uncorrected refractive error, cataract, and corneal opacity. This physical finding warrants immediate ophthalmologic consultation. Binocular diplopia is more common in the traumatic setting and may result from an alteration in globe position, such as proptosis or enophthalmos, or from limitation of globe movement through entrapment of orbital soft tissues. Alternatively, nerve injury may occur intracranially or within the orbit as a result of compression from hematoma or bone fragments. Surgical repair of the bony orbit and decompression of affected nerves result in correction of diplopia.

16. What is a blowout fracture of the orbit?

A blowout fracture of the orbit results from direct trauma to the globe resulting in distortion of the globe and increased intraorbital pressure. The orbital rim generally stays intact, and the force is transmitted to the interior area of the orbital cavity. The force is dissipated by outward fracture of the weaker bones of the orbital floor and medial wall. As force increases, the fractures may extend both posteriorly and circumferentially. A thorough physical examination and diagnostic imaging, specifically CT scanning, are required to evaluate the size of the defect and possible entrapment of orbital structures. Significant defects require operative repair to prevent post-traumatic enophthalmos.

17. What are the differences between superior orbital fissure syndrome and orbital apex syndrome?

Superior orbital fissure syndrome results from compression of the contents found in the superior orbital fissure by hematoma or bony fragment. Clinical findings include:
  • Pupillary dilation through dysfunction of cranial nerve (CN) III innervation of pupillary constrictor muscles

- Ophthalmoplegia secondary to palsy of CN III, IV, and VI
- Upper eyelid ptosis from levator palpebrae paresis
- Anesthesia of the forehead and loss of corneal reflex from ophthalmic division of the trigeminal nerve compression
- Proptosis secondary to edema from obstruction of the ophthalmic vein and lymphatic system

Orbital apex syndrome usually results from retrobulbar hematoma with compression of the optic canal and superior orbital fissure. Clinical findings include tense proptosis and periorbital swelling, retro-orbital pain, pupillary dilation, ophthalmoplegia, and, most importantly, a change in vision. Funduscopy reveals a pale disc with cherry red maculae. Prompt surgical decompression via lateral canthotomy is required to prevent permanent vision loss.

18. Why is the placement of a nasogastric tube sometimes contraindicated in a midface fracture patient?

Midface fractures commonly extend through the nasal cavity and may result in soft tissue disruption in the nasopharynx with concomitant cranial injuries. Inadvertent placement of a nasogastric tube in these patients may result in the intracranial placement of the tube or soft tissue dissection in a previously traumatized region.

19. Describe the different management considerations for frontal sinus fractures.

Management considerations following frontal sinus fractures include assessment of the following:

Fracture displacement defined as > 1 table-width

Injury to the nasofrontal duct

CSF leak

Displaced fractures of the outer table require reduction and fixation to prevent cosmetic deformities. Displaced fractures of only the inner table are seldom treated if no CSF leak exists. If CSF leak is present, cranialization (removal of inner table allowing the brain to expand forward and occupy the sinus space) and repair of the dura are recommended. If the frontonasal duct is injured, the sinus must be obliterated with an appropriate material such as fat, muscle, or bone. All sinus mucosa must be removed with a rotary instrument to prevent future potential mucocele or mucopyocele formation. The orifice of the frontonasal duct must also be packed to prevent ingrowth of the epithelium or migration of microorganisms from the nasal cavity.

20. What is the bowstring test and for what type of fracture assessment is it useful?

The bowstring test is a means of assessing the status of the medial canthal ligament in NOE fractures. Commonly, the ligament remains intact and attached to the lacrimal bone, which may be fractured and displaced. The bowstring test is performed by placing gentle lateral traction over the lateral canthus while palpating the medial canthal region to assess mobility. A positive test confirms bony fracture with displacement of the medial canthal ligament or traumatic telecanthus.

21. Describe the relationship between orbital volume changes as they relate to orbital trauma.

The normal volume of the bony orbit is approximately 30 cc. Fractures of orbital bones may increase or decrease this volume with resultant changes in the position of the orbital contents. Fractures that decrease orbital volume compress the orbital contents and may create exophthalmos. Increases in orbital volume provide more room for the globe and may result in dystopia or a change in the vertical position of the globe. Enophthalmos is a change in anterior-posterior position of the globe. Alterations in globe position as a function of orbital volume change are dependent on two factors: disruption of Lockwood's suspensory ligament and the relationship of the change in volume relative to the axis of the globe. The axis is defined as a line connecting the lateral orbital rim to an area just in front of the lacrimal bone. Volume changes behind this line can produce significant alterations in globe position. It is estimated that 1 ml of volume loss behind the axis produces 1.5 mm of enophthalmos. Anterior orbital floor and medial wall fractures are usually in front of the axis and produce minimal changes in globe position.

22. What is hyphema and how is it managed?

Hyphema is the layering of blood in the anterior chamber of the globe, usually from the tearing of blood vessels at the root of the iris. It may present with pain, blurred vision, and photophobia. Retinal hemorrhage is also found in over 50% of hyphemas. Management of hyphema is directed toward prevention of rebleeding, which occurs in 3–30% of cases. Rebleeds generally occur 3–5 days after injury, are usually more severe than the original injury, and may result in impaired vision, corneal staining, and glaucoma formation. Patients are usually admitted for bed rest and daily ophthalmologic evaluation. An eye patch is applied, and increased intraocular pressure is treated with topical beta-blockers and carbonic anhydrase inhibitors or mannitol if necessary. Aspirin is absolutely contraindicated in these patients.

23. What is a saddle nose deformity?

Saddle nose deformity is the concave appearance of the nasal dorsum that sometimes follows significant nasal trauma. It results from fracture and inferior displacement of the nasal bones, resulting in buckling of the cartilaginous septum and disruption of the upper lateral cartilage position. Late effects of the injury that amplify the deformity include septal collapse, which may result from septal hematoma formation, asymmetric septal growth, and scar contractures.

24. What is the appropriate management of dentoalveolar fractures?

Alveolar fractures are typically treated with reduction and verification of occlusion followed by fixation with arch bars or composite splints for 4–6 weeks. Maxillomandibular fixation is not required unless adequate stability cannot be achieved with single arch stabilization. Patients should eat a soft, non-chew diet throughout the period of fixation. Antibiotics are recommended because these fractures commonly involve the periodontal ligament space and are, therefore, classified as compound open fractures. Endodontic evaluation of the involved teeth is recommended because of their possible devitalization after trauma.

25. What is the management of avulsed teeth in the primary and permanent dentition?

Avulsed primary teeth usually require no treatment and are not replanted. Dental radiographs of the injured area are recommended to rule out retained root fragments and assess potential damage to the developing permanent dentition. Avulsed permanent teeth should be replanted as soon as possible because reimplantation success declines exponentially after 2 hours. If immediate reimplantation is not possible, Hank's balanced salt solution is recommended as a storage medium. Cool milk is an acceptable substitute followed by saline, saliva, and water in decreasing order of utility. The teeth should be inspected for any gross pathology or fractures prior to reimplantation, and the root surfaces and alveolar socket should be irrigated gently with no mechanical manipulation prior to reimplantation. After reimplantation and verification of occlusion, teeth should be splinted with a light passive wire and composite splint for 7–10 days. Antibiotic coverage for 5–10 days is generally recommended because these are open injuries. Initiation of endodontic therapy should begin 7–14 days after injury to minimize root resorption.

26. Describe the differences among subdural, subarachnoid, and epidural hemorrhages.

The central nervous system and the brain are enveloped by three layers known as the meninges. The outermost layer is the dura mater, the middle layer is the arachnoid mater, and the inner layer is the pia mater. Intracranial hemorrhages are named by their anatomic position relative to these structures. An epidural hematoma is blood collection between the inner cortex of the skull and the dura that results from a high-pressure bleed such as the middle meningeal artery. It is characterized by a period of unconsciousness followed by a lucid interval and then gradual worsening of neurologic status until coma. CT scan reveals a biconvex, lens-shaped, high-density lesion between the skull and brain with possible mass effect due to the increased pressure.

A subdural hematoma results from the accumulation of blood between the dura and arachnoid and usually occurs from acceleration-deceleration injuries with shearing of the bridging veins between the cerebral cortex and dural sinuses. Patients commonly present with signs of increasing intracranial pressure including lethargy, headache, altered consciousness, hemiparesis, or ipsilateral pupil dilation. Findings on CT scan include a crescent-shaped, high-density lesion over the cerebral cortex producing a mass effect if large enough. Prompt surgical decompression is indicated for symptomatic lesions.

Subarachnoid hemorrhage occurs when there is bleeding between the arachnoid and pia mater, usually resulting from a ruptured aneurysm or arteriovenous malformation. Patients report "the worst headache of my life" and present with neck stiffness, vomiting, hypertension, and loss of consciousness. CT scan demonstrates a diffuse, high-density signal in the cerebrospinal fluid (subarachnoid space). Neurosurgical intervention is the treatment of choice.

27. Describe the differences between primary and secondary healing in bone and soft tissue.

Primary healing in bone and soft tissue occurs when direct apposition of wound edges is present, whereas secondary healing occurs across an open wound or avulsive injury. In soft tissues, primary healing involves minimal re-epithelialization and collagen formation, allowing the wound to be "sealed" within 24 hours, which results in a lower incidence of infection and scar formation. Secondary healing involves re-epithelialization via migration from the wound edges, collagen deposition in the connective tissue, contracture, and remodeling. Healing is slower and results in scarring and wound depression.

Primary healing in bone is seen when the gap between bony edges is less than 1 mm and involves minimal fibrous tissue formation and no callus formation. Union occurs via bone remodeling units in which osteoclasts traverse the fracture site removing a core of bone through the fracture site and into the bone on the other side. Vessel ingrowth and eventual osteoblast deposition of bone follow until the fracture site is bridged with new bone. Secondary bone healing occurs in four stages:

1. Initial reaction in which a hematoma is formed and periosteal cells give rise to osteoblasts, fibroblasts, and chondroblasts. Collagen and cartilage are formed and capillary ingrowth begins.

2. Cartilaginous callus formation in which there is an increase in blood vessels, external cartilage begins calcification, osteoblasts proliferate, and osteoclasts become present. Internally, no fibrocartilage is formed and osteoblasts form a direct bony callus. This stage serves to stabilize the involved area.

3. Hard callus formation in which the cartilaginous callus undergoes calcification into woven bone.

4. Remodeling in which woven bone is replaced with more organized lamellar bone.

28. What are the most common facial fractures in an adult and child?

In an adult, the location of facial fractures is influenced by both the resistance of the bone to fracture and how prominent its position on the facial skeleton is. Adult facial fractures are most commonly seen in the nasal bones followed by the zygoma, mandible, and maxilla. In children, early growth in the cranium and orbits predisposes young children to frontal bone and orbital fractures. The mandible and maxilla are more elastic because of a high cancellous-to-cortical bone ratio. As a result, more greenstick and nondisplaced fractures are seen. The mandible becomes more susceptible to fracture in the mixed dentition stage because of weakening by the developing tooth buds. The zygoma and maxilla remain relatively protected until the paranasal sinuses aerate.

29. What is the most likely position of a displaced condylar fracture and why?

Condylar displacement usually occurs in an anteromedial direction secondary to the pull of the lateral pterygoid muscle. The patient will deviate to the side of the fracture upon opening because of the unbalanced action of the contralateral lateral pterygoid muscle.

30. What is the appropriate management of tongue lacerations?

The tongue has a very rich blood supply that can lead to significant bleeding. After local anesthesia administration, the wound is closed in layers with resorbable sutures. Large lacerations merit a thorough evaluation of the airway because of the possibility of significant swelling and posterior displacement of the tongue. Wounds should be explored and radiographs taken to rule out the presence of foreign bodies such as dental fragments.

31. What are the zones of the neck and how are they assessed in penetrating neck injuries?

Penetrating trauma to the neck carries significant risk of vascular injury. In an attempt to standardize management, three zones of the neck have been defined. Zone 1 extends from the clavicle to cricoid cartilage, zone 2 extends from the cricoid cartilage to mandibular angle, and zone 3 extends from the mandibular angle to base of skull. Diagnosis of vascular injury by physical examination or exploratory surgery is most easily accomplished in zone 2, whereas zone 1 and 3 injuries often remain obscure. Similarly, surgical repair of zone 2 injuries is frequently successful while repair of zones 1 and 3 is often fraught with danger. Consequently, arteriography and possible embolization are the recommended treatment modalities for wounds in zones 1 and 3.

32. Describe the management of epistaxis in the emergency department.

Anterior nasal epistaxis usually involves Kiesselbach's plexus, which is the confluence of the terminal ends of the superior labial, anterior ethmoid, and sphenopalatine arteries. Packing of this area with phenylephrine-soaked cotton pledgets is frequently successful. Direct visualization with a nasal speculum may allow direct cauterization with either electrocautery or silver nitrate sticks to be performed. Excessive cauterization should be avoided, however, in order to prevent subsequent septal perforation. Most commonly, sterile petrolatum-impregnated gauze is carefully packed in a layered manner and left in place for 2–5 days. Broad-spectrum antibiotic coverage should be initiated to prevent maxillary sinus infections caused by blockage of the middle meatus.

Posterior nose bleeds are more difficult to manage because the lack of posterior stops prevents creation pressure with packing. This frequently is managed by placing a Foley urinary catheter into the affected nares, inflating the balloon with saline, and pulling the balloon back to seal the nasopharynx and to allow packing to be placed around the Foley. Tension is maintained on the catheter by placing an umbilical clip on the catheter at the entrance of the nose. Commercially available posterior nasal balloons are also available.

33. What is Battle's sign and what is its clinical significance?

Battle's sign is ecchymosis posterior to the ear. It is generally indicative of a basilar skull fracture involving the middle cranial fossa. It is a relatively late sign presenting approximately 24 hours after injury. "Raccoon eyes" (bilateral periorbital ecchymosis) is commonly seen after fracture of the base of the anterior cranial fossa or maxillary fractures.

34. How do animal and human bites differ from other traumatic injuries?

Animal and human bites differ from other traumatic injuries because they are contaminated by the oral flora. Thorough cleansing and debridement of the wound with the use of copious normal saline irrigation is essential prior to closure. Facial wounds can then be closed in routine layered fashion. Wound infections from human bites are frequently caused by *Streptococcus* and *Staphylococcus* organisms. Serious infections may also be associated with *Eikenella*. Prophylactic antibiotic coverage with penicillin or amoxicillin–clavulonic acid is recommended. Unlike human bites, 50–75% of infections in animal bites are caused by *Pasteurella multocida*. Amoxicillin–clavulonic acid is recommended for prophylaxis in animal bites. Tetanus immunization is required for all bites, and rabies prophylaxis may be required when animals exhibit suspicious behavior.

35. How does muscle pull affect displacement of mandibular fractures?

Muscles involved in displacing mandibular fractures include the medial and lateral pterygoid, temporalis, masseter, digastric, geniohyoid, genioglossus, and mylohyoid. The lateral pterygoid displaces the condyle anteriorly and medially because of its insertion on the pterygoid fovea. Muscles attached to the ramus (i.e., temporalis, masseter, and medial pterygoid) result in superior and medial displacement of the proximal segment. As fractures progress anteriorly toward the cuspid region, the digastric, geniohyoid, genioglossus, and mylohyoid exert a posterior-inferior force on the distal segment.

36. When treating mandible fractures, what is a tension band?

During mandibular functioning, stress forces are exerted on the bone in different vectors depending on the location. The superior border is under tension while the inferior border is compressed. A rotational force is found in the parasymphyseal region. A tension band in mandibular fracture management refers to a mechanical means of resisting fracture displacement in the tension zone. This may be accomplished by a superior border plate if teeth are not in the way (i.e., a plate over the external oblique ridge in an angle fracture), an arch bar if stable teeth are present on both sides of the fracture, a superior border wire, or an eccentric dynamic compression plate at the inferior border.

37. Explain dynamic compression, eccentric dynamic compression, and passive plating in rigid fixation.

The concept of rigid internal fixation was designed to allow primary bone healing even under functional loading. In an effort to enhance stability, plates were developed that provide compressive forces across fracture lines. Passive plating provides rigid fixation without compression. Dynamic compression plates compress the fracture site by providing axial guiding inclines for the screw heads to slide down as the screw is tightened. The screws first engage the bone, and as they are tightened they are moved 0.8 mm toward the fracture site by the guiding incline. This produces a compressive force of approximately 300 kPa. Eccentric dynamic compression plates provide compressive forces in more than one direction by changing the direction of the guiding incline in the outer holes of the plate. This concept is useful when plating mandibular body fractures. A compression plate at both the superior and inferior border would ideally provide compression throughout the fracture but is usually not possible because of the presence of teeth superiorly and other vital structures. A single eccentric dynamic compression plate placed at the inferior border serves the same purpose by angling the guiding inclines of the outer holes toward the superior border of the mandible and eliminating the need for a superior border tension plate.

38. Name the possible etiologies of extraocular movement disorders following trauma.

Extraocular movements are controlled by the six extraocular muscles. The inferior, superior, medial rectus, and inferior oblique muscles are all innervated by CN III (oculomotor). The superior oblique muscle is innervated by the trochlear nerve (CN IV), and the lateral rectus muscle is supplied by the abducens nerve (CN VI). Traumatic disruption of either muscle or nerve continuity would likely result in a movement disorder manifested by limited gaze in the direction of affected muscle pull and binocular diplopia. Entrapment of muscle in traumatic bony defects (e.g., orbital floor blowout fracture) also may lead to restricted gaze.

39. What are the causes of traumatic ptosis?

Ptosis refers to the drooping of the upper eyelid. Normal resting eyelid position is mediated by the sympathetic nervous system by the superior cervical ganglion. The muscle endpoint of these nerves is Mueller's muscle, a smooth muscle that inserts on the upper tarsal plate. Disruption of the sympathetic fibers (e.g., in Horner's syndrome) leads to ptosis. The levator palpebrae superioris is responsible for voluntary eye opening and is innervated by CN III. Injury to this nerve or muscle also results in ptosis. Alteration in globe position may result in the appearance of ptosis despite full function of related nerves and muscles.

BIBLIOGRAPHY

1. Aminoff MJ, Greenberg DA, Simon RP: Clinical Neurology, 3rd ed. Stamford, CT, Appleton & Lange, 1995.
2. Assael LA: Maxillofacial Trauma. Part 1: Applying Science to Practice. Oral and Maxillofacial Surgery Clinics of North America. Vol. 10, no. 4. Philadelphia, W.B. Saunders, 1998.
3. Deangelis AJ, Backland LK: Traumatic dental injuries: Current treatment concepts. J Am Dental Assoc 129:1401–1414, 1998.
4. Ellis E 3rd: Treatment methods for fractures of the mandibular angle. J Craniomaxillofac Trauma 2:28–36, 1996.
5. Fonseca RJ, Walker RV, Betts NJ, Barber HD: Oral and Maxillofacial Trauma, 2nd ed. Philadelphia, W.B. Saunders, 1997.
6. Graper C, Milne M, Stevens MR: The traumatic saddle nose deformity: Etiology and treatment. J Craniomaxillofac Trauma 2:37–49, 1996.
7. Kaban LB (ed): Oral and Maxillofacial Surgery in Children and Adolescents. Oral and Maxillofacial Surgery Clinics of North America. Vol. 6, no. 1. Philadelphia, W.B. Saunders, 1994.
8. Posnick JC (ed): Craniomaxillofacial Fractures in Children. Oral and Maxillofacial Clinics of North America. Vol. 6, no. 1. Philadelphia, W.B. Saunders, 1994.
9. Schendel SA (ed): Orbital Trauma. Oral and Maxillofacial Surgery Clinics of North America. Vol. 5, no. 3. Philadelphia, W.B. Saunders, 1993.

29. ODONTOGENIC INFECTIONS

A. Omar Abubaker, D.M.D., Ph.D., and Kenneth J. Benson, D.D.S.

1. What is the source of the bacteria that cause most odontogenic infections?

Odontogenic infections are caused mostly by indigenous bacteria that normally live on or in the host. When such bacteria gain access to deeper tissues, they cause odontogenic infection.

2. What are the predominant bacteria found in the oral cavity?

AEROBES	ANAEROBES
Gram-positive rods	Gram-positive rods
Corynebacterium	*Actinomyces*
Rothia	*Lactobacillus*
Diphtheroids	*Propionibacterium acnes*
Gram-negative rods	*Bifidobacterium*
Eikenella corrodens	*Eubacterium*
Haemophilus	Clostridia
Enterobacteriaceae	Gram-negative rods
Klebsiella	*Bacteroides*
Pseudomonas	*B. gingivalis*
Escherichia	*B. intermedius*
Gram-positive cocci	*B. endontalis*
Streptococcus	*B. oralis*
Alpha hemolytic	*B. melaninogenicus*
Strep. salivarius	*Fusobacterium*
Strep. mitior	*F. nucleatum*
Strep. sanguis	*Wollinella*
Strep. mutans	*Capnocytophaga*
Strep. milleri	Gram-positive cocci
Beta hemolytic	*Peptostreptococcus*
Strep. pyogenes	*Streptococcus*
Enterococci	Gram-negative cocci
Staphylococcus	*Veillonella*
Staph. aureus	
Staph. epidermidis	
Gram-negative cocci	
Neisseria	
Branhamella	
Spirochetes	
Treponema	
Fungi	
Candida	

Adapted from Peterson LJ: Microbiology of head and neck infections. Oral Maxillofacial Surg Clin 3:247–258, 1991.

3. Which species of bacteria cause odontogenic infection?

Most of the micro-organisms associated with odontogenic infections are gram-negative rods (fusobacteria, bacteroides). Some are gram-positive cocci (streptococci and peptostreptococci), and 25% are aerobic, mostly gram-positive streptococci. About 60% are anaerobic

207

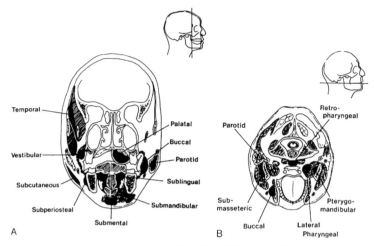

Anatomy of the deep space infections. **A**, Coronal and **B**, axial sections of the head showing most of the deep fascial spaces of the head and neck. (From Flynn TR, Topazian C: Infections of the oral cavity. In Wait DE (ed): Textbook of Practical Oral and Maxillofacial Surgery, 3rd ed. Philadelphia, Lea & Febiger, 1987; with permission.)

bacteria. Almost all odontogenic infections are caused by multiple bacteria (an average of five species). *Fusobacterium* spp. is associated with severe infections.

Species of Bacteria Responsible for Odontogenic Infections

ORGANISM	PERCENTAGE
Aerobic[†]	25
Gram-positive cocci	85
Streptococcus spp.	90
Streptococcus (group D) spp.	2
Staphylococcus spp.	6
Eikenella spp.	2
Gram-negative cocci (*Neisseria* spp.)	2
Gram-positive rods (*Corynebacterium* spp.)	3
Gram-negative rods (*Haemophilus* spp.)	6
Miscellaneous and undifferentiated	4
Anaerobic[*]	75
Gram-positive cocci	30
Streptococcus spp.	33
Peptococcus spp.	33
Peptostreptococcus spp.	33
Gram-negative cocci (*Viellonella* spp.)	4
Gram-positive rods	14
Eubacterium spp.	
Lactobacillus spp.	
Actinomyces spp.	
Clostridia spp.	
Gram-negative-rods	50
Bacteroides spp.	75
Fusobacterium spp.	25
Miscellaneous	6

[†] 49 different species.   [*] 119 different species.
Adapted from Peterson LJ: Principles of management and prevention of odontogenic infection. In Peterson LJ, Ellis E, Hupp J, Tucker M (eds): Contemporary Oral and Maxillofacial Surgery, 2nd ed. St. Louis, Mosby, 1998, pp 392–417.

4. Which staphylococci are clinically important to orofacial infections?

Of the 23 species of staphylococci, only three are clinically important to orofacial infections: *Staphylococcus aureus*, *Staphylococcus epidermidis*, and *Staphylococcus saprophyticus*.

5. What is coagulase? Which *Staphylococcus* species produces coagulase?

Coagulase is an enzyme that coats the bacteria with fibrin and reduces the ability of the host cell to phagocytize it. *S. aureus* is the only coagulase-positive staphylococci.

6. What is the basis for microbiologic diagnosis of odontogenic infection?

Initially, an empirical diagnosis of the causative organism of odontogenic infection is made, based on the presumption of involvement of bacteria typical for the site (oral flora). The microbiologic diagnosis stems from this presumption, and can be confirmed via Gram stain and culture.

7. What is Gram staining? What is its clinical significance?

Each specimen obtained from a patient with an infectious process initially should be stained according to the protocol developed by Hans Christian Joachim Gram. The process involves staining, decolorizing, and restaining the specimen with a different stain. The organisms are categorized into one of four groups based on their stain retention and morphology: gram-positive cocci, gram-negative cocci, gram-negative rods, or gram-positive rods. Because Gram staining can be completed within a few minutes, it usually narrows the list of likely causative organisms immediately, whereas culture and sensitivity testing and biochemical identification may take 1–5 days to complete.

8. Describe the Gram stain process.

- The smear of specimen is heat-fixed to the slide and stained with crystal violet. The cells will appear dark blue or purple.
- The slide is placed in a dilute solution of iodine, which further fixes the violet stain to the cell by forming a crystal-violet-iodine complex.
- The slide is rinsed in a 95% solution of alcohol, or alcohol and acetone. The cell walls of micro-organisms with high lipid contents develop porosities, allowing for loss of the violet stain. In organisms with more carbohydrates in their cell walls, the violet stain-iodine complex is further fixed by the alcohol.
- The specimen is counterstained with a red dye, safranin. Organisms that retained their initial stain will remain violet (gram positive), whereas those that lost the initial stain will be restained red (gram negative).

9. How do morphologic findings relate to bacterial categories?

MORPHOLOGIC FINDINGS	BACTERIAL SPECIES
Gram-positive cocci, single or clumps	Micrococcus, Peptococcus, Staphylococcus
Gram-positive cocci, pairs and chains	Enterococcus, Peptostreptococcus, Streptococcus
Gram-positive rods, large	Bacillus, Clostridium
Gram-positive rods, small	Arachnia, Bacterionema, Bifidobacterium, Corynebacterium, Erysipelothrix, Eubacterium, Lactobacillus, Listeria, Propionibacterium
Gram-positive rods, branching	Actinomyces, Nocardia
Gram-negative rods, large	Enterobacteriaceae
Gram-negative rods, thin, uniform	Pseudomonas

(Table continued on next page.)

MORPHOLOGIC FINDINGS	BACTERIAL SPECIES
Gram-negative rods, small, coccobacillary	Bacteroides, Bordetella, Brucella, Capnocytophaga, Cardiobacterium, Eikenella, Fusobacterium, Haemophilus, Pasteurella
Gram-negative rods, nonspecific morphology	Alcaligenes, Campylobacter, Cardiobacterium, Chromobacterium, Flavobacterium, Helicobacter, Pectobacterium, Vibrio, Yersinia
Gram-negative cocci, pairs	Acinetobacter, Moraxella, Neisseria
Gram-negative cocci	Veillonella

Adapted from Bartlett RC: Laboratory diagnostic techniques. In Tobazian RG, Goldberg MH (eds): Oral and Maxillofacial Infections, 3rd ed. Philadelphia, W.B. Saunders, 1994, p 88.

10. Describe the progression of odontogenic infections.

Early infection is often initiated by high-virulence aerobic organisms (commonly streptococci), which cause cellulitis, followed by mixed aerobic and anaerobic infections. As the infections become more chronic (abscess stage), the anaerobic bacteria predominate, and eventually the infection becomes exclusively anaerobic.

11. What is cellulitis?

Cellulitis is a warm, diffuse, erythematous, indurated, and painful swelling of the tissue in an infected area. Cellulitis can be easy to treat, but can also be severe and life threatening. Antibiotics and removal of the cause are usually sufficient. Surgical incision and drainage are indicated if no improvement is seen in 2–3 days, or if evidence of purulent collection is identified.

12. What is an abscess?

An abscess is a pocket of tissue containing necrotic tissue, bacterial colonies, and dead white cells. The area of infection may or may not be fluctuant. The patient is often febrile at this stage. Cellulitis, which may be associated with abscess formation, is often caused by anaerobic bacteria.

13. What is the difference between an abscess and cellulitis?

	CELLULITIS	ABSCESS
Duration	Acute	Chronic
Pain	Severe and generalized	Localized
Size	Large	Small
Localization	Diffuse borders	Well circumscribed
Palpation	Doughy to indurated	Fluctuant
Presence of pus	No	Yes
Degree of seriousness	Greater	Less
Bacteria	Aerobic	Anaerobic

Adapted from Peterson LJ: Principles of management and prevention of odontogenic infection. In Peterson LJ, Ellis E, Hupp J, Tucker M (eds): Contemporary Oral and Maxillofacial Surgery, 2nd ed. St. Louis, Mosby, 1998.

14. List the signs and symptoms of a serious orofacial infection.

Serious infection occurs when the infection extends beyond the local area of infection and presents life-threatening systemic manifestations, including airway compromise, bacteremia,

septicemia, fever, lethargy, fatigue, malaise, and dehydration. Presence of swelling, induration, fluctuation, trismus, rapidly progressing infection, involvement of secondary spaces,
dysphagia, odynophagia, and drooling are also signs and symptoms of serious orofacial infection.

15. What factors influence the spread of odontogenic infection?
- Thickness of bone adjacent to the offending tooth
- Position of muscle attachment in relation to root tip
- Virulence of the organism
- Status of patient's immune system

16. What are the *primary* fascial spaces?
The spaces directly adjacent to the origin of the odontogenic infections. Infections spread
from the origin into these spaces, which are:

Vestibular	Submental
Canine	Sublingual
Buccal	Submandibular

17. What are the *secondary* fascial spaces?
Fascial spaces that become involved following spread of infection to the primary spaces.
The secondary spaces are:

Pterygomandibular	Infratemporal
Masseteric	Lateral pharyngeal
Superficial and deep temporal	Retropharyngeal
Masticator	Prevertebral

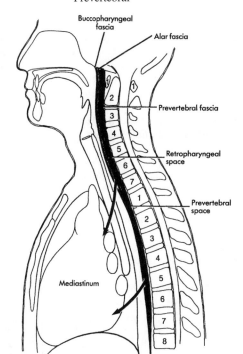

Retropharyngeal and prevertebral spaces, with the potential for spread of infection to the mediastinum
from these spaces. (From Cumming CW, et al (eds): Otolaryngology: Head and Neck Surgery, Vol. 2. St.
Louis, Mosby, 1986; with permission.)

18. What is the danger space?

Also called space 4 of Grodinsky and Holyoke, it is the potential space between alar and prevertebral fascia. Its superior limit is the skull base, and it extends inferiorly into the posterior mediastium.

19. List the seven spaces of Grodinsky and Holyoke in the head and neck.

Space 1	Between platysma and investing fascia
Space 2	Between investing and infrahyoid fascias
Space 2a	Space among infrahyoid muscles
Space 3	The pretracheal and retrovisceral spaces
Space 4	Danger space and B/W prevertebral and alar fascia
Space 4a	Between prevertebral and investing fascia above clavicle
Space 5	Space within prevertebral fascia

20. Which teeth are likely to be the cause of space infections? What are the surgical approaches for incision and drainage of these spaces?

See the table on the following pages.

21. What imaging and laboratory studies are used for diagnosis of odontogenic infections?

- Radiographs to identify the cause of infection: periapical, occlusal, and panoramic views.
- Imaging studies to identify the extent of infection and presence of purulent collection: computed tomography (CT), magnetic resonance imaging (MRI), soft tissue films, and ultrasound.
- Laboratory studies to evaluate the immune system: white cell and differential counts.

22. What are the principles of therapy for odontogenic infection?

The important components in treatment of odontogenic infection are:
- Determining the severity of infection
- Determining whether the infection is at the cellulitis or abscess stage
- Evaluating the state of the patient's host defense mechanisms.

Odontogenic infection is treated surgically, pharmacologically, or by medical support of the patient, including removing the source of infection, incision and drainage, and use of antibiotics, fluids, analgesics, and nutritional support.

23. How is the severity of odontogenic infection determined?

By analyzing the history, the physical findings, and the results of laboratory and imaging studies.

24. List the different methods of drainage of odontogenic infections.

- Endodontic treatment
- Extraction of the offending tooth
- Incision and drainage of soft tissue collection

25. What are the surgical principles of incision and drainage?

- Prior to incision, obtain fluid for culture through aspiration of pus using a syringe and needle.
- Incise the abscess in healthy skin or mucosa and in a cosmetically or functionally acceptable place, using blunt dissection and thorough exploration of the involved space.
- Use one-way drains in intraoral abscesses; use through-and-through drainage for extraoral cases.
- Remove the drain gradually from deep sites.

Teeth Likely to Cause Fascial Space Infections, With Surgical Approaches

FASCIAL SPACE	ANATOMIC BOUNDARIES OF SPACE	LIKELY SOURCE OF INFECTION	SWELLING SITE	SITE OF I & D
Canine	Between canine fossa, zygomaticus, orbicularis oris, levator labii superiors and levator anguli oris	Maxillary canines, especially with very long roots and apex situated above attachment of muscles. May also be caused by central, lateral or premolar teeth	Extraoral swelling just lateral to nose, obliterating nasolabial fold and may extend upwards causing periorbital cellulites. May be in labial sulcus	Intraoral incision in horizontal direction in mucobuccal fold. Rarely, space is drained extraorally
Buccal	Check area between buccinator and buccopharyngeal fascia medially, overlying skin laterally, zygomatic muscle and depressor muscles anteriorly, zygomatic arch superiorly, lower border of mandible inferiorly, and pterygomandibular raphe posteriorly	Upper premolars Upper molars and lower premolars	Extraoral swelling over cheek area between inferior border of mandible and zygomatic arch. Typically, if inferior border of mandible palpable, it is buccal space; if inferior border not palpable, then involved space is submandibular	Intraoral by a transverse incision to depth of buccinator muscle passing through mucosa, submucosa, and buccinator muscle, avoiding injury to important anatomical structures such as parotid duct. Drainage also accomplished by extraoral incision near point of fluctuance below Stenson's duct
Sublingual	Above mylohyoid muscle. Roof of space is mucosa of floor of mouth; floor is made by mylohyoid, genioglossus, geniohyoid, and styloglossus muscles, tongue, and lingual frenum (medial raphe).	From teeth of root apices above mylohyoid muscle attachment, namely lower premolars and sometimes first molars	Infection spread lingual in floor of mouth causing sublingual swelling involving contralateral side (because barrier between two sides is very weak)	Intraoral incision parallel to Worton's duct and lingual cortex in anteroposterior direction, as close as possible (within 1 cm) to lingual cortical bone because sublingual fold contains sublingual gland and duct of submandibular gland. Intraoralextraoral approach may be used.

(Table continued on next page.)

Teeth Likely to Cause Fascial Space Infections, With Surgical Approaches (cont.)

FASCIAL SPACE	ANATOMIC BOUNDARIES OF SPACE	LIKELY SOURCE OF INFECTION	SWELLING SITE	SITE OF I & D
Submandibular	Below mylohyoid muscle. Lies inferior to mylohyoid muscle; inferior boundary is anterior and posterior bellies of diagastric muscles. Medially, mylohyoid hyoglossus, and styloglossus muscles bound space. Lateral boundary is skin, superficial fascia, platysma muscle, superficial layer of deep cervical fascia, and lateral border of mandible.	Lower molars, especially lower second and third molars	Swelling mostly extraoral due to pus accumulation between skin and mylohyoid muscle. Swelling begins by obliterating inferior border of mandible, then extends medially to anterior belly of diagastric and posterior to hyoid bone.	Through extraoral incision parallel to inferior border of mandible, kept at least 1 cm from border to avoid injury to mandibular branch of facial nerve, submandibular gland, facial artery, and lingual nerve
Submental	Between hyoid bone and symphysis, at site of attachment of anterior belly of diagastric muscle. Roof of space is mylohyoid muscle, floor is skin, laterally is anterior belly of digastric muscle.	Lower incisors and canines, or from trauma such as symphyseal fracture	Mostly extraoral. Submentally, chin and sub-mental areas swollen. Pus situated between diagastric muscle, mylohyoid muscle, and skin. Rarely, there is submental swelling only. Usually submandibular and submandibular swelling because boundaries between two spaces is not definitive (only digastric muscle), so pus travels posteriorly to submandibular region.	Extraoral transverse incision midway between symphysis and hyoid bone.
Masseteric	Between outer surface of ascending ramus medially and masseter muscle laterally	Can spread from a buccal space infection at site of attachment of buccinator muscle. Also from	Extraoral swelling over area occupied by masseter muscles, which is over ascending ramus and	Approximately 4 cm long incision made below and behind angle of ascending ramus. Dis-

(Table continued on next page.)

Teeth Likely to Cause Fascial Space Infections, With Surgical Approaches (cont.)

FASCIAL SPACE	ANATOMIC BOUNDARIES OF SPACE	LIKELY SOURCE OF INFECTION	SWELLING SITE	SITE OF I & D
Masseteric (cont.)		pericoronitis of lower third molars, or from fracture of angle of mandible.	angle of mandible. Infection of this space characterized by trismus due to involvement of muscles of mastication.	section carried through skin, superficial fascia, and platysma muscles. When inserting, artery forceps should remain in contact with outer aspect of ascending ramus. Incision can be used to approach 2 spaces (masseteric and pterygoid mandibular). Masseteric space can also be drained through an intraoral incision or a combined intraoral-extraoral approach.
Pterygoidmandibular	Between ascending ramus and medial pterygoid muscle medially; laterally is inner surface of ascending ramus. Superiorly, space bound by lateral pterygoid muscle, posteriorly by parotid gland, and anteriorly by pterygoid mandibular raphe and superior constrictor of pharynx	Can result from infection of molar teeth, especially third molar; spread from infratemporal space which communicates freely with pterymandibular space; septic inferior dental nerve block with contaminated needle or solution; pericoronitis; spread from submandibular space infection; spread from sublingual space.	Intraoral swelling of mucosa over medial aspect of the ascending ramus. Extraorally, swelling extremely rare, but if seen is found near mandibular angle area. Sometimes no extraoral swelling at all, only trismus due to involvement of medial pterygoid muscle, especially when infection caused by inferior dental nerve block.	Can be drained extraorally at angle of mandible. When inserting, artery forceps should remain in contact with inner surface of ascending ramus. This space can also be drained through intraoral incision placed just medial to pterygomandibular raphe and by dissecting posteriorly along medial surface of ramus of mandible. Incision can also be used to drain lateral pharyngeal space and inferior portion of infratemporal space.

(Table continued on next page.)

Teeth Likely to Cause Fascial Space Infections, With Surgical Approaches (cont.)

FASCIAL SPACE	ANATOMIC BOUNDARIES OF SPACE	LIKELY SOURCE OF INFECTION	SWELLING SITE	SITE OF I & D
Temporal	Muscle divides into two spaces: superficial temporal between temporalis muscle and temporal fascia, and deep temporal space (infratemporal space) between temporalis muscle and bony wall of skull medially. Temporal space is contiguous pterygomandibular and masseteric spaces.	Infection usually originates from upper and lower molars, or from extension of infection from masseteric or pterygomandibular spaces through infratemporal space, or from spread of infection from posterior superior alveolar nerve block.	Extraoral swelling just behind lateral orbital rim and above zygomatic arch	Infection of this space almost always associated with trismus; thus is difficult to approach intraorally. Extraoral approach more practical, but intraoral is preferred. Intraoral site for I&D is placed at anterior border of ascending ramus, with forceps inserted on outer aspect of ascending ramus and directed up. Extraoral incision is through transverse incision starting slightly superior to zygomatic arch extending posteriorly between lateral orbital rim and hairline. Incision is made parallel to it to avoid zygomatic branch of facial nerve.
Lateralpharyngeal	Inverted cone shape extending from base of skull to hyoid bone. Situated just medial to pterygoid mandibular space. Lateral wall made up of medial pterygoid muscle and superior constrictor muscle. Posteriorly, boundary is parotid gland, and anteriorly is pterygoid mandi-	Infection can result from infection of lower and upper molars by way of neighboring spaces such as submandibular or pterygomandibular spaces. Can also result from non-odontogenic sources such as palatine tonsils, infected parotid gland, and infected lymph nodes. If infection	Most common site is an intraoral swelling of lateral pharyngeal wall (very characteristic). Medial displacement of uvula and palatal draping may also be present. Extraoral lateral swelling of neck immediately below angle of mandible and anterior to anterior border of sternocleidomas-	Intraoral drainage of anterior compartment via a similar incision to that of intraoral incision for drainage of pterygomandibular space. Incision made through mucosa, and dissection directed medially and posteriorly along medial side of medial pterygoid muscle. Extra-

(Table continued on next page.)

Teeth Likely to Cause Fascial Space Infections, With Surgical Approaches (cont.)

FASCIAL SPACE	ANATOMIC BOUNDARIES OF SPACE	LIKELY SOURCE OF INFECTION	SWELLING SITE	SITE OF I & D
Lateralpharyngeal (cont.)	bular raphe. Medial wall is continuous with carotid sheath. Styloid process divides this space into 2 compartments: anterior compartment, which contains mainly muscles, and posterior compartment, which contains several important structures, namely carotid sheath inside which are external carotid artery, internal jugular vein, and cranial nerve X. Outside sheath are CN IX, XI, and XII	of this space is not treated at early stage, it can readily spread to retropharyngeal and prevertebral spaces	toid muscle also possible	oral approach through horizontal incision made at level of hyoid bone just anterior to sternocleidomastoid. Dissection made superiorly and medially between submandibular gland and posterior belly of diagastric muscle until medial surface of medial pterygoid muscle reached. Dissection carried along surface of muscle into space. Space can also be drained using through-and-through drainage.
Retropharyngeal	Extending from base of skull superiorly to upper mediastinum inferiorly (level of C6 or T1 behind posterior pharyngeal wall). Anteriorly, space is bounded by posterior wall of pharynx and posterior to it lies "danger space" which communicates with posterior mediastinum.	Spreads from upper and lower molars by extension from lateral pharyngeal space by way of pterygomandibular, submandibular, or sublingual spaces. Retropharyngeal and lateral pharyngeal spaces separated by thin layer of fascia, which can easily rupture and cause spread of infection. Infection of retropharyngeal space may also result from nasal and pharyngeal infection in children, esophageal trauma, foreign bodies, and TB.	If able to visualize pharynx, bulge of posterior pharyngeal wall will be noticed—usually unilateral. Lateral soft-tissue radiographs or CT will better delineate extent of swelling.	Extraoral approach by incision parallel to and along anterior border of sternocleidomastoid muscle below hyoid bone. Muscle and carotid sheath are retracted laterally, and a finger is inserted posterior to inferior constrictor. A soft noncollapsable rubber drain is preferred because of deep location of this space

I & D = incision and drainage

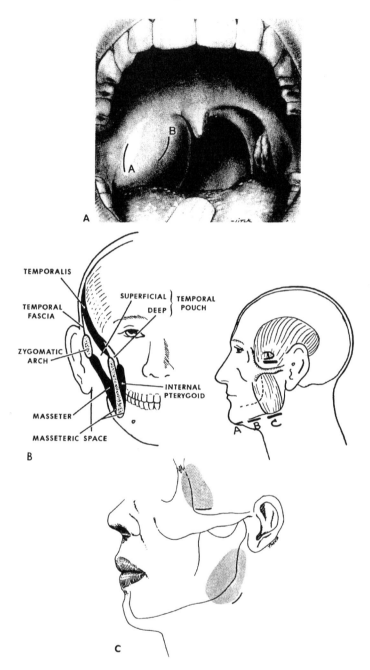

Typical sites of incision and drainage for various fascial space infections. **A**, Intra-oral drainage of pterygoid compartment of masticator space (A), and lateral pharyngeal space (B). **B**, Masseteric, pterygoid,
and temporal compartments of the masticator space. Incisions at (B) and (C) can be used to drain the submandibular space. **C**, Suggested locations for incision for extra-oral drainage of temporal and lateral pharyngeal space infections. (From Goldberg MH, Topazian RG: Odontogenic infections and deep fascial
space infections of dental origin. In Topazian RG, Goldberg MH (eds): Oral and Maxillofacial Infections,
3rd ed. Philadelphia, W.B. Saunders, 1994; with permission.)

26. What is the percentage of oral bacteria resistant to commonly used antibiotics for treatment of odontogenic infection?

	ORAL BACTEROIDS	FUSO-BACTERIA	ANAEROBIC COCCI	ALPHA STREPTOCOCCI
Penicillin	15–30	6	4	0
Erythromycin	0	85	18	0
Clindamycin	4	0	2	0
Metronidazole	0	0	24	100
Cephalexin	10	0	6	18

Adapted from Peterson LJ: Microbiology of head and neck infections. Oral Maxillofacial Surg Clin 3:255, 1991.

27. What should you look for on the follow-up appointment after treating a patient for odontogenic infection?
- Response to treatment
- Recurrence of infection
- Presence of allergic reactions
- Toxicity reactions to antibiotics
- Secondary infection (e.g., *Candida*)

28. What are the principles of antibiotic use?
When choosing a specific antibiotic as part of treatment of odontogenic infection, adhere to the following principles:
- Use the correct and narrow-spectrum antibiotic.
- Use the least toxic drug with the fewest side effects.
- Use bactericidal drugs whenever possible.
- Be aware of drug cost.
- Ensure effective oral administration through the use of proper dose and proper dosage interval.
- Continue the antibiotic for an adequate length of time.
- Administer the antibiotics through the proper route.

29. Name the most commonly used antibiotic formulations for oral and maxillofacial infections.

DRUG	TYPES	FORMULATIONS	UNIT DOSE
Penicillin G			
Potassium	Generic, Pfizerpen	Vial for IM, IV	1-, 5-, and 20-million units
Sodium	Generic	Vial for IM, IV	5-million units
Repository	Bicillin CR	Vial for IM	300–600,000 units/ml
Penicillin V	Generic, Betapen VK, Pen Vee K, Veetids	Tablets Oral solution	250, 500 mg 125, 250 mg/5 ml
Ampicillin	Generic, Omnipen, Poly-cillin, Principen	Capsules Oral suspension Pediatric drops Vial	250, 500 mg 250 mg/5 ml 100 mg/ml 125, 250, 500, 1000, 2000 mg
Amoxicillin	Generic, Amoxil, Polymox, Trimex, Wymox	Capsule Oral suspension Pediatric drops	250, 500 mg 125, 250 mg/5 ml 50 mg/ml

(*Table continued on next page.*)

DRUG	TYPES	FORMULATIONS	UNIT DOSE
Amoxicillin-clavu-lanate	Augmentin	Tablets Tablets (chewable) Oral suspension	250, 500 mg 125, 250 mg 125, 250 mg/5 ml
Oxacillin	Generic, Prostaphlin	Capsules Oral solution Vials for IM, IV	250, 500 mg 250 mg/5 ml 250, 500, 1000 mg
Dicloxacillin	Generic, Dynapen, Pathocil	Capsules Oral suspension	250, 500 mg 62.5 mg/5 ml
Cefalexin	Generic, Keflex	Capsules/Pulvules Tablets Oral suspension Pediatric drops	250, 500 mg 250, 500, 1000 mg 125, 250 mg/5 ml 100 mg/ml
Cephradine	Generic, Anspor, Velosef	Capsules Oral suspension Vial for IM, IV	250, 500 mg 125, 250 mg/5 ml 250, 500, 1000 mg
Cefazolin	Generic, Ancef, Kefzol	Vial for IM, IV	250, 500, 1000 mg
Cefaclor	Ceclor	Pulvules Oral suspension	250, 500 mg 125, 250 mg/5 ml
Cefoxitin	Mefoxin	Vial for IM, IV	1000 mg
Erythromycin			
Base	Generic, ERYC, Ilotycin, E-mycin, Ery-Tab	Tablets	250, 500 mg
Estolate	Generic, Ilosone	Tablets Tablets (chewable) Oral suspension Pediatric drops	250, 500 mg 125 mg 125, 250 mg/5 ml 100 mg/ml
Ethylsuccinate	Generic, EES, Ery Ped, Eryzole, Pediamycin	Tablets Tablets (chewable) Oral suspension Pediatric drops	400 mg 200 mg 200, 400 mg/5 ml 100 mg/2.5 ml
Clindamycin	Generic, Cleocin	Capsules Oral solution Vial for IM, IV	75, 150, 300 mg 75 mg/5 ml 250, 500, 750 mg
Chloramphenicol	Chloromycetin	Capsule Oral suspension Vial for IV	250 mg 150 mg/5 ml 1000 mg
Vancomycin	Generic, Vancocin	Capsules Oral solution Vial for IV	125, 250 mg 250 mg/5 ml 500, 1000 mg
Metronidazole	Generic, Flagyl, Protostate	Tablets Vial for IV	250 mg 500 mg
Nystatin	Generic, Mycostatin, Nilstate	Tablets Oral suspension Pastilles	500,000 units 100,000 units/ml 200,000 units
Clotrimazole	Mycelex	Troche	10 mg
Ketoconazole	Nizoral	Tablets	200 mg
Acyclovir	Zovirax	Capsules Ointment Vial for IV	200 mg 5% concentration 500 mg

Adapted from Hupp JR: Antibacterial, antiviral, and antifungal agents. Oral Maxillofacial Surg Clin 3:275, 1991.

30. Describe minimal inhibitory concentration (MIC) of antibiotics.

MIC is a measure of sensitivity of bacteria. For an antibiotic to have maximum antibiotic efficacy in treatment of specific infections, the concentration of the antibiotic at the site of infection should be 3–4 times the MIC. Concentrations > 4 times the MIC are not more effective.

31. What is the β-lactam group of antibiotics?

These antibiotics, which have in common a β-lactam ring in their structures, comprise three classes: penicillins, cephalosporins, and carbapenems. Penicillins and cephalosporins encompass many different antibiotics that are commonly used for odontogenic infection. Imipenem is an example of the carbapenems.

32. What was the first carbapenem to be used clinically?

Imipenem was the first clinically available carbapenem. It has the broadest antibacterial activity of any currently used systemic antibiotic and, therefore, is reserved for use in treatment of severe head and neck infections.

33. Describe the mode of action of penicillin.

Penicillin affects bacteria by two mechanisms:
1. It inhibits bacterial cell wall synthesis.
2. It activates endogenous bacterial autolytic processes that cause cell lysis. The bacteria must be actively dividing, and the cell wall must contain peptidoglycans for this action. The penicillin inhibits enzymes necessary for cell wall synthesis.

34. How do bacteria build up resistance to antibiotics?

An antibiotic's ability to penetrate cell walls and bind to enzymes plays an essential role in resistance of antibiotics. Specifically, bacteria build resistance by two mechanisms:
1. Alteration in cell wall permeability to prevent antibiotics from inhibiting peptidoglycan synthesis
2. Bacterial production of β-lactamase that causes β-lactams to become ineffective.

35. What are the pediatric and adult dosages for the most commonly used antibiotics?

ANTIBIOTIC	ROUTE(S) OF ADMINISTRATION	ADULT DOSE	PEDIATRIC DOSE PER DAY
Penicillin G	IM, IV	6–12 x 10 units/4h	100,000 units/kg ÷ 3
Penicillin V	PO	500 mg qid	50 mg/kg ÷ 3 or 4
Ampicillin	PO, IM, IV	500 mg qid PO	25 mg/kg ÷ 4
Amoxicillin	PO	250 mg qid PO	25 mg/kg ÷ 3
Amoxicillin-Clavulanate	PO	250–500 mg tid	20 mg/kg 3
Oxacillin	IM, IV	500–1000 mg q 6h	50–200 mg/kg ÷ 4
Dicloxacillin	PO	250–500 mg q 6 h	12.5–50 mg/kg ÷ 4 or 5
Cephalexin	PO	500 mg qid	25–50 mg/kg ÷ 4
Cephradine	PO, IV	500 mg qid	25–50 mg/kg ÷ 3
Cefazolin	IM, IV	1 gm q 8 h	25–50 mg/kg ÷ 3 or 4
Cefaclor	PO	500 mg q 6 h	20 mg/kg ÷3
Cefoxitin	IM, IV	500 mg q 6 h	80–160 mg/kg ÷ 4 or 5
Erythromycin	PO, IV	500 mg qid	40 mg/kg ÷ 4
Clindamycin	PO, IM, IV	300–450 mg q 6 h	10–20 mg/kg ÷ 4
Chloramphenicol	PO, IV	500–750 mg q 6 h PO	75–100 mg/kg ÷ 4

(Table continued on next page.)

ANTIBIOTIC	ROUTE(S) OF ADMINISTRATION	ADULT DOSE	PEDIATRIC DOSE PER DAY
Vancomycin	IV	500 mg q 6 h	50 mg/kg ÷ 4
Metronidazole	PO	500 mg tid	30–40 mg/kg
Nystatin	Topical, PO	0.5–2 million units/day ÷ 2–4	Infants: 800,000 units ÷ 4 Older children: 1.6 million units ÷ 4
Clotrimazole	Topical	10 mg 5 times/day	< 3 yrs: safety not established ≥ 3 yrs: 10 mg 5 times/day
Ketoconazole	PO	200–400 mg q d	3.3–6.6 mg/kg
Acyclovir	Topical, PO, IV	600 mg ÷ 3 oral 15 mg/kg ÷ 3 IV	Safety in children not established

Adapted from Hupp JR: Antibacterial, antiviral, and antifungal agents. Oral Maxillofacial Surg Clin 3:276, 1991.

36. What is the antimicrobial spectrum of the most common antibiotics used in treatments for oral and maxillofacial infections?

Penicillin	*Streptococcus* (except group D) *Staphylococcus* (non–beta-lactamase producing *Treponema* *Actinomyces* Oral anaerobes	Erythromycin	*Streptococcus* *Staphylococcus* *Mycoplasma* *H. influenzae* *Legionella* Oral anaerobes
Ampicillin and amoxicillin	Same as penicillin plus: *E. coli* *H. influenzae* *Proteus mirabilis*	Clindamycin	*Streptococcus* *Staphylococcus* *Actinomyces* *Bacteroides fragilis* Oral anaerobes
Amoxicillin plus clavulanate	Same as ampicillin plus: *Klebsiella* *Staph. aureus* *Staph. epidermidis* Enterococci Gonococci	Chloramphenicol	*Streptococcus* *Staphylococcus* *H. influenzae* *E. coli* *Salmonella* *Shigella* *Rickettsia*
Oxacillin and dicloxacillin	Beta-lactamase-producing staphylococci		*Bacteroides fragilis* Oral anaerobes
Cephalexin, cephradine, and cefazolin	*Streptococcus* (except group D) *Staphylococcus* *E. coli* *Proteus mirabilis* *Klebsiella*	Vancomycin Metronidazole	*Streptococcus* *Staphylococcus* Oral anaerobes
Cefaclor	Same as cephalexin plus: *H. influenzae*		
Cefoxitin	Same as cephalexin plus: *Enterobacter* *Bacteroides fragilis* Oral anaerobes		

37. When should antibiotics be used?
- Acute-onset infection
- Infection with diffuse swelling
- Patients with compromised host defenses
- Involvement of fascial spaces
- Severe pericoronitis
- Diagnosed osteomyelitis of the jaw

38. When are prophylactic antibiotics for prevention of odontogenic infections not necessary?
Antibiotics have minimal or no benefits in the treatment of chronic well-localized abscess, minor vestibular abscess, dry socket, and root canal sterilization.

39. What are the indications for prophylactic antibiotics?
- To prevent local wound infection
- To prevent infection at the surgical site causing local wound infection
- To prevent metastatic infection at a distant susceptible site due to hematogenous bacterial seeding from the oral flora (e.g., subacute bacterial endocarditis, infection of prosthetic joint replacement of the oral surgical procedure).

40. When are prophylactic antibiotics indicated for prevention of local wound infection?
- When the procedure to be performed has a high incidence of infection
- When infections may have grave consequences
- When the patient's immune system is compromised
- When the surgical procedure lasts longer than 3 hours
- When the surgical procedure has a high degree of contamination

41. What is the antibiotic of choice for treatment of odontogenic infection?
The empiric therapy is **penicillin** or penicillin plus metronidazole, if the patient is not allergic to antibiotics and is not immunocompromised. In patients who are allergic to penicillin, **clindamycin** is an excellent alternative. Definitive antibiotic therapy should be based on culture and sensitivity.

42. What are the mechanism of action, route of excretion, and spectrum of the most commonly used antibiotics for oral and maxillofacial infection?
See table on next page.

43. List the possible causes of failure of antibiotic therapy.
- Inadequate surgical treatment
- Depressed host defenses
- Presence of foreign body
- Problems associated with use of antibiotics (e.g., patient compliance, inadequate dose, antibiotic-related infection, use of wrong antibiotic)

44. What antibiotic is associated colitis (AAC)?
AAC is a toxic reaction associated with the use of an antibiotic that causes alteration of colonic flora leading to the overgrowth of *Clostridium difficile*. The toxins from *C. difficile* cause pseudomembranous colitis or ACC, which is manifested clinically as profuse, watery diarrhea that may be bloody, cramping, abdominal pain, fever, and leukocytosis.

45. What are the risk factors for AAC?
Risk factors associated with AAC are related to the type of antibiotic and patient-related factors. Clindamycin, which originally was thought to be the main antibiotic associated with ACC, has now been recognized to be associated with only one-third of cases. Ampicillin is associated with one third, and the cephalosporins are associated with the last third. Patient-related factors for ACC include previous gastrointestinal procedures, medically compromised patients, advanced age, female gender, inflammatory bowel disease, cancer chemotherapy, and renal disease.

Profiles of the Most Commonly Used Antibiotics for Oral and Maxillofacial Infection

	PENICILLIN V	ERYTHROMYCIN	CLINDAMYCIN	CEPHALEXIN	CEFADROXIL	METRONIDAZOLE	DOXYCYCLINE	AMOXICILLIN	NYSTATIN
Bactericidal or bacteriostatic	Bactericidal	Bacteriostatic	Both	Bactericidal	Bactericidal	Bactericidal	Bacteristatic	Bactericidal	Bactericidal
Spectrum	Streptococci, oral anaerobes	Gram-positive cocci, oral anaerobes	Gram-positive cocci, anaerobes	Gram-positive cocci, some gram-negative rods, oral anaerobes	Gram-positive cocci, some gram-negative rods, oral anaerobes	Anaerobes	Gram-positive cocci, some gram-negative rods, oral anaerobes	Gram-positive cocci, E. coli, H. influenzae, oral anaerobes	Candida organisms
Dose-interval	250–500 mg qid	250–500 mg qid	150–300 mg q 6 h	500 mg qid	500 mg bid	250 mg qid	100 mg bid	250 mg tid	200,000 U lozenge qid
Metabolized	Kidney	Liver	Liver	Kidney	Kidney	Liver	Liver	Kidney	—
Toxicity and side effects	Allergy	Nausea, vomiting, cramping, diarrhea	Nausea, vomiting, cramping, diarrhea, antibiotic associated colitis	Allergy, antibiotic-associated colitis	Allergy, antibiotic-associated colitis	Nausea, vomiting, cramping, diarrhea, disulfram-like effect	Teeth discoloration, photosensitivity, nausea, vomiting, diarrhea	Allergy, antibiotic-associated colitis	—
Primary indication	Drug of choice	Useful alternative for mild infection	Useful alternative, especially for resistant anaerobes	Bactericidal drug required	Bactericidal drug required	Only anaerobic bacteria involved	Broad-spectrum in mild infections	Broader-spectrum needed	Candidosis

Adapted from Peterson LJ: Principles of management and prevention of odontogenic infection. In Peterson LJ, Ellis E, Hupp J, Tucker M (eds): Contemporary Oral and Maxillofacial Surgery, 2nd ed. St. Louis, Mosby, 1993, pp 426–427.

46. Describe the diagnosis of and treatment for AAC.

In addition to the clinical signs and symptoms, the diagnosis of AAC is usually made based on positive *C. difficle* culture and *C. difficle* toxin in the patient's stool. Sigmoidoscopy is occasionally used to confirm the diagnosis. Treatment includes discontinuation of the causative antibiotics, use of alternate antibiotics if necessary, restoration of fluid and electrolytes balance, and administration of anticlostridia antibiotics. The usual choice is oral vancomycin or oral metronidazole.

47. What is Ludwig's angina?

Ludwig's angina is bilateral, brawny, board-like induration of the submandibular, sublingual, and submental spaces due to infection of these spaces. The term *angina* is used because of the respiratory distress caused by the airway obstruction. This obstruction can occur suddenly owing to the possible extension of the infection from the sublingual space posteriorly to the epiglottis, causing epiglottis edema.

48. How is Ludwig's angina treated?

The principles of treatment of Ludwig's angina are early diagnosis, prompt surgical intervention, and definitive airway management. After securing an airway, surgical drainage of each individual space should begin even before flactuace becomes palpable externally. Appropriate antibiotics and management of the host defense mechanism are also important.

49. What is erysipelas?

Erysipelas is a superficial cellulitis of the skin by that is caused by β-hemolytic streptococcus and by group B streptococcus. It usually presents with warm, erythematous skin and spreads rapidly from release of hyalaronidase by the bacteria. It is associated with lymphadenopathy and fever and has an abrupt onset with acute swelling. It may affect the skin of the face. Treatment consists of parenteral penicillin.

50. Define cervicofacial necrotizing fasciitis.

Cervicofacial necrotizing fasciitis is a very aggressive infection of the skin and superficial fascia of the head and neck and is commonly seen in diabetic and immunocompromised patients. It carries a mortality rate of 30–50% from sepsis of the dead tissue in the affected area. The etiologic factors of the cervicofacial necrotizing fasciitis include odontogenic infections, burn, cuts, abrasions, contusions, periotonsillar abscess and boils of the head and neck region, surgery, and trauma.

51. Which organisms are involved in necrotizing fasciitis of the head and neck?

The causative organisms of necrotizing fasciitis include aerobes and obligate anaerobes in synergistic combinations. In a study of 16 patients with necrotizing fasciitis, two distinctive types of bacterial findings were found. Both types had identical clinical presentations. **Type I** patients had anaerobic and facultative anaerobic bacteria such as Enterobacteriaceae and streptococci other than group A. **Type II** patients had group A streptococcus (pyogenous) alone or in combination with anaerobic bacteria. Group A streptococci and staphylococci were not isolated from Type I patients.

52. What are the clinical features of necrotizing fasciitis of the head and neck?

The initial presentation of necrotizing fasciitis is usually deceivingly benign, although the extent of tissue and fascial destruction far exceeds the external evidence of infection. The rate of infection is usually rapid, and the patient often has a concomitant systemic disease such as diabetes mellitus, arteriosclerosis, obesity, malnutrition, and/or alcoholism.

The clinical features of this condition are usually manifested as smooth, tense, and shiny skin, with no sharp demarcation in the area involved. As the disease progresses, the pathognomonic signs of the condition include dusky purplish discoloration of the skin, small purplish patches with ill-defined borders, formation of blisters or bullae, subcutaneous fat, necrosis of the fascia, and gangrene of the overlying skin. Typically, the drainage in these patients yields "dishwater"—purplish, foul-smelling discharge. Systemic features of necrotizing fasciitis include sepsis, hypotension, hypertension, hyperpyrexia, jaundice, and hemoglobinuria.

53. Describe the treatment of necrotizing fasciitis.

Treatment of necrotizing fasciitis includes antibiotics, fluid replacement, nutrition, and daily debridement to remove devitalized tissues. However, the cornerstone of treatment is debridement of the necrotic tissue and daily monitoring to assure adequate removal. Appropriate antibiotics and medical support are also important. Medical support includes fluid and electrolyte replacement, monitoring of the intravascular volume, and management of the underlying medical condition. Hyperbaric oxygen treatment has also been suggested for promotion of vascularization of infected tissue.

After resolution of infection, the resulting soft tissue defect is reconstructed with a skin graft and/or regional or local tissue flaps. Penicillin, clindamycin, and aminoglycosides are also effective antimicrobial agents for this condition.

54. What are the common granulomatous infections with recognized head and neck manifestations?

DISEASE	CAUSATIVE ORGANISM	TYPICAL CLINICAL APPEARANCE
Actinomycosis	*Actinomyces israelii* (anaerobic gram-positive bacillus)	Painless, slowly enlarging soft-tissue cervico-facial infection with fistulae
Cat scratch disease	Unnamed gram-negative bacillus	Indolent regional lymphadenitis
Glanders	*Pseudomonas mallei* (gram-negative bacillus)	Farcy: draining facial abscesses, lymphadenopathy
Leishmaniasis	Leishmania (protozoal parasite)	Mucocutaneous ulcerations
Leprosy	*Mycobacterium leprae* (acid–alcohol-fast bacillus)	Facial leproma, nasomaxillar destruction, paresthesia of V2 and VII
Scleroma	*Klebsiella rhinoscleromatis* (gram-negative bacillus)	Chronic destructive lesion of naso-maxillary complex
Syphilis (tertiary)	*Treponema pallidum* (spirochete)	Gumma of soft tissue or bone
Tuberculosis	*Mycobacterium tuberculosis* (acid-fast aerobic bacillus)	Scrofula: indolent cervical lymphadenitis, ulcerations of palate or tongue
Tularemia	*Francisella tularensis* (gram-negative coccobacillus)	Oropharyngeal ulcerations

Adapted from Wood RS: Chronic granulomatous infections. Oral Maxillofacial Surg Clin 3:408, 1991.

55. What are the classifications of salivary gland infections?

Salivary gland infection can be classified based on clinical, microbiological, or mechanical causes. Accordingly, they are classified as **acute or chronic**, bacterial or viral, obstructive or nonobstructive (involvement by systemic granulomatous diseases). The **bacterial and viral** include mumps, acute, chronic and recurrent sialadenitis. The **obstructive** include silolithiasis, mucous plugs, stricture/stenosis, and foreign bodies. Systemic granulomatous infections (**nonobstructive**) include tuberculosis, actinomycosis, fungal infections, and sarcoid.

56. Which studies should be included in evaluation of chronic salivary gland infection?

Complete blood count with differential, Gram stain, and culture and acid-fast staining of the salivary secretions are all useful in evaluation of patients with salivary gland infection.

Plain films (occlusal and panoramic view), sialography, CT, MRI, ultrasonography, and scintigraphy of the gland are useful in showing tissue changes of the salivary gland tissue. Chest x-ray, tuberculin test, and salivary gland biopsy may be necessary when involvement of the gland by systemic disease is suspected.

57. What is the treatment of sialodenitis?

If stones are present in the submandibular gland duct, a ductoplasty is indicated. If the stone is large, beyond the mylohyoid flexure of the duct, or intraglandular, the gland must be removed. Parotid gland infection is more serious and must be drained or treated by superficial parotidectomy. Antibiotics should be administered to cover Streptococcus and Staphylococcus species. *Escherichia coli* and *Haemophilus influenzae* are also occasionally implicated. Hydration with intravenous fluid, especially in the elderly and children, is often a necessary part of the treatment of acute sialodenitis.

58. What are the most commonly used antibiotics for treatment of salivary gland infection?

Empirically or if Gram stain shows gram-positive cocci, administration of penicillinase-resistant antistaphylococcal antibiotics such as methicillin is advisable. In patients who have a history of allergy to penicillin, cephalosporins can be used. Aminoglycosides (gentamicin) could also be used. Antibiotics should be administered in high doses and intravenously in patients who are hospitalized or seriously ill.

59. Which cranial nerves pass through the cavernous sinus?

Cranial nerves III, IV, V (ophthalmic division of V), and VI pass through the cavernous sinus.

60. What is the cavernous sinus thrombosis?

It is an uncommon but potentially lethal extension of odontogenic infection. Valveless veins in the head and neck allow retrograde flow of the infection from the face to the sinus. The pterygoid plexus of veins and angular and ophthalmic veins may contribute to retrograde flow. The first clinical signs of cavernous sinus thrombosis include vascular congestion in periorbital, scleral, and retinal veins. Other clinical signs include periorbital edema, proptosis, thrombosis of the retinal vein, ptosis, dilated pupils, absent corneal reflex, and supraorbital sensory deficits.

61. What are the pathways of odontogenic infection to the cavernous sinus?

An orofacial infection can reach the cavernous sinus through two routes: an **anterior route** via the angular and inferior ophthalmic, and a **posterior route** via the transverse facial vein and the pterygoid plexus of veins.

62. What is the flora of acute and chronic sinusitis?

Acute sinus infections are due to *Streptococcus pneumoniae* (30–50%) and *Haemophilus influenzae* (20–40%). Other organisms associated with acute sinusitis include *Moraxella catarrhalis*, *Staphylococcus aureus*, *Streptococcus pyogenes*, and beta and alpha hemolytic streptococci.

Chronic sinusitis is due to *S. aureus*, alpha hemolytic streptococci, Peptostreptococcus, Pseudomonas, *S. proteus*, and Bacteroides. The flora of chronic sinusitis is usually a mixture of aerobic and anaerobic organisms.

63. What is the treatment of maxillary sinus infections?

Treatment of maxillary sinus is based on a combined approach of medical treatment and, if necessary, surgical treatment. The medical treatment includes use of antibiotics, topical or oral decongestants, antihistamines, and topical or oral steroids. Commonly prescribed antibiotics for the treatment of maxillary sinusitis include ampicillin, amoxicillin, amoxicillin and clavulanic acid, cefaclor, cepfuroxime axetil, and trimethoprim-sulfmethoxazole.

Surgical treatment is indicated when the underlying cause of the infection cannot be corrected by medical therapy. The goal is to re-establish drainage and remove the underlying cause (if identified) using minimally invasive techniques such as functional endoscopic surgery.

64. What are the most common bacterial and fungal infections affecting patients with diabetes mellitus?

Mucormycosis (phycomycosis) is the most common infection in patients with diabetes mellitus, especially those with diabetic ketoacidosis. Of patients with rhinocerebral mucormycosis, 75% have ketoacidosis. Mucormycosis is a fungal disease, possibly caused by phycomycetes organisms of the zygomycetes class.

65. Which organisms are associated with infections from a human and animal bite?

Approximately 25% of animal bite infections are caused by *Pasteurella multicida*. Approximately 10% are caused by *S. aureus*, 40% are caused by alpha-hemolytic streptococci, and 20% are caused by bacteroides and fusobacteria. About 25% of human bite infections are caused by *S. aureus* from the skin of the victim; 10% are caused by alpha-hemolytic streptococci; 50% are caused by anaerobic bacteria including gram-positive cocci, fusobacteria, and Bacteroides species; and 15% are caused by *Eikenella corrodens*. The latter organisms are mostly associated with severe infections.

66. Describe the treatment for animal and human bites.

Treatment includes antibiotic therapy and surgical intervention. Good surgical technique involves debridement of the devitalized tissue and thorough irrigation with copious quantities of saline. Oral ampicillin or amoxicillin are the antibiotics of choice for both types of bites. Also provide prophylaxis against rabies virus, if deemed necessary.

67. What is actinomycosis?

Actinomycosis is a bacterial infection caused by a gram-positive, facultative, anaerobic rod bacteria called *Actinomyces israeli*. The organism is part of the normal oral flora. The infection presents as a hard swelling of the jaw and drainage characterized by sulfur granules. The treatment of actinomycosis includes 10–20 million units of PCN daily for 2–4 weeks, followed by 5–10 million units for 3–4 months. Surgical debridement of the area may accelerate resolution of the infection.

68. Which diseases are associated with Epstein-Barr virus?

Mononucleosis, Burkitt's lymphoma, nasopharyngeal carcinoma, and hairy leukoplakia are associated with the Epstein-Barr virus.

69. What is a Jarisch-Herxheimer reaction?

It is a transient, increased discomfort in an erythematous skin lesion plus temperature elevation occurring within 2 hours after starting antibiotic therapy in treatment of secondary syphilis and Lyme disease (penicillin or tetracycline).

70. List the various fungal infections that may affect the head and neck.

The various fungal infections of the head and neck include candidiasis, zygomycosis, histoplasmosis, blastomycosis, aspergillosis, and coccidiomycosis.

71. What are the common *antifungal* agents?

The most common antifungal agents are nystatin, clotrimazole, ketoconazole, and amphotericin B.

72. What are the common *antiviral* agents?

The common antiviral agents are acyclovir, zidovudine, vidarabine (ara-A), and idoxuridine.

73. What are the most common agents used in HIV-positive patients?

IMMUNOSUPPRES-SIVE DRUG	MAIN ACTION	COMPLICATIONS
Glucocorticoids	Decrease circulating lymphocytes Impair delayed hypersensitivity Alter lymphocyte-macrophage interaction Cause monocytopenia Impair neutrophil chemotaxis	Infection Diabetes mellitus Adrenal suppression Peptic ulcer disease Impaired wound healing
Azathioprine	Interferes with DNA/RNA synthesis, leading to lymphocytopenia	Hepatitis Agranulocytosis Infection

Antithymocyte
  globulin
	Lymphocyte-selective immunosuppression	Infection
		Predisposition to tumor
		  development
		Thrombocytopenia
		Hemolysis
		Leukopenia

Cyclosporine	Inhibits T-cell proliferation and activation	Nephrotoxicity Hepatotoxicity Lymphoma Gingival hyperplasia
Cyclophosphamide	Depletes circulating T-lymphocyte pools Inhibits T-cell function and proliferation	Leukopenia

Adapted from Miyasaki SH, Perrott D, Kaban LB: Infections in immunocompromised patients. Oral Maxillofacial Surg Clin 3:393–402, 1991.

74. True or false: Osteomyelitis can be classified into three major groups.

False. Osteomyelitis is generally classified into two major groups: suppurative and non-suppurative.

75. What is the most common classification of osteomyelitis of the jaws?

Suppuritive osteomyelitis is classified into acute, chronic, or infantile osteomyelitis. Nonsuppurative osteomyelitis is classified into chronic sclerosing (focal and diffuse), Garre's sclerosing osteomyelitis, and actinomycotic osteomyelitis.

76. What is Garre's osteomyelitis?

Garre's osteomyelitis is characterized by localized, hard, nontender, and bony swelling of the lateral and inferior aspects of the mandible. It is primarily present in children and young adults and is usually associated with carious molar and low-grade infection. The radiographic features of Garre's osteomyelitis include a focal area with proliferative periosteal formation—most often seen as a carious mandibular molar opposite to the hard bony mass—and periosteal bony outgrowth seen on occlusal films. Treatment of this condition includes extraction of the tooth and removal of potential sources, which leads to gradual remodeling of the area involved. Long-term postoperative antibiotics generally are not necessary.

77. Which conditions are associated with periosteal thickening?

In addition to Garre's osteomyelitis, infantile osteomyelitis, cortical hyperostoses (Caffey's disease), syphilis, leukemia, Ewing's sarcoma, metabolic neuroblastoma, and fracture callus are all associated with periosteal thickening.

78. What are the general treatment principles of osteomyelitis of the jaws?

Treatment of osteomyelitis of the jaws usually includes both surgical intervention and medical management of the patient, as well as sensitivity testing. Medical management involves culture administration of empirical antibiotics, performing Gram stain, administration of culture-guided antibiotics, use of appropriate imaging to rule out other causes such as tumors, and evaluation and correction of the patient's immune defenses. Surgical treatment includes removal of loose teeth, sequestra, and foreign bodies; sequestectom; debridement; decortication; resection; and reconstruction, if necessary.

BIBLIOGRAPHY

1. Bartlett RC: Laboratory diagnostic techniques. In Tobazian RG, Goldberg MH (eds): Oral and Maxillofacial Infections, 3rd ed. Philadelphia, W.B. Saunders, 1991, pp 79–112.
2. Flynn TR: Anatomy and surgery of deep fascial space infections of the head and neck. Oral Maxillofac Surg Knowl Update 1:79–105, 1994.
3. Hupp JR: Antibacterial, antiviral and antifungal agents. Oral Maxillofac Surg Clin 3:273–286, 1991.
4. Lieblich SE: Clinical microbiology and taxonomy. Oral Maxillofac Surg Knowl Update 1:11–21, 1994.
5. Miyasaki SH, Perrott DH, Kaban LB: Infections in immunocompromised patients. Oral Maxillofac Surg Clin 3:393–402, 1991.
6. Peterson LJ: Microbiology of head and neck infections. Oral Maxillofac Surg Clin 3:247–258, 1991.
7. Peterson LJ: Principles of management and prevention of odontogenic infection. In Peterson LJ, Ellis E, Hupp J, Tucker M (eds): Contemporary Oral and Maxillofacial Surgery, 2nd ed. St. Louis, Mosby, 1998, pp 392–417.
8. Rogerson KC: Microbiology of the maxillary sinus antrum: Treatment of infections. Oral Maxillofac Surg Knowl Update 1:49–60, 1994.
9. Topazian RG: Osteomyelitis of the jaws. In Topazian R, Goldberg M (eds): Oral and Maxillofacial Infections, 3rd ed. Philadelphia, W.B. Saunders, 1994, pp 251–288.
10. Wood RS: Chronic granulomatous infections. Oral Maxillofac Surg Clin 3:405–422, 1991.

30. TEMPOROMANDIBULAR JOINT ANATOMY, PATHOPHYSIOLOGY, AND SURGICAL TREATMENT

Renato Mazzonetto, D.D.S., Ph.D., Steven G. Gollehon, D.D.S., M.D., and Daniel B. Spagnoli, D.D.S., Ph.D.

1. What is the main function of cartilage?

Cartilage is aneural, avascular, and alymphatic. Its main function is to withstand compressional forces during frictional joint loading. The articular cartilage functions to resist forces of compression and joint friction between the condyle and fossa. Chondrocytes within the cartilage also secrete important biochemicals for joint function such as lubricin, which acts to maintain joint integrity and reduce functional wear.

2. What is the difference between temporomandibular joint (TMJ) articular cartilage and cartilage of other synovial joints?

Most synovial joints have hyaline cartilage on their articular surface; however, a number of joints, such as the sternoclavicular, acromioclavicular, and temporomandibular joints, are associated with bones that develop from intramembranous ossification. These have fibrocartilage articular surfaces.

3. Discuss the unique properties of the TMJ articular disc as it relates to the temporal bone and dentition.

The articular disc is tightly attached to the lateral and medial poles of the condyle. Therefore, during mouth opening, the condyle-articular disc complex moves in a sliding movement relative to the temporal bone to or beyond the apex of the articular eminence, while the condyle rotates underneath the disc. Because the TMJ has characteristics of both a hinge joint (ginglymus) and a gliding joint (articulatio plana), it is classified as a ginglymoarthrodial joint. A unique feature of the TMJ is that it is rigidly connected to both the dentition and the contralateral TMJ.

4. What are the main protective and functional responsibilities of the articular disc of the TMJ?

The main functions of the disc are to absorb shocks and to resist stretching and compressional forces by transforming them into tension stresses in the collagen fibers. These stresses are dispersed throughout the collagen network and consequently reduced. Another function of the articular disc is to establish joint stability while translatory movements of the condyle occur.

5. What causes internal derangements of the TMJ specifically?

The causes of internal derangements are classified as macrotrauma or microtrauma. External factors such as clenching, grinding, bruxing, nail biting, and other parafunctional habits can cause excessive joint loading and lack of motion. These actions lead to inflammatory biochemical alterations in the joint that promote degradation, synovial inflammation, and formation of adhesions.

6. Explain the relationship between osteoarthritis and TMJ disc displacement.

The relationship between osteoarthritis and disc displacement is a subject of debate. Disc displacement may be a sign as well as a cause of TMJ osteoarthritis. However, it often is a concomitant phenomenon with an initial disturbance of molecular and cellular processes leading to osteoarthritis in cartilaginous tissues. The concomitant manifestation of both osteoarthritis and disc displacement comprises a substantial portion of all TMJ disorders, although both conditions may manifest separately and may be mutually independent. Currently, osteoarthritis, alone or in combination with disc displacement, is one of the most prevalent TMJ disorders.

7. How do external factors lead to anatomic alterations in the TMJ?

Acute **macrotrauma** to the joint, such as direct or coup-contracoup injuries, may result in displacement, contusion, hemorrhage, and irreversible deformation of the joint tissues with the potential for intracapsular interferences, restrictive fibrosis, and inflammation.

Functional overload, or **microtrauma**, is another frequent cause of internal derangements. Chronic microtrauma is associated with parafunctional activities such as chronic clenching habits, grinding, nail biting, and gum chewing that alter the lubricating properties of the joint, introduce friction between the disc and the condyle causing degenerative changes, and result in gradual anterior displacement and eventual perforation of the disc.

8. Describe the sensitive balance between anabolism and catabolism that exists in the TMJ synovium and articular disc.

Because the articular cartilage is avascular and alymphatic, nutrition and elimination of waste products are dependent on diffusion through the cartilage matrix from and to the synovial fluid. Joint loading significantly stimulates disc diffusion and is essential to chondrocyte nutrition. Because cartilage is avascular, chondrocytes have to function under almost anaerobic conditions. Consequently, they have relatively low metabolic activity, which renders them vulnerable to toxic influences. Chondrocytes are unable to regenerate after major trauma, but they have considerable recuperative abilities. Although once thought of as an inert tissue, articular cartilage is now recognized as a dynamic system that is capable of remodeling under functional demands and turnover of extracellular matrix components. As long as the environment of the TMJ synovium and articular cartilage exists in a balance between net breakdown and net buildup, most destructive processes in the TMJ remain subclinical. It is when the net catabolism (breakdown) exceeds the anabolic buildup (reparative processes) that most chronic inflammatory conditions begin to become symptomatic.

9. What is synovitis and how does it occur?

Synovitis is an inflammatory disorder of the synovial membrane that is characterized by hyperemia, edema, and capillary proliferation in the synovial membrane. Synovitis occurs when the level of cellular debris and the concentration of biochemical mediators of inflammation and pain produce levels that the synovial membrane is unable to ingest, absorb, or process.

10. Biochemically, what compounds have been linked to the pathogenic pathway in TMJ osteoarthritis?

In osteoarthritic cartilage, which is characterized by tissue degradation, an imbalance between protease and protease inhibitor levels or activities has been postulated as a possible pathogenic pathway in osteoarthritis. In support of this, high levels of active metalloproteases, in particular MMP-2, MMP-9, and MMP-3, were found in lavage fluids of affected TMJs.

11. What is "weeping lubrication"? Explain its origin and function in maintaining TMJ homeostasis.

Loading of cartilage during joint movement results in an increase of the internal hydrostatic pressure. If the hydrostatic pressure exceeds the osmotic pressure exerted by the proteoglycans, water is squeezed out of the extracellular matrix, contributing to the lubrication of the joint surfaces during joint movement. This so-called weeping lubrication occurs particularly under high loads. Under low loads, the so-called boundary lubrication functions through a lubricating glycoprotein, lubricin. The proteoglycans, in collaboration with the collagen network, determine the viscoelastic properties of the cartilage and provide it with its resilience, elasticity, shear strength, and self-lubrication. In addition, proteoglycans can function as internal membrane receptors.

12. What are the goals of nonsurgical management of TMJ disorders?

Some patients with TMJ disorders can be managed successfully without surgery. Between 2% and 5% of all patients treated for TMJ disorders undergo surgery. Physical therapy, occlusal splint therapy, pharmacologic therapy, occlusal adjustments, and patient counseling can treat joint pain and limitation in mouth opening. The goals are:
- To eliminate pain or at least decrease it to a level that the patient can manage
- To decrease or eliminate symptoms of jaw dysfunction
- To restore jaw movements to normal levels
- To counsel the patient about habits that tend to decrease TMJ function

13. What are the indications to proceed with TMJ surgery?

Patients with pain and dysfunction whose signs and symptoms do not respond satisfactorily to nonsurgical therapy within a period of 3 months may be candidates for surgery, particularly if they are diagnosed with advanced internal derangement caused by ankylosis, rheumatoid arthritis, or severe degenerative osteoarthritis. Patients with no improvement in range of motion and mouth opening despite conservative treatment are also candidates for surgical therapy.

14. When is TMJ arthrocentesis indicated?

Arthrocentesis is used to manage TMJ problems in patients who do not respond well to nonsurgical therapy. The major indications for its use are (1) acute or chronic limitation of motion due to an anterior displaced disc without reduction and (2) hypomobility due to restriction of condylar translation in the upper joint space. Patients with normal range of motion despite an anterior disc displacement with reduction who nonetheless have chronic pain also respond favorably to arthrocentesis. Arthrocentesis may also be used to manage pain and dysfunction in patients who have undergone previous invasive procedures that have failed to relieve pain with limitation of function. The alteration of the biochemical environment within the intracapsular space by arthrocentesis to relieve various vasoactive pain mediators is also another strong indication for treatment. Arthrocentesis may bridge the gap between nonsurgical therapy or nonsurgical and pharmacologic therapy and invasive TMJ surgery.

15. What are the major advantages of TMJ arthroscopic surgery above invasive open joint surgery?

Direct visualization of the anatomic structures in the pathologic tissue with a minimally invasive surgical procedure, biopsy of pathologic tissue, and removal of osteoarthritic fibrillation tissue as well as direct injection of steroid into inflamed synovial tissues and correlation of clinical findings with the actual joint pathology or previous imaging studies has given arthroscopic TMJ surgery a distinct advantage over invasive open joint surgery with decreased patient morbidity, decreased recovery time, and decreased intra-articular inflammation and destruction.

16. When is arthroscopic surgery contraindicated?

Contraindications to arthroscopy are similar to those for other elective procedures, such as any medical condition that places the patient at an increased risk from general anesthesia or the surgical procedure itself. Local contraindications include skin or ear infections, possible tumor seating, and severe or advanced fibrous ankylosis resulting in severe limitations and movement of the condyle. Emotional instability, obesity that prevents the joints from being palpated adequately, and other circumstances unique to the patient are also considerations.

17. Why is preservation of the synovial membrane, articular cartilage, and disc important during arthroscopic procedures?

The synovial membrane must be maintained to provide joint lubrication. Excessive removal of synovial tissue with shavers, cautery, or laser should be avoided to prevent scar formation and the subsequent formation of dense connective tissue. Articular cartilage should be preserved when possible to maintain resiliency and compressibility of the joint; moreover, only the fibrillated osteoarthritic tissue should be removed conservatively during arthroscopy. Disc preservation is important because it gives the joint a biochemical advantage by facilitating intracapsular boundaries and hydrostatic weeping lubrication.

18. Do lasers have advantages over conventional rotary instruments in arthroscopic procedures?

Yes. The effectiveness of joint surgery has improved greatly with the application of laser technology. Diseased tissues can be removed without mechanical contact, thus minimizing trauma to the articular cartilage and surrounding synovial surfaces. Coagulation of bleeding occurs instantly without thermal damage. Bone spurs are easily removed, minimizing the use of larger mechanical instruments in narrow places, which further reduce local tissue insult.

19. List the indications for total joint reconstruction.
- Fibrous or bony ankylosis with severe anatomic abnormalities
- Failed autogenous grafts in multiply operated patients
- Destruction of autogenously grafted tissues by pathology
- Failed Proplast-Teflon implants that result in severe anatomic joint mutilation
- Failed Vitek-Kent total or partial joints
- Severe inflammatory disease such as rheumatoid arthritis that results in anatomic mutilation of the joint components and functional destabilization

20. In the total joint reconstruction surgery, what is the best way to reproduce the patient's anatomy and create an accurate and long-lasting custom joint prosthesis?

Currently, conventional computed tomography (CT) is used to create a three-dimensional stereolithographic model from epoxy resin material that reproduces a functional model of the patient's cranium, temporal bones, and mandible. Recontouring "model surgery" can be done to simulate the surgical changes needed to provide a stable, accurate replica of the patient's anatomy and increase the chances for successful fit and placement of prosthetic components. Accurate reproduction of the patient's occlusion and centric relation positions of the mandible can be obtained, and prosthetic joint components can then be fabricated using diagnostic wax-ups. Once accuracy is maintained and diagnostic wax-ups are verified, customized TMJ prostheses using chrome, cobalt, and molybdenum can be fabricated with or without high-molecular-weight polyethylene fossa components. In total TMJ reconstruction, these techniques have become the standard of care for providing a long-lasting, stable prosthesis in patients who require total joint rehabilitation.

21. What are the stages of osteoarthritis?
   I. Initial stage
   II. Repair stage
   III. Degradation stage
      Early
      Progressive
   IV. Late stage

22. Describe the initial and repair stages of osteoarthritis.

If a primary insult, whether biochemical, biomechanical, inflammatory, or immunologic, disturbs the chondrocyte control balance between synthesis and degradation of extracellular matrix components in normal tissue turnover, cartilage degradation ensues. Initially, cartilage degradation caused by increased proteolytic activity will be counteracted by attempts at repair. In the repair stage, an increased degradation of extracellular matrix components by protease is counteracted by an increased anabolic cytokine-mediated synthesis of these components by chondrocytes. This results in a new balance between increased degradation and increased synthesis of extracellular matrix components. Histologically, the repair stage is characterized by the proliferation of chondrocytes. Clinically, the cartilage changes in the repair stage of osteoarthritis may remain asymptomatic for many years. In general, osteoarthritis is progressive and ultimately manifests clinically. However, what causes the established balance to tip, resulting initially in a focal net degradation of extracellular matrix components, is still not known.

23. How does the early degradation stage of osteoarthritis differ from the initial and repair stages?

In early stages of osteoarthritis, the degradation that is caused by the increased synthesis and activity of protease exceeds the increases of extracellular matrix components by the chondrocytes. This results in an initial focal degradation and loss of articular cartilage. The key feature of disease progression is the enzymatic breakdown of the cartilage. Consequently, the content of several extracellular matrix components is reduced focally, whereas the composition and distribution of the other extracellular matrix components are altered. The collagen network shows signs of electron-microscopic disorganization. The fibrils, of the articular surface in particular, appear disoriented and separated more widely than normal. In addition, the histochemical stains for proteoglycans show uneven staining with focally increased affinity, especially in areas of swelling and focal loss of metachromasia. Also, the chondrocytes may produce free radicals that will cause cleavage of extracellular matrix molecules. The content of proteolytic enzymes, including acid phosphatase, serine protease, and metalloprotease such as collagenase and stromelysin-1, is increased in early osteoarthritic cartilage proportional to the severity of the disease process.

24. What role does synovial clearance play in the initial clinical manifestations of osteoarthritis?

The degradation products of the extracellular matrix components are further degraded by the chondrocytes or diffused into synovial fluid, where they are removed by the circulation or are phagocytosed by synovial A lining cells. This latter phenomenon is called synovial clearance and frequently induces a secondary synovitis. Often, the osteoarthritic process becomes manifest only when a secondary synovitis develops, causing joint pain and, frequently, a limitation of joint movement. Moreover, the involvement of the synovial tissues in the osteoarthritic process initiates a cascade of secondary events, creating a vicious circle that leads to further cartilage damage by the synthesis of inflammatory and pain mediators.

25. What is the clinical importance of interleukin-1 and prostaglandins in the early breakdown stages of osteoarthritis?

Interleukin 1 induces increased synthesis of prostaglandins, prostaglandin E_2 (PGE_2) in particular, by synoviocytes. This increase in prostaglandins may be responsible for several of the symptoms observed in this stage of osteoarthritis. Prostaglandins and leukotrienes are mediators of inflammation. In response to inflammatory changes, nonmyelinated sensory neurons in the synovial tissues may release substance P and other pain mediators. Among other effects, substance P may enhance the synthesis of collagenase and PGE_2 by the synovial lining cells, thereby perpetuating the catabolic process.

26. Describe the progressive degradation stage of osteoarthritis.

In this stage, the anabolic process has become increasingly defective relative to catabolic effects. The synthesis of extracellular matrix components fails or, as the synthesis and activity of protease remains increased, results in a progressive degradation, erosion, and loss of articular cartilage. Histologically, the progressive degradation stage of osteoarthritis is characterized by fibrillation, detachments, and thinning of the cartilage from mechanical wear. Irregularities and reduplication of the tide mark have been observed, although less often in the TMJ than in other osteoarthritic synovial joints.

27. What are the hallmark arthroscopic features of the progressive degradation stages of osteoarthritis?

Arthroscopically, the articular cartilage of the TMJ may appear fibrillated or eroded. Fibrillation of the cartilage of the articular eminence may be focal or extensive. Because of the reduced smoothness of the articular cartilage surface, articular disc displacement, either reducing or nonreducing, may develop. Angiogenesis of the cartilage of the articular eminence may be observed, while creeping synovitis may be seen on the posterior wall of the glenoid fossa and the articular disc. The synovial tissues may appear hypervascularized and redundant or may show fibrotic changes in local areas. In addition, adhesion formation may result in a reduction of the anterior and posterior joint recesses.

28. Describe the late stages of osteoarthritis.

The content of several extracellular matrix components including water, proteoglycans and collagen is further reduced. The synthesis and activity of protease may remain increased or may be finally reduced when the articular cartilage is nearly destroyed resulting in so-called residual osteoarthritis. Histologically, the late stage of osteoarthritis is characterized by an extensive fibrillation of the cartilage, eventually resulting in severe thinning of the articular cartilage layer or even denudation of the subchondral bone. Chondrocyte necrosis often occurs. The collagen network is severely disorganized and disintegrated, while histochemical stains for proteoglycans show severe depletion of proteoglycans. Biochemically, the late stage of osteoarthritis is characterized by continuous increased syntheses of protease or by decreased synthesis of protease in the case of residual osteoarthritis. The content of several extracellular matrix components is further reduced to levels in residual osteoarthritis.

29. What arthroscopic findings are seen in the late stage of osteoarthritis?

Cartilage may appear severely fibrillated and eroded. Denudation of subcondylar bone is seen, and angiogenesis of the cartilage of the articular eminence may be present. Disc displacement or disc perforation may have developed. The synovial tissues may appear hypervascularized and redundant or may have become fibrotic. In the latter stages of this disease, adhesion formation with opposing surfaces frequently results in limited joint recesses.

30. List the clinical manifestations of the late stages of osteoarthritis.

- Clinically, the late stage of osteoarthritis may be manifest by joint pain and limitation of joint movement.
- Joint noises may be present if the disc displacement or proliferation has developed or may be caused by articular cartilage surface irregularities.
- In the case of residual osteoarthritis of the TMJ, clinical signs and symptoms may have ceased.

31. Correlate the activity of the osteoarthritis process with clinical signs and symptoms. What test has the potential to yield even more information in this regard?

Arthroscopically observed synovitis was found to correlate with the presence of joint pain. Recent studies using synovial fluid analysis have shown a correlation of pain with PGE_2 and leukotriene B_4, tumor necrosis factor alpha, neuropeptides, serotonin, and interleukin-1 beta. A limitation of joint mobility was found to correlate with the presence of adhesions, whereas the pain mediators neuropeptide Y and serotonin were also associated with restricted mandibular mobility. The presence of cartilage degradation observed arthroscopically was associated with elevated keratin sulfate levels and with high concentrations of chondroitin 4-sulfate and chondroitin 6-sulfate, especially compared with the amount hyaluronic acid.

Of all these tests, synovial fluid analysis, despite its limitations, offers the most possibilities to monitor the presence and progression of existing osteoarthritic processes in the TMJ.

BIBLIOGRAPHY

1. Dijkgraaf LC, Milam SB: Osteoarthritis: Histopathology and biochemistry of the TMJ. Oral Maxillofac Surg Knowledge Update. 3:1–20, 2000.
2. Dijkgraaf CL, Spijkervet FK, de Bont LG: Arthroscopic findings in osteoarthritic temporomandibular joints. J Oral Maxillofac Surg 57:255–268, 1999.
3. Frost DE, Kendell BD: The use of arthrocentesis for treatment of temporomandibular joint disorders. J Oral Maxillofac Surg 57:583–587, 1999.
4. Hall DH: The role of discectomy for treating internal derangements of the temporomandibular joint. Oral Maxillofac Surg Clin North Am 6:287–296, 1994.
5. Hoffmann KD: Differential diagnosis and characteristics of TMJ disease and disorders. Oral Maxillofac Surg Knowledge Update 1:43–66, 1994.
6. Israel HA: The use of arthroscopic surgery for treatment of temporomandibular joint disorders. J Oral Maxillofac Surg 57:579–582, 1999.
7. Laskin DM: Etiology and pathogenesis of internal derangements of the temporomandibular joint. Oral Maxillofac Surg Clin North Am 6:217–229, 1994.
8. Quinn JH: Arthroscopic histopathology. Oral Maxillofac Surg Knowledge Update 1:115–132, 1994.
9. Sanders B: Arthroscopic management of internal derangements of the temporomandibular joint. Oral Maxillofac Surg Clin North Am 6:259–269, 1994.
10. Spagnoli DB: Anatomy of the TMJ. Oral Maxillofac Surg Knowledge Update 1:1–41, 1994.
11. Wilkes CH: Internal derangements of the temporomandibular joint. Pathological variations. Arch Otolaryngol Head Neck Surg 115:469–477, 1989.

31. TEMPOROMANDIBULAR DISORDERS AND FACIAL PAIN: BIOCHEMICAL AND BIOMECHANICAL BASIS

Steven G. Gollehon, D.D.S., M.D., and Daniel B. Spagnoli, D.D.S., Ph.D.

1. How are the treatment modalities to manage temporomandibular joint (TMJ) pain and dysfunction classified?

The treatment of pain and dysfunction originating from derangements in the TMJ is divided into irreversible and reversible modalities. **Reversible therapy** consists of patient education, medication, physical therapy, and splint therapy. Occlusal adjustments, prosthetic restoration, orthodontic treatment, orthognathic surgery, and TMJ surgery are **irreversible therapies** that involve permanent changes in the function or morphology of the masticatory system.

2. What is the most common form of pain and discomfort associated with TMJ disorders?

Masticatory myalgia or myofascial pain.

3. How is the etiology of muscle pain categorized?

1. Muscle hyperactivity (functional and dysfunctional)
2. Muscle inflammation (myositis) secondary to injury or infection
3. Myalgia associated with muscle hyperactivity

In contrast to episodic myofascial pain, myofascial pain dysfunction syndrome (MPD) is chronic and self-perpetuating. Sustained muscular hyperactivity results in increased loading of the articular surfaces, and microtrauma leads to inflammation, arthralgia, reflex muscle splinting, and continued myospasm.

4. What clinical sign is pathognomonic for the first stage of internal derangement of the articular disc and is not associated with severe pain?

Reciprocal clicking is considered pathognomonic for the first stage of disc displacement. In the first stage of internal derangement, clicking begins suddenly and spontaneously or after an injury. The noise is often loud and may be audible to others. The patient may be aware of a feeling of obstruction within the joint during movement until the click occurs. The mandible frequently deviates toward the affected side until the click occurs and then returns to the midline after the click.

5. What are the hallmarks of the second stage of internal derangement?

The second stage of disc derangement is reciprocal clicking with intermittent locking. The typical patient complains that the jaw becomes locked and there is usually, but not always, severe pain over the affected joint. Patients may describe a feeling of obstruction to opening within the joint. Patients may be able to manipulate the joint to restore function. In some cases, the jaw may unlock spontaneously. In nearly all cases, there is a prior history of clicking of the affected joint.

6. Compare and contrast stages 3 and 4 of internal derangements of the articular disc.

The third stage of disc derangement is associated with limited opening and has been termed **closed lock**. A limited opening of < 27 mm and severe pain over the affected joint are characteristic findings. A deviation of the mandible on opening is also a seen. Again, the patient often describes a feeling of fullness or obstruction. In contrast to stage 2, few patients are able to unlock or relocate their closed lock and restore normal function.

7. Why is the fourth stage of internal derangement less painful when compared to earlier stages of disc derangement?

The fourth and final stage in the classification of internal derangement involving the articular disc is characterized by an increase in opening and crepitus occurring within the joint during movement due to disc perforation. This stage appears to be less painful than previous stages because the neurovascular tissue is no longer impinged between the condyle and the glenoid fossa.

8. What is the relationship between disc displacement and clinical symptoms of pain and discomfort?

Despite the clinical evidence supporting the existence of TMJ disc derangement, many questions remain unanswered, raising doubts about its clinical significance. Because pain is usually aggravated by functional and parafunctional movements, it would appear that pain originates from pressure and traction on the disc attachments. However, many, and perhaps the majority of, patients with displaced discs have no pain while some have severe pain. Studies by Kircos et al. (1987), Westesson et al. (1989), and Kozeniauskas and Ralph (1988) show a 30% incidence of disc displacement in asymptomatic patients with normal TMJ examinations and an 88% incidence of disc displacement in the contralateral asymptomatic joint in patients with unilateral pain and discomfort, respectively. These findings make it clear that disc displacement is not necessarily related to pain.

9. Does "preemptive" analgesia reduce postsurgical pain and chronic pain following surgery in patients with TMJ disorders?

Recent studies have demonstrated that dynamic processing by neurons in the affected pathway may facilitate nociception. The old view that nociceptive pathways are merely static conductors of signals generated by noxious stimuli appears to be invalid. As a result, preemptive analgesic techniques may reduce postsurgical pain and, perhaps, reduce the possibility of chronic pain in the operated patient.

10. What is the main goal in the postoperative management of patients with TMJ dysfunction?

Chronic pain and restricted jaw movement are the most common complaints of multiply operated TMJ dysfunction patients. Typically, pain restricts the patient's ability to comply with postsurgical physical therapy, contributing to a gradual decline in jaw mobility. Therefore, the major management objective should be adequate pain control coupled with effective physical therapy to maintain jaw function.

11. Describe the management strategies used to treat pain and discomfort in the multiply operated patient with TMJ dysfunction.

Strategies include pharmacologic approaches, behavioral modification techniques, psychiatric counseling, and physical therapy. Obviously, the success of any approach will depend on an accurate assessment of the patient's physical and emotional status. Furthermore, combination therapies (provided by a coordinated, multidisciplinary team of qualified health care providers) are often required to optimize the patient's condition.

12. Define the term *peripheral sensitization* and describe its role in hyperalgesia in facial pain.

According to Hargreaves et al., small-diameter group III and IV afferent nerve fibers innervate joints and muscles and respond to stimuli that can be perceived as noxious such as pressure, algesic chemicals, and inflammatory agents. Ischemia is also an effective stimulus if present for significant amounts of time and is associated with muscle contractions. These nociceptors may be excited by a variety of stimuli, and their sensitivity may be increased following mild, persistent injury. As a result, this "peripheral sensitization" is thought to be a major factor in the production of hyperalgesia. In conjunction with central sensitization, peripheral sensitization explains the persistent, chronic nature of myofascial pain and the pain of TMJ disorders.

13. What subnucleus of the trigeminal tract seems to be related to reception and processing as a second-order sensory neuron in the modulation of facial and TMJ-derived pain?

Electrophysiologic data acquired in the last two decades generally support the view that subnucleus caudalis of the V spinal tract nucleus is an essential V brain stem relay for orofacial pain. Neurons responsive to noxious mechanical stimuli or to algesic chemicals applied to articular and muscular tissues predominate in the superficial and deep laminae of subnucleus caudalis, where anatomic studies indicate projections of deep afferent inputs terminate. Evidence is emerging that the role of subnucleus caudalis in pain is related primarily to processing of nociceptive information from facial skin and deep tissues; whereas, the more rostral components such as subnucleus oralis may be more involved in intraoral and perioral pain mechanisms.

14. What are the main types of neurons that perceive and transmit nociceptive stimuli from the orofacial region?

Second-order nociceptive-specific and wide dynamic range neurons in the nucleus caudalis of V receive nociceptive input from peripheral nociceptors in skin and deep muscle tissues. It is the transmission, interaction, and feedback mechanisms at the level of higher order sensory neurons in the thalamus and somatosensory cortex that remain unknown and are an intense area of research.

15. How do ischemia and subsequent reperfusion mediate inflammation, degeneration, and the pain associated with these processes?

With persistent muscle tension, pressures generated within the joint and surrounding muscles exceed normal capillary perfusion pressure, which results in an overall net hypoxic state. During this period, significant alterations in metabolism occur in the affected cells. When joint pressures decline with muscular relaxation, tissue perfusion is reestablished. Metabolically transformed cells may then generate free radicals from the replenished oxygen substrate. This type of injury is known as the **hypoxia-reperfusion injury**. Superoxide and OH-radicals degrade hyaluronic acid from synovial fluid, thereby reducing its viscosity. Free radicals also may damage the cartilage matrix by both direct and indirect actions. These findings suggest that oxygen-derived free radicals may contribute to the degenerative processes in affected joints by degrading important molecules and reducing the synthetic reparative functions of chondrocytes resulting in a net catabolic breakdown of resident tissues, formatting inflammation and thus pain.

16. What role does estrogen play in the female predilection for TMJ dysfunction?

In general, women tend to report more pain and exhibit a higher incidence of joint noise and mandibular deflection with movement than do men. Functional estrogen receptors have been identified in the female TMJ but not in the male TMJ. Estrogen may also promote degenerative changes in the TMJ by increasing the synthesis of specific cytokines, whereas testosterone may inhibit these cytokines. It is likely that sex hormones profoundly influence several cell activities that may be associated with remodeling or degenerative processes in the human TMJ.

17. What is the incidence of TMJ dysfunction and pain in patients with rheumatoid arthritis?

The occurrence of TMJ pain caused by rheumatoid arthritis depends on the severity of the systemic disease. According to several clinical investigations, about one-third to one-half of patients with rheumatoid arthritis will experience pain in this joint at some time, with nearly 60% of patients suffering from bilateral joint dysfunction. For more than one-third of patients, temporomandibular dysfunction symptoms begin within 1 year after the onset of general disease. Fifteen percent to 16% of these patients will develop great functional disability.

18. Describe the progression of rheumatoid arthritis in the TMJ.

The progression of this disease in the temporomandibular joint follows a general scheme with exudation, cellular infiltration, and pannus formation. The articular surfaces of the temporal and condylar components are destroyed, the disc becomes grossly perforated, and the subchondral bone is resorbed. Complete ankylosis of the joint seldom occurs, although most persons have reduced mandibular mobility and loss of posterior height resulting in apertognathia. The progression of rheumatoid arthritis is slow in most people, although a few experience severe joint destruction within a few months. The presence of a high erythrocyte sedimentation rate is a negative prognostic factor.

19. Define the term *chondromalacia* as it applies to the TMJ.

Chondromalacia is a term used rather loosely by the medical profession to describe a clinically distinctive post-traumatic softening of the articular cartilage of the patella in young people. The term is now also applied to the TMJ and mimics lesions of early osteoarthritis. Osteoarthritis starts focally in a joint; clinical symptoms occur when it is present to a certain degree or when a certain area is affected.

20. Compare and contrast primary and secondary osteoarthritis as it applies to the TMJ.

Primary osteoarthritis will result in degenerative changes, disc displacement, and finally changes in joint morphology. All signs and symptoms seem to be the result of this primary, idiopathic process. **Secondary osteoarthritis** shows degenerative changes due to joint afflictions, such as rheumatoid arthritis, but also may be due to disc displacement. Osteoarthritis of the TMJ deals with synovial joint pathology, primarily with a connective tissue disease.

BIBLIOGRAPHY

1. Dolwick MF: Temporomandibular joint disk displacement: Clinical perspectives. In Sessle BJ, Bryant PS, Dionne RA (eds): Temporomandibular Disorders and Related Pain Conditions: Progress in Pain Research and Management, 4th ed. Seattle, IASP Press, 1995.
2. Hoffmann KD: Differential diagnosis and characteristics of TMJ disease and disorders. Oral Maxillofac Surg Knowl Update 1:43, 1994.
3. Kopp S: Degenerative and inflammatory temporomandibular joint disorders: Clinical perspectives. In Sessle BJ, Bryant PS, Dionne RA (eds): Temporomandibular Disorders and Related Pain Conditions: Progress in Pain Research and Management, 4th ed. Seattle, IASP Press, 1995.
4. Lambert GM, et al: Degenerative and inflammatory temporomandibular joint disorders: Basic science perspectives. In Sessle BJ, Bryant PS, Dionne RA (eds): Temporomandibular Disorders and Related Pain Conditions: Progress in Pain Research and Management, 4th ed. Seattle, IASP Press, 1995.
5. Milam SB: Nonsurgical management of the multiply operated TMD patient. Selected Readings Oral Maxillofac Surg 6:4, 1999.
6. Milam SB: Articular disk displacements and degenerative temporomandibular joint disease. In Sessle BJ, Bryant PS, Dionne RA (eds): Temporomandibular Disorders and Related Pain Conditions: Progress in Pain Research and Management, 4th ed. Seattle, IASP Press, 1995.
7. National Institutes of Health: Management of Temporomandibular Disorders: National Institutes of Health Technology Assessment Conference Statement. Bethesda, MD, NIH, 1996.
8. Sessle BJ: Masticatory muscle disorders: Basic science perspectives. In Sessle BJ, Bryant PS, Dionne RA (eds): Temporomandibular Disorders and Related Pain Conditions: Progress in Pain Research and Management, 4th ed. Seattle, IASP Press, 1995.
9. Stohler CS: Clinical perspectives on masticatory and related muscle disorders. In Sessle BJ, Bryant PS, Dionne RA (eds): Temporomandibular Disorders and Related Pain Conditions: Progress in Pain Research and Management, 4th ed. Seattle, IASP Press, 1995.

32. DIAGNOSIS AND MANAGEMENT OF DENTOFACIAL ABNORMALITIES

A. Omar Abubaker, D.M.D., Ph.D., and Kenneth J. Benson, D.D.S.

1. What are the two types of mandibular anteroposterior (AP) deficiencies?

1. Low mandibular plane angle type
2. High mandibular plane angle type

Each has distinct morphologic and occlusal presentations, but in both types the mandible is small.

2. Describe the features of AP mandibular deficiencies.

The features of the **low mandibular plane angle** type include small mandible, short facial height, curled-over lower lip, and deep labiomental crease. The angles of the mandible and the masseters are usually well-developed and well-defined, and the maxilla may be vertically deficient. The occlusion shows a curve of Spee, which is generally excessive in both arches. The mandibular anterior teeth may occlude with the palate along with an excessively deep bite. Radiographically, the ramus height is usually normal, and the angular and linear cephalometric measurements are usually smaller than normal.

The **high mandibular plane angle** variety is characterized by normal or excessive face height, a small and retropositioned chin, flattened labiomental fold, and excessive activity of the mentalis muscles. The mandibular ramus is short, the condyles are usually small, and the angles of the mandible are obtuse and hypoplastic. The occlusion is characterized by protrusive maxillary teeth, narrow arch form, constricted mandibular arch, and class II canine and molar relationships. There may be an open bite, which is indicative of conditions such as rheumatoid arthritis, temporomandibular joint (TMJ) ankylosis, and condylar resorption. If mandibular AP deficiency of the high mandibular plane angle type exists along with vertical maxillary excess, all of the features of vertical maxillary excess are present, and the features of mandibular deficiency are exaggerated.

3. How is mandibular deficiency treated?

Treatment of isolated mandibular deficiency usually involves mandibular advancement. Bilateral sagittal split osteotomy (BSSO) with rigid fixation is the most frequently performed procedure to accomplish this advancement, while inverted-L osteotomy with rigid fixation and bone grafting is recommended for advancement greater than 1 cm. In general, stability of mandibular advancement is better with smaller amounts of advancements than with large ones. Augmentation genioplasty procedures using an alloplastic or osteoplastic technique with and without BSSO technique occasionally is used to disguise significant mandibular deficiency. Also, mandibular subapical osteotomy may help in leveling the mandibular arch.

4. What are the features of mandibular prognathism?

Although isolated mandibular prognathism is a rare condition, mandibular prognathism often is associated with maxillary deficiency. When the two conditions are present together, the appearance on mandibular prognathism is exaggerated. Overclosure of the vertical dimension and centric relation-centric occlusion slides also may coexist and exaggerate such appearance. The chin and lower lip in patients with these conditions are forward relative to the upper lip, often making them the dominant facial feature. The mandibular body and mandibular angle are well-defined, often with an obtuse angle. The occlusion is class III, and often the skeletal discrepancy is greater than the occlusal discrepancy because of the dental compensations.

242

Such compensation is manifested as flared maxillary anterior teeth and upright mandibular anterior teeth.

5. How is mandibular prognathism treated?

Sagittal split osteotomy with rigid fixation is the procedure of choice for correction of mandibular prognathism. Transoral vertical ramus osteotomy is advocated by some, especially for large posterior movement and when there is a need for an asymmetric setback. However, problems with control of the proximal segment and adverse postsurgical occlusal changes have been reported with this procedure. Surgery should be undertaken only after dental compensations are eliminated with presurgical orthodontics and, preferably, after mandibular growth is completed.

6. Describe the clinical and radiographic features of condylar hyperplasia.

Condylar hyperplasia (hemimandibular elongation) is typically a postpubertal-onset, gradually developing asymmetry. The clinical features of this condition include asymmetry affecting the lower facial third, deviation of the mandible away from the affected side, and a secondary compensatory vertical growth of the maxilla on the affected side. There is also a shift of the mandibular dental midline away from the affected side, with asymmetric canine and molar relationships and lateral crossbite. The canine and molars are always in class III occlusion on the affected side. Associated mandibular prognathism or maxillary deficiency also may be present.

The radiographic features include a longer condylar neck on the affected side with a condylar head that may or may not be normal in morphology, depending on the rate of growth when the condition begins. The cephalometric radiograph always demonstrates asymmetry of the mandibular ramus and angle with varying degrees of dental compensation. Similarly, the AP cephalogram often shows mandibular asymmetry, with varying degrees of dental compensation and enlargement of the affected ramus and condyle.

7. How is mandibular condylar hyperplasia treated?

An important component of planning the treatment of condylar hyperplasia is determining the status of growth of the mandibular condyle prior to intervention. This can be done by eliciting a careful history of asymmetric growth. A history of recent change suggests active growth, whereas a history of lengthy presence without change indicates inactivity. Scintigraphic studies also are helpful in confirming active growth, although false-positive interpretations of this study are possible.

Once growth status of the mandibular condyle is determined, a decision on the treatment and its timing should be made. If active growth is present, the condylectomy may be performed or may be delayed until growth has ceased. When condylectomy is performed, reconstruction of the ramus may be necessary. Maxillary and mandibular osteotomies, with and without condylectomy, to correct the facial asymmetry and malocclusion are also often part of the treatment of this condition.

8. What is hemimandibular hypertrophy?

Hemimandibular hypertrophy, like condylar hyperplasia, causes facial asymmetry. Unlike condylar hyperplasia, however, development of hemimandibular hypertrophy usually occurs earlier, sometimes even during childhood. With this condition the maxilla can be affected secondarily, with a downward cant of the occlusion on the affected side. Depending on the degree of compensation, there may or may not be a malocclusion or shifting of the mandibular dental midline. The nonaffected side of the face is commonly small, and, therefore, the exact pathology is difficult to identify. The major distinguishing feature of this condition is an overall elongation of the side of the face, affecting both the osseous and soft tissue components.

The radiographic features of hemimandibular hypertrophy always show an enlargement of all parts of the mandible on the affected side including the condyle, ramus, body of the mandible, and sometimes even the teeth. The enlargement may terminate short of the facial midline or may cross the midline and gradually taper with an abrupt stop in the inferior mandibular border. The inferior alveolar neurovascular bundle is often displaced inferiorly toward the inferior border of the mandible.

9. What is the treatment of hemimandibular hypertrophy?

As with condylar hyperplasia, a careful history of the growth pattern is necessary. Scintigraphic studies may be helpful in identifying growth activity and are critical for planning treatment. Surgical treatment generally consists of combined maxillary and mandibular osteotomies, to elongate the short side and shorten the long side of the face, and inferior border osteotomy and bone grafting. Condylectomy with reconstruction of the ramus also may be indicated if the condyle is actively growing.

10. What are the clinical features of vertical maxillary excess (VME)?

VME is characterized by excessive tooth display at lip repose, excessive gingival exposure on smiling, and lip incompetency. An open bite is almost always present, especially when there are steps in the maxillary occlusal plane. The face height is always long, and the chin is rotated downward and posteriorly. This condition is exaggerated by the presence of a short upper lip or maxillary protrusion. VME can be seen with class I, II, or III occlusions.

11. How is VME treated?

VME can be treated with orthodontic intervention early in life (8–12 years) with high-pull head gear or open bite bionator to control vertical growth of the maxilla. If successful, such treatment may resolve the skeletal abnormalities, and ultimately the soft tissues and other facial structures grow accordingly. However, when an adult presents with this condition, it usually is treated with Le Fort I osteotomy and superior repositioning of the maxilla.

12. Are there any special factors that should be considered when treating VME?

Yes. Because the vertical growth of the maxilla is the last vector to cease, the excessive vertical development may continue growing later than expected. If significant vertical growth occurs, postsurgical relapse can result. Accordingly, as with most deformities characterized by excessive growth, delaying surgery until growth has slowed or completed is recommended. However, if VME is severe, early surgery may be justified on the basis of psychosocial benefits.

13. What are the causes of posterior VME?

1. When opposing posterior mandibular teeth have been extracted, passive eruption of the maxillary teeth results.

2. Posterior VME may also be caused by excessive maxillary vertical growth, which is usually associated with anterior open bite.

14. What are the clinical and radiographic features of posterior VME?

A distinct step in the maxillary occlusal plane is usually present. When posterior maxillary vertical excess occurs due to passive eruption of teeth, the condition is usually associated with inadequate interarch space, which poses a serious prosthetic challenge. Facial change is not apparent because the passive eruption ceases when the teeth contact the mandibular ridge. When posterior VME occurs in the dentate state, there is an increased facial height with lip incompetency secondary to downward and backward rotation of the mandible. The maxillary incisor-to-lip relationship may be normal, but during animation excessive gingiva show in the posterior region. In both conditions,

Radiographic features of both conditions include excessive distance from the palatal plane to the first molar cusp. In the partially edentulous patient, excessive pneumatization of the maxillary sinus may be seen.

15. How is posterior VME treated?

Treatment of posterior VME involves an interdental osteotomy and superior positioning of the posterior segment. If inadequate space exists between the teeth, orthodontic movement or extraction of a tooth is necessary to avoid damage to adjacent teeth.

In the partially edentulous patient, the anterior occlusion should not change if isolated posterior maxillary osteotomy is performed. In the dentate state, superior repositioning of the posterior maxilla results in closure of the open bite, shortening of the face height, improved lip competency, improved mandibular rotation, and forward projection of the chin.

16. What are the clinical and cephalometric features of maxillary vertical deficiency?

- Maxillary vertical deficiency is often present with other skeletal abnormalities, such as AP or transverse maxillary deficiency or mandibular prognathism.
- The lower face height is always reduced, and the freeway space is excessive.
- Often, the maxillary incisors are completely covered by the upper lip at rest, with only a portion of the crowns exposed when smiling, and a proper sized mandible will appear prognathic because of the overclosed position.
- The occlusion is typically class III with differences between centric relation–centric occlusion.
- Cephalometrically, the palatal plane to first molar distance is always reduced.

17. How is vertical maxillary deficiency treated?

Treatment of vertical maxillary deficiency usually involves Le Fort I osteotomy with downgrafting, often in combination with mandibular osteotomy.

18. What are the features of maxillary AP deficiency? How is it treated?

AP deficiency of the maxilla is typically characterized by paranasal deficiencies, deficiency of the infraorbital region, and lack of zygomatic prominence. The upper lip behind the lower lip is the soft tissue characteristic. The occlusion is class III with compensatory flaring of the maxillary anterior incisors in the true condition and is overly retracted if premolars have been removed previously to compensate orthodontically for mandibular deficiency.

Cephalometrically, the maxillary unit length measurements may confirm the diagnosis.

Treatment of maxillary AP deficiency usually consists of Le Fort I advancement with or without bone grafts, depending on the extent of advancement.

19. What are the possible complications of a Le Fort I osteotomy?

1. **Intraoperative complications:**
   Unfavorable osteotomy
   Bleeding
   Improper maxillary repositioning
   Inability to stabilize the maxilla
   Other minor technical difficulties
2. **Postoperative complications:**
   Relapse
   Bleeding
   Neurologic dysfunction
   Unfavorable facial aesthetics
   Ophthalmic injury (rare)
   Condylar malpositioning (rare)
   Avascular necrosis of segment (rare)

20. What are the possible complications of a BSSO?

As with maxillary procedures, complications of BSSO are classified as either intraoperative or postoperative complications. The most common complications of mandibular procedures in general and BSSO in particular include unfavorable osteotomy splits, nerve injury, bleeding, proximal segment malpositions, mandibular dysfunction including TMJ symptoms, and relapse. Wound infection, wound dehiscence, and vascular injury are some other possible complications.

21. What is the incidence of neurosensory dysfunction after Le Fort I osteotomy?

Injury to cranial nerve V2 is the most common injury with 25% of patients experiencing reduced nociceptive response to pinpricks. Injury also has been reported to cranial nerve IV and the parasympathetic fibers of the lacrimal gland.

22. What is the incidence of unfavorable split osteotomy during BSSO? How is this complication treated?

An unfavorable split between the proximal and distal segments occurs in 3.1–20% of cases. The use of heavy osteotome and twisting technique is believed to be the main cause. Unfavorable split should be treated by completing the osteotomy and using plates and screws to fix the fractured segments.

23. What is the incidence of neurosensory deficits following BSSO?

Neurosensory deficits of the inferior alveolar nerve following BSSO is one of the most significant concerns with this procedure. Complications occur in 20–85% of surgeries. However, the incidence is only 9% at 1 year after surgery. This complication is more common in patients older than 40 years and in patients who undergo simultaneous genioplasty.

24. Name the different mandibular procedures for correction of mandibular deficiency and prognathism.

For treatment of mandibular deficiency, BSSO and inverted-L osteotomy with bone grafting are the preferred procedures. For treatment of mandibular prognathism, BSSO and vertical subcondylar osteotomy are the most widely used procedures. Other procedures for treatment of mandibular deficiency and prognathism include C-ramus, subapical, and segmental osteotomies. More recently, distraction osteogenesis has become a popular procedure for treatment of mandibular deficiency and hypoplasia.

25. Which orthognathic procedure has the highest degree of relapse?

According to Proffit et al., transverse expansion of the maxilla is the most unstable orthognathic procedure. The greatest relapse is seen in the second molar region with an average of 50% loss of surgical expansion. After 1 year, inferior maxillary positioning and mandibular setbacks were also found to be less predictable than in other surgical techniques.

26. What is idiopathic condylar resorption?

Condylar resorption of the mandibular condyle is a progressive dissolution of the condylar head without a history of apparent direct cause. The condition is seen mostly following orthognathic surgery although it has been reported in patients who are undergoing or finished orthodontic treatment.

27. What are the causes of idiopathic condylar resorption?

Several clinical and radiographic risk factors have been reported in the literature, but the exact causes and pathogenesis of the condition remain unclear.

   1. **Patient-related risk factors:**
      - Age (young)
      - Gender (female)
      - Preoperative TMJ dysfunction symptoms
      - Mandibular hypoplasia
      - High mandibular plane angle

- Short posterior height
- Small posterior-to-anterior facial height ratio
2. **Surgery-related risk factors:**
   - Counterclockwise rotation of the proximal and distal segments
   - Surgically induced posterior condylar displacement in patients with extremely high mandibular plane angle
   - Type of fixation (wire osteosynthesis and IMF; controversial)
   - Direction and degree of mandibular movement (severe magnitude mandibular advancement; controversial)
   - Condylar displacement after orthognathic surgery (controversial)

28. What are the clinical manifestations of condylar resorption?

The clinical signs of occlusal relapse after orthognathic surgery or orthodontic treatment develop before the radiographic sign of condylar resorption. The resorptive process can occur unilaterally or bilaterally and usually starts within the first year following treatment. Clinically, idiopathic condylar resorption is manifested by progressive development of anterior open bite and posterior rotation of the mandible with class II canine and molar relation. The patient often begins to appear retrognathic and occludes mostly on the posterior teeth. The patient may have pain or changes in range of motion. In some patients, the clinical presentation of condylar resorption is similar to that of rheumatoid arthritis. If pain is present, it usually is mild in proportion to the degree of radiographic changes in the joint.

The radiographic features of condylar resorption include generalized resorption of the condylar head, often bilaterally with anterior rotation of the condylar stump in the glenoid fossa. The resorption process often continues regardless of the treatment until the entire condylar head resorbs. Bone scintigraphy often shows an increased uptake throughout the resorptive process that may not be interrupted by a period of decrease or cessation of uptake.

29. What are the treatment options of condylar resorptions?

As with other progressive condylar changes, a critical step in treatment planning for condylar resorption is to determine whether the condition is still progressing or has ceased. History of recent occlusal changes and scintigraphy are important to determine the stage of this condition. Most authors agree on delaying surgical intervention, especially orthognathic surgery, until the resorptive activity has stopped. During such activity, nonsurgical measures such as nonsteroidal anti-inflammatory drugs (NSAIDs) and splint therapy are recommended. Once the resorptive process ceases, orthognathic surgery or condylar replacement with alloplastic or costochondral graft (the two most common surgical modalities) is performed. Recent reports show higher stability following costochondral graft than with orthognathic surgery alone.

30. Name the commonly used systems of cephalometric bony analysis.

Arnett	Ricketts
Steiner	McNamara
Tweed	Harvold
Sassouni	Witts

31. List the most common soft tissue facial measurements.

Facial contour angle
Nasolabial angle
Upper lip length
Lower lip length
Ricketts E-line
Upper face height-to-total face height ratio

32. What is the most likely source of profuse bleeding during internal vertical ramus osteotomy (IVRO)?
- Internal maxillary artery, which lies just deep to the ramus at the level of the condylar neck (most likely)
- Masseteric artery
- Inferior alveolar artery
- Retromandibular vein

33. What is the most likely source of profuse bleeding following Le Fort I incision but prior to bony osteotomy?

The posterior superior alveolar artery, which is located at the posterolateral surface of the maxilla, is often encountered during reflection of the periosteum off the bone prior to making the bony cut. If these vessels are lacerated, they bleed profusely. This bleeding can easily be controlled with pressure packing.

34. What muscles are freed with a suprahyoid myotomy and advancement of the mandible?

     Genioglossal
     Geniohyoid
     Anterior fibers of the mylohyoid
     Anterior bellies of the digastrics

BIBLIOGRAPHY

1. Arnett GW, Tamborello JA: Progressive class II development: Female idiopathic condylar resorption. Oral Maxillofac Surg Clin North Am 2:699, 1990.
2. Bell WH, Proffit WR, White RP: Surgical Correction of Dentofacial Deformities, vol 2. Philadelphia, W.B. Saunders, 1980.
3. Crawford FG, Stoelinga PJ, Blijchop PA, Brouns JJ: Stability after reoperation for condylar resorption after orthognathic surgery: Report of 7 cases. J Oral Maxillofac Surg 52:460–466, 1994.
4. Epker BN, Wolford LM: Surgical Correction of Dentofacial Deformities. St. Louis, Mosby, 1980.
5. Hoppenreijs TJ, Freihfer M, Stoelinga PJ, et al: Condylar remodeling and resorption after Le Fort I and bimaxillary osteotomies in patients with anterior open bite. A clinical and radiographic study. Int J Oral Maxillofac Surg 27:81–91, 1998.
6. Huang YL, Pogrel MA, Kaban LB: Diagnosis and management of condylar resorption. J Oral Maxillofac Surg 55:114–119, 1997.
7. Hwang SJ, Haers PE, Zimmermann A, et al: Surgical risk factors for condylar resorption after orthognathic surgery. Oral Surg Oral Med Oral Pathol Oral 89:542–552, 2000.
8. O'Ryan F: Complications of orthognathic surgery. Oral Maxillofac Surg Clin North Am 2:593–613, 1990.
9. Proffit W, Turvey TA, Phillips C: Orthognathic surgery: A hierarchy of stability. Int J Adult Orthodon Orthognath Surg 11:191–204, 1996.
10. Turvey TA, Simmons KE: Recognition and management of dentofacial and craniofacial abnormalities. In Kwon PH, Laskin DM (eds): Clinician Manual of Oral and Maxillofacial Surgery, 2nd ed. Chicago, Quintessence, 1996, pp 375–386.

33. CLEFT LIP AND PALATE

A. Omar Abubaker, D.M.D., Ph.D., and Kenneth J. Benson, D.D.S.

1. How many pharyngeal arches are in the human embryo?

There are six pharyngeal arches: arch I or the maxillomandibular arch, arch II or hyoid arch, arches III–IV, and arches V–VI or the rudimentary arches.

2. What structures (including muscles and nerves) are derived from each arch?

First arch: all muscles of mastication; the mylohyoid, anterior digastric, tensor veli palatini, and tensor tympani muscles; and the fifth cranial nerve. **Second (hyoid) arch:** the muscles of facial expression; posterior digastric, stylohyoid, and stapedius muscles; and the facial nerve, including the chorda tympani to the anterior two-thirds of the tongue. **Third arch:** the stylopharyngeus and the glossopharyngeal nerves. **Fourth arch:** the pharyngeal constrictors, levator veli palatini, cricothyroid, larynx, and vagus nerve. **Fifth arch:** laryngeal muscles and recurrent laryngeal branch of the vagus nerve.

3. Which processes merge to form the upper lip and anterior maxillary alveolus, the nose, and the mouth?

The merger of the maxillary and medial nasal processes forms the upper lip and anterior maxillary alveolus. The merger of maxillary and mandibular processes forms the mouth, while the merger of the lateral nasal process forms the ala of the nose.

4. What structures are formed by the merger of the medial nasal process and the intermaxillary segment?

This merger forms the philtrum of the lip, the premaxilla, and the primary palate.

5. What does the merger of the mandibular processes form?

The merger of the mandibular processes forms the mandible, lower lip, and lower part of the face.

6. Differentiate the primary and secondary palates.

The primary palate comprises the lip, alveolar arch, and palate anterior to the incisive foramen (the premaxilla). The secondary palate comprises the soft palate and hard palate posterior to the incisive foramen. The primary and secondary palates are separated by the incisive foramen (see figure, top of next next page).

7. How is the secondary palate formed?

The secondary palate is formed by fusion of the palatine processes of the maxillary arches, which involves fusion of the palatine processes of the maxilla, fusion of the palatine bones, the soft palate, and uvula.

8. How does cleft lip develop?

Cleft lip develops from failure of fusion of the medial nasal process and the maxillary process.

9. What is the anatomy of cleft lip and palate?

A cleft lip and palate is a disruption of the facial anatomy that may involve the lip and its muscles, nose, alveolar segments, palate (hard and soft), nose septum, and the soft palate palatini muscles.

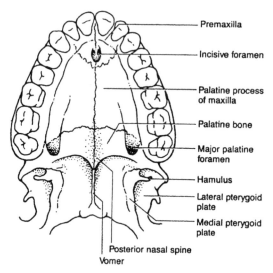

Anatomy and divisions of the palate into primary and secondary palate. (From Randall P, La Rosa D: Cleft palate. In McCarthy JG (ed): Plastic Surgery. Philadelphia, W.B. Saunders, 1990, p 2726, with permission.)

10. Embryologically, when do cleft lips and/or palates develop?

The upper lip, nose, and palate form in two phases. Anterior to the incisive foramen, the upper lip, nose, and premaxilla develop during the second month of gestation. Posterior to the incisive foramen, the palate develops during the third month. Accordingly, the time when a cleft develops depends on the type of cleft.

11. Which orofacial muscles are anatomically abnormal in cleft lip and palate?

In cleft lip, the main muscle involved is the orbicularis oris muscle. In cleft palate, several muscles are usually involved, depending on the extent of the cleft. In *complete* cleft palate, the levator veli palatini, tensor veli palatini, uvular, palatopharyngeus, and palatoglossus muscles are involved.

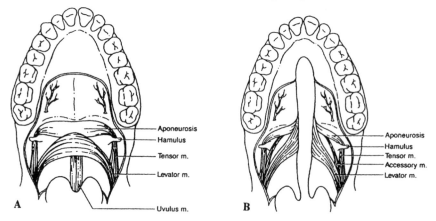

Musculature of the normal (A) and cleft (B) soft palate. Note that in the normal musculature, the elevator muscles are oriented transversely and insert in the midpalate. In the cleft palate, the musculature is disrupted and the muscles are oriented more longitudinally, inserting on the posterior edge of the palatal bone and along the bony edges of the cleft. (From Randall P, La Rosa D: Cleft palate. In McCarthy JG (ed): Plastic Surgery. Philadelphia, W.B. Saunders, 1990, pp 2726 and 2730, with permission.)

12. What are the most common nasal deformities associated with cleft lip?

Most patients with cleft lip have nasal deformities that become more apparent and severe with age. These deformities include: (1) a shortened columella with its base angled to the noncleft side, (2) septal deviation and distortion to the noncleft side, with a similar deflection of the caudal septum toward the noncleft side and a compensatory hypertrophy of inferior turbinate on the cleft side, (3) collapse of medial crura of lower lateral cartilage inferomedially on the cleft side, (4) lateral crura of lower lateral cartilage collapsed and buckled on the cleft side, and (5) flaring of the alar base.

13. What are the most common skeletal jaw deformities in the cleft palate patient?

The skeletal deformities associated with cleft lip and palate vary, but generally include one or more of the following: midface deficiency, maxillary transverse deficiency, class III skeletal and occlusal deformity, and prognathic mandible.

14. What is Passavant's ridge?

Passavant's ridge is a transverse ridge or a bulge produced by the forceful contraction of the superior pharyngeal constrictor on the posterior pharynx opposite to the arch of the atlas. This ridge is observed during gagging and pronunciation of vowels. It is an important mechanism in velopharyngeal closure.

15. Why are left-sided secondary or palatal clefts more common than right-sided clefts?

Up to the 7th week of gestation, the two palatal shelves of the human embryo lie almost vertically. As the neck straightens from its flexed position, the tongue drops posteriorly, and the shelves rotate superiorly to the horizontal position; they fuse from anterior to posterior to form the palate by 12 weeks. In rodents, the right palatal shelf reaches the horizontal position before the left one, leaving the left side susceptible to developmental interruption for a longer period than the right. It is believed that this sequence of changes occurs in humans as well, and may account for the higher incidence of left-sided clefts.

16. How can clefts be classified?

Clefts can be described as **complete** or **incomplete**, and prepalatal (cleft of the primary palate) or palatal (cleft of the secondary palate). **Prepalatal** can be further divided into unilateral or bilateral; each may be further subdivided into involving one-third, two-thirds, or all (complete cleft) of the lip. Similarly, **palatal** clefts may be described as involving one-third, two-thirds, or all of the soft palate and one-third, two-thirds, or all of the hard palate, extending up to the incisive foramen (see figure, top of next page).

A cleft can also be classified as a submucosal cleft palate or a bifid uvula (see Questions 18 and 19).

17. Differentiate complete and incomplete cleft lips.

A complete cleft lip is a cleft of the entire lip and the underlying premaxilla, or alveolar arch. An incomplete cleft lip involves only the lip.

18. What is a submucous cleft?

A submucous cleft is a deficiency in the musculature of the palate due to failure of the levator muscle fibers to fuse completely in the midline. However, clinically the palate looks intact because the overlying oral and nasal mucous membranes are present. A submucous cleft is characterized by a bifid uvula, loss of the posterior nasal spine, and a bluish midline streak on the soft palate due to muscular diastases. A notch may be present in the posterior hard palate.

This type of cleft usually leads to difficulties with speech and to velopharyngeal incompetence because the muscles of the soft palate are unable to function normally. A congenital absence of the muscularis uvulae may also occur—with or without a bifid uvula—and is often associated with palatal incompetence.

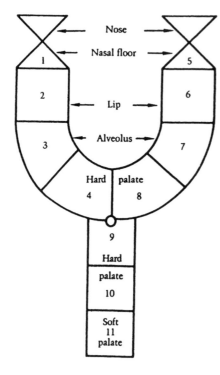

Millard's modified classification of Kernahan's and Elsahy's classification of cleft lip and palate. The small circle indicates the incisive foramen. (From Randall P: Cleft palate. In Smith JW, Aston SJ (eds): Grabb and Smith's Plastic Surgery, 4th ed. Boston, Little, Brown, 1991, p 291, with permission.)

19. What is a bifid uvula?

A bifid uvula is another variation of cleft palate seen in 2% of the normal U.S. population. It may be associated with palatal incompetence, and patients should be followed for possible speech problems.

20. What factors are known to cause cleft deformities?

Less than 40% of clefts of lip and palate are of genetic origin, and less than 20% of isolated cleft palates are of genetic origin. Corticosteroids and diazepam taken during the first 8 weeks of pregnancy are also believed to be etiologic factors. Viral infections, lack of certain vitamins, and other factors during the first trimester of pregnancy are suspected as well.

21. What is the incidence of cleft lip with or without cleft palate in the general population? In different ethnic groups?

The incidence of cleft lip worldwide is approximately 1 in every 700 to 800 live births. Incidence is highest in the Japanese, about 2.1 to 3.2 in every 1000 births. In Caucasians, incidence is 1.4 in every 1000 births; in Africans, it is 0.3 to 0.43 in every 1000 births.

The incidence of isolated cleft palate in general is 1:2000.

22. What is the familial risk for developing cleft palate?

Newborns are at greatest risk when both parents are affected. Risk for a newborn developing cleft palate when one parent has cleft versus neither parent with cleft varies depending on the number of normal siblings. When one parent and one child are affected, the chance of a second child having a cleft palate is 13%. When both parents are normal (without cleft), but two of the children have clefts, the chance of a third child being affected is 19%. When one parent has a cleft palate and two offspring are normal, the chance of the third child being born with a cleft palate is the lowest (3.5%).

23. When is a cleft palate associated with a cleft lip?

The most frequent combination is a unilateral cleft of the lip and palate, which is seen more often in boys than girls, and predominantly on the left side. The hereditary incidence in these patients is fairly high. The next most common cleft is isolated cleft palate, which is seen more frequently in girls; the hereditary incidence in these patients is fairly low. Bifid uvula has an incidence of about 2%, but most cases are asymptomatic. However, as many as 20% of patients with bifid uvula have some degree of velopharyngeal incompetence.

24. What is the incidence of clefts affecting the left side versus the right side, and males versus females?

Cleft palate alone occurs in females 2:1 compared to males. The left side cleft occurs 2:1 versus the right side. The incidence of cleft lip *and* palate is 2:1 in males versus females.

25. Which disciplines should be included in a cleft palate team?

The team should include a pediatrician, a surgeon experienced in cleft management such as a plastic and/or maxillofacial surgeon, a speech pathologist, a pediatric otolaryngologist, an orthodontist, a pediatric dentist, and an audiologist. The team also should have access to a geneticist, a prosthodontist, an ophthalmologist, a clinical psychologist and/or psychiatrist, a social worker, and a nurse experienced in cleft problems.

26. What are the criteria for timing of cleft lip repair?

Surgical repair of cleft lip is generally carried out at 10–14 weeks of age. However, traditionally the time of repair of cleft lip often is based on the **Rule of Tens**. According to this rule, cleft lip can be closed when the infant is ≥ 10 weeks old, the hemoglobin is ≥ 10 g/dl, and the child's weight is ≥ 10 pounds.

27. At what age should cleft palate be surgically repaired?

Some authors advocate repair at 6–9 months of age. Others even suggest a slight improvement with closure at 3–6 months of age. However, in most centers, repair of cleft palates is carried out when the child is 10–18 months of age, the age at which articulate speech skills are beginning to develop. In contrast, some centers prefer repair to be delayed until 18–24 months of age, after eruption of the first molars. The differences in timing of cleft palate repair are mostly based on different opinions regarding the balance between needs for normal speech vs. normal palate growth and occlusion.

28. List the goals of successful cleft palate repairs.

• Separation of the nasal and oral cavities through closure of both mucosal surfaces
• Construction of a water-tight velopharyngeal valve
• Preservation of facial growth
• Good development of aesthetic dentition and functional occlusion

29. What are the basic techniques for repairing cleft lip?

These techniques are lip adhesion procedure, the Millard rotation-advancement flap, and the Tennison-Randall triangular flap.

30. Describe the lip adhesion procedure.

This technique is most commonly used for a wide, internal cleft with protrusive premaxilla and when there is inadequate tissue available for primary repair. The primary repair is completed after 6 months. The advantage of this procedure is that it turns a wide, complete cleft into an easier-to-correct incomplete cleft.

31. What is the Millard rotation-advancement flap?

The Millard rotation-advancement flap is a modified Z-plasty technique placed at the top of the cleft so that the point of greatest tension is placed at the base of the nares. It is the most popular method of cleft lip repair. It is used for complete, incomplete, and wide cleft repairs and is ideal for closing incomplete or narrow clefts. The technique involves downward rotation of the philtrum of the lip as a flap into normal symmetrical position, while the lateral lip segment is advanced across the cleft and into the space behind the central lip. The final scar from the suture line closely recreates the philtrum of the lip on the cleft side.

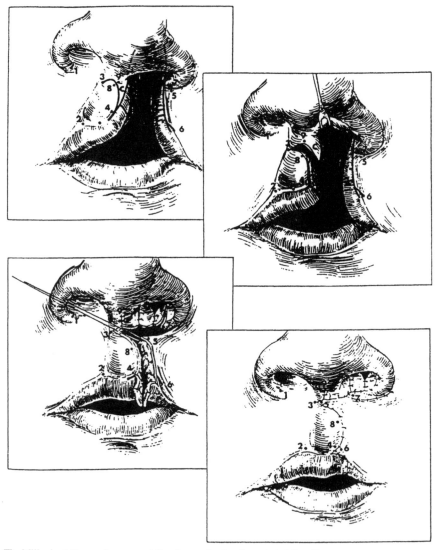

The Millard rotation—advancement flap for repair of unilateral cleft lip. (From Musgrave RH: General aspects of the unilateral cleft lip repair. In Grabb WC, Rosenstein SW, Bzoch KR (eds): Cleft Lip and Palate: Surgical, Dental and Speech Aspects. Boston, Little, Brown, 1971, pp 197–200, with permission.)

32. What is the Tennison-Randall method?

This technique uses a Z-plasty of the cleft lip edges to position the Cupid's bow. It produces an unnatural lip scar across the philtrum column and partial flattening of the philtrum dimple.

33. Describe the basic techniques of cleft palate closure.

The V-Y pushback and two-flap palatoplasties are the most commonly used techniques for repairing incomplete and complete clefts of the palate, respectively. Other techniques include von Langenbeck, the vomer flap, four-flap palatoplasty, Furlow palatoplasty, Wardill-Kilner operation, and Schweckendiek's primary veloplasty.

34. What is the V-Y pushback repair?

It is used for repair of complete and incomplete clefts of the palate. The procedure involves elevation of most of the palatal mucosa as posteriorly based flaps over the greater palatine vessels and repositioning of these flaps posteriorly. This technique provides adequate closure of the palate and additional palatal length.

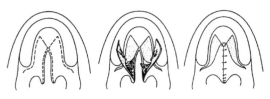

The The V-Y pushback palatoplasty. (From Randall P., LaRosa D: Cleft palate. In McCarthy JG (ed): Plastic Surgery. Philadelphia, W.B. Saunders, 1990, p 2744, with permission.)

35. Describe the von Langenbeck operation.

The von Langenbeck operation involves long, relaxing incisions laterally, with elevation of large mucoperiosteal flaps from the hard palate, which is bipedicled anteriorly and posteriorly. The cleft margins of both the hard and soft palates are approximated at the midline. The levator muscles are completely detached from their abnormal bony insertion, and the soft palate musculature is repaired in the midline. A palatal lengthening procedure is not included in this operation.

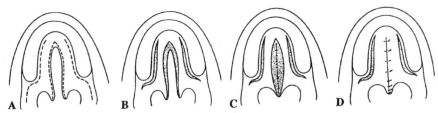

The von Langenbeck operation. A, Flap design. B, The relaxing incisions. C, Elevation of the mucoperiosteal flap. D, Closure of the nasal mucosa and closure of the oral mucosa. (From Randall P, LaRosa D: Cleft palate. In McCarthy JG (ed): Plastic Surgery. Philadelphia, W.B. Saunders, 1990, p 2743, with permission.)

36. What is a vomer flap?

This procedure consists of elevation of a wide, superiorly based flap of nasal mucosa from the vomer to close the hard palate. In bilateral clefts, vomer flaps can be obtained from each side of the vomer. This technique avoids the need for elevating large mucoperiosteal flaps from the hard palate and the potential risk of resultant maxillary growth disturbances.

37. What are the most common postoperative complications of cleft palate?

Hypernasal speech is the most common complication following cleft palate repair, occurring in up to 30% of patients. Oral-nasal fistulas are the second most common complication and occur in 10–21% of cleft repairs. These fistulas typically occur at either end of the hard palate (i.e., at the anterior alveolus or at the junction of the soft and hard palate).

38. List the major sequelae of an unrepaired cleft palate.

The problems associated with an unrepaired cleft palate are numerous, and they begin at birth and continue for the patient's lifetime:
- An inability to build up suction and nasal regurgitation
- Poor Eustachian tube function, which may lead to fluid in the middle ear space and is prone to recurrent otitis media
- Breathing problems, particularly if the chin is short and the tongue falls backward, causing inspiratory obstruction as in Pierre Robin sequence
- Speech problems, including hypernasality with vowel sounds and distortion of the pressure consonants
- Adjacent teeth angled into the cleft and possibly malformed or absent, if the alveolar ridge is involved
- Dental caries and severe malocclusion.

39. What are the goals of successful alveolar grafting?

The goals for alveolar grafting are providing alveolar continuity for eruption of the maxillary anterior teeth and/or for fabrication of acceptable prosthesis; establishing continuity of the maxillary arch; and providing bony support for the nasal structures. In addition, any residual oronasal fistula, if present, is often successfully closed during the alveolar grafting.

40. What is the ideal age for alveolar cleft repair?

Most studies indicate that the bone graft should be placed prior to the eruption of the permanent canine and when the canine root is one-forth to one-half or one-half to two-thirds developed. Root resorption and graft failure are common when bone grafts are placed after eruption of the canine. Traditionally, bone grafts are placed at ages 9–11, although early grafting at ages 5–7 is becoming more popular. Orthodontic treatment to stimulate growth and tooth eruption should be instituted within 3 months before bone graft. Orthodontic expansion of the maxillary arch *after* grafting instead of before grafting, at approximately ages 7–12, has also been advocated.

41. Which is the ideal bone for alveolar cleft repair?

Particulate bone with cancellous marrow is the best choice for grafting an alveolar cleft because its osteoinduction and osteoconduction qualities are most predictable.

42. What is velopharyngeal incompetence (VPI)?

VPI is the inability of the soft palate to make contact with the posterior pharyngeal wall to achieve full velopharyngeal closure. Such deficiency leads to speech problems and hypernasality. Evaluation of palatal function should begin as speech development occurs and continue through puberty. Various diagnostic tools are used to evaluate VPI, including speech articulation tests, cinefluoroscopy, lateral neck x-rays, manometry, and nasopharyngoscopy.

43. Which muscles are the most important in achieving VP closure?

The levator palatini muscles contribute the most to VP closure, by pulling the middle third of the soft palate superiorly and posteriorly to produce firm contact with the posterior pharyngeal wall at about the level of the adenoidal pad. Other muscles that contribute to VP closure include the paired palatopharyngeus muscles, which pull the soft palate posteriorly; the muscularis uvulae, which cause the uvula to thicken centrally with contraction; and the superior pharyngeal constrictors, which move the lateral pharyngeal walls medially or the posterior pharyngeal wall anteriorly with contraction.

44. How is velopharyngeal incompetence managed?

Speech therapy usually begins with parental counseling when the child is 6 months old, and individual child therapy should begin when the child is about 4 years of age or when the definitive diagnosis is made. Dental prosthesis may also be helpful. About 20–25% of VPI cases require surgery. Surgical methods include secondary palatal lengthening, pharyngeal augmentation using soft tissue or implants, and pharyngeal flaps. Such flaps convert the incompetent nasopharynx into two lateral "ports," and are most successful in patients with good lateral pharyngeal wall motion.

45. What is the traditional sequence of treatment for cleft lip and palate?
- At birth, the cleft lip and palate team evaluates the child.
- At 10 weeks old, the cleft lip is repaired.
- At 1 year of age, the child is re-evaluated by the cleft lip and palate team.
- At 12–18 months, the soft and hard palates are repaired.
- At 5–8 years, interceptive orthodontics are employed.
- At 5–7 years, the pharyngeal flap (if necessary) is done.
- At 7–8 years, maxillary expansion is done, if needed.
- At 9–11 years, alveolar cleft bone grafting is performed.
- At 12–13 years, comprehensive orthodontics are initiated.
- At 14–16 years, orthognathic surgery and nasal surgery are done, if needed.

BIBLIOGRAPHY

1. American Cleft Palate-Craniofacial Association: Parameters for evaluation and treatment of patients with cleft lip or palate and other craniofacial anomalies. In Philips BJ, Warren DW (eds): The Cleft Palate and Craniofacial Team. Chapel Hill, NC, American Cleft Palate Association, 1993.
2. Grabb WC, Rosenstein SW, Bzoch KR (eds): Cleft Lip and Palate: Surgical, Dental, and Speech Aspects. Boston, Little, Brown, 1971, pp 197–200.
3. Hendrick DA: Cleft lip and palate. In Jafek BW, Stark AK (eds): ENT Secrets. Philadelphia, Hanley & Belfus, 1996, pp 338–344.
4. Johnson MC, Bronsky PT, Millicorsky G: Embryogenesis of cleft lip and palate. In McCarthy JG (ed): Plastic Surgery. Philadelphia, W.B. Saunders, 1990, pp 2515–2552.
5. Kernahan DA: The striped Y-A symbolic classification for cleft lip and palate. Plast Reconstr Surg 47:469, 1971.
6. Millard DR Jr: Combining the Von Langenbeck and the Wardill-Kilner operations in certain clefts of the palate. Cleft Palate J 29:85–86, 1992.
7. Millard DR Jr: Cleft lip. In Weinzweig J (ed): Plastic Surgery Secrets. Philadelphia, Hanley & Belfus, 1996, pp 60–65.
8. Millard DR Jr, Latham RA: Improved primary surgical and dental treatment of clefts. Plast Reconstr Surg 86:856, 1990.
9. Natsume N, Kawai T: Incidence of cleft lip and palate in 39,696 Japanese babies born in 1983. Int J Oral Maxillofac Surg 15:565–568, 1986.
10. Randall P: Cleft palate. In Smith JW, Aston SJ (eds): Grabb and Smith's Plastic Surgery, 4th ed, Boston, Little, Brown, 1991, p 291.
11. Randall P, LaRosa D: Cleft palate. In Weinzweig J (ed): Plastic Surgery Secrets. Philadelphia, Hanley & Belfus, 1996, pp 66–72.
12. Randall P, LaRosa D: Cleft palate. In McCarthy JG (ed): Plastic Surgery. Philadelphia, W.B. Saunders, 1990, pp 2723–2751.

34. DIAGNOSIS OF SALIVARY GLAND DISEASES

Chris A. Skouteris, D.M.D., DRDENT (Path)

1. What are the signs and symptoms suggestive of salivary gland malignancy?
Rapid tumor growth or a sudden growth acceleration in a long-standing salivary mass, pain, and peripheral facial nerve paralysis.

2. Can peripheral facial nerve paralysis be a sign of nonmalignant conditions affecting the parotid gland?
Yes. It has been reported that peripheral facial nerve paralysis can be associated with acute suppurative parotitis, nonspecific parotitis with inflammatory pseudotumor, amyloidosis, and sarcoidosis of the parotid.

3. What are the appropriate diagnostic methods in evaluating salivary obstruction?
Clinical examination:
• Palpation of the gland
• Bimanual palpation along the course of the duct
• Visual confirmation of diminished or absent salivary flow
• Assessment of the type of any ductal discharge
Salivary endoscopy: used for diagnosis and treatment of sialolithiasis
Imaging techniques:
• Plain films: occlusal, frontal, lateral, lateral oblique, and panoramic views
• Sialography: contraindicated in the presence of acute sialadenitis and when sialoliths have been positively identified on clinical examination and plain films
• Ultrasonography
• Computed tomography (CT): useful in identifying parenchymal or extraparenchymal masses that can cause obstruction by pressure or ductal invasion
• Radionuclide scanning: evaluates the effect of the obstruction on glandular dynamics and function

4. Are sialoliths always visible on radiographs?
No. Sialoliths in early stage of development are quite small and not adequately mineralized to be visible radiographically. It has also been reported in the literature that 30–50% of parotid and 10–20% of submandibular sialoliths are radiolucent. These radiolucent sialoliths can be visualized indirectly by the imaging defect that they produce on sialography.

5. Is fine needle aspiration (FNA) biopsy efficacious in the diagnosis of salivary gland pathology?
Refinements in sampling techniques and specimen preparation, as well as improvements in cytologic interpretation, have considerably increased the diagnostic value of FNA biopsy in the evaluation of salivary pathology. The specificity of the procedure ranges from 88% to 99% and the sensitivity is 71–93%.

6. What are the contemporary imaging modalities for visualizing tumors of the major salivary glands?

Ultrasound	CT sialography
CT	MR sialography
Magnetic resonance imaging (MRI)	Positron emission tomography (PET)

7. Is there an association between salivary disease and AIDS?

Yes. Conditions affecting the salivary glands in AIDS patients include parotid lymphoepithelial lesions, cysts, lymphadenopathy, Kaposi's sarcoma, AIDS-related intraglandular lymphoma, salmonella and cytomegalovirus parotitis, and a Sjögren's syndrome-like condition with xerostomia.

8. What is the incidence of tumors affecting the sublingual salivary glands?

Sublingual salivary gland tumors comprise less than 1% of all salivary gland neoplasms. These tumors are predominantly malignant (> 80%) and are usually adenoid cystic or mucoepidermoid carcinomas.

9. Are there any imaging techniques for visualization of the facial nerve?

High-resolution MRI using a three-dimensional Fourier transform gradient-echo sequence is able to visualize the facial nerve in its course from the stylomastoid foramen to the level of the retromandibular vein. However, this technique as well as others has not been successful in visualizing the intraparotid divisions and course of the nerve, which is of great clinical importance.

10. Can ultrasonography, CT, MRI, and PET scanning distinguish between benign and malignant salivary gland tumors?

Ultrasonography can be useful in differentiating between benign and malignant tumors. Recent evidence suggests that malignant tumors (with the exception of lymphomas) are characterized sonographically by attenuation of posterior echoes, whereas benign tumors exhibit distal echo enhancement. CT can effectively differentiate among benign, malignant, and inflammatory lesions in approximately 75% of cases. MRI appears to be the most suitable for evaluation of salivary gland tumors, especially malignant tumors. However, PET scanning is not able to distinguish between benign and malignant tumors.

11. What is the role of radionuclide imaging in the diagnosis of salivary gland pathology?

In addition to assessing salivary function, salivary scintigraphy can be useful in the diagnosis of acute and chronic sialadenitis of specific or nonspecific etiology, abscesses, lymphomas, and tumors. In salivary neoplasia, radionuclide imaging can identify glandular masses greater than 1 cm in diameter, distinguish between certain tumor types based on their specific uptake characteristics, and, in some instances, differentiate benign from malignant disease.

12. Name the most common non-neoplastic salivary gland pathoses in children.

Acute viral sialadenitis
Acute bacterial sialadenitis
Sialolithiasis
Mucoceles

13. How can one differentiate between viral and bacterial parotitis?

Viral parotitis infection is bilateral and is preceded by prodromal signs and symptoms of 1–2 days' duration including fever, malaise, loss of appetite, chills, headache, sore throat, and preauricular tenderness. Purulent discharge from Stensen's duct is rare but, if present, might be the result of the development of secondary bacterial sialadenitis. Laboratory investigations reveal elevated serum titers for mumps or influenza virus, leukopenia, relative lymphocytosis, and high levels of serum amylase.

14. What syndromes can affect the salivary glands?

Primary Sjögren's syndrome is usually characterized by parotid and lacrimal gland enlargement, xerostomia, and xerophthalmia. **Secondary Sjögren's syndrome** involves autoimmune parotitis that occurs with rheumatoid arthritis, lupus, systemic sclerosis, thyroiditis, primary biliary cirrhosis, and mixed collagen disease. **Sarcoidosis** may involve the parotid gland. Sarcoidosis of the parotid gland along with fever, lacrimal adenitis, uveitis, and facial nerve paralysis is called **Heerfordt's syndrome**. Recently, a **sicca syndrome–like condition** has been recognized in HIV-positive children. This condition presents with parotid gland enlargement, xerostomia, and lymphadenopathy.

15. What is the incidence of metastatic neck disease in patients with malignant salivary tumors?

In a large series of patients with malignant tumors of the parotid, submandibular, sublingual, and minor salivary glands, the reported overall incidence of metastatic cervical lymphadenopathy was 15.3%. Parotid cancer is associated with metastatic lymph node involvement in 18–25% of cases.

16. How is acute bacterial parotitis diagnosed?

- History—with emphasis on diabetes, dehydration, malnutrition, immunosuppressive therapy, antisialic drugs, debilitating systemic disease, and recent surgery
- Physical examination—palpation and observation for purulent ductal discharge
- Imaging—ultrasound, CT
- Culture of purulent discharge and antibiotic sensitivity testing

17. What types of lesions can result from mucus escape?

Mucoceles
Ranulas
Plunging ranulas
Pure cervical ranulas without an intraoral component

18. What are the most common causes of xerostomia?

Xerostomia can be idiopathic, drug-induced, radiation-induced, or the principal manifestation of primary and secondary Sjögren's syndrome.

19. Is incisional biopsy indicated for the diagnosis of pathologic conditions of the parotid gland?

Yes, for the diagnosis of suspected systemic disease with parotid involvement particularly when FNA biopsy findings are inconclusive. Systemic conditions in which incisional parotid biopsy can be of great diagnostic value include sarcoidosis, Sjögren's syndrome, lymphoma, and sialosis.

20. Describe the clinical manifestations of a tumor involving the deep lobe of the parotid.

Tumors of the deep parotid lobe can grow undetected until they are large and clinically evident. In cases where the tumor has grown into the lateral pharyngeal space, a bulging in the lateral pharyngeal wall can be seen. Extensive tumors in this anatomic location can displace the soft palate and uvula with resultant difficulties in speech, breathing, and deglutition.

21. Name the most common benign tumor of minor and major salivary glands.

Pleomorphic adenoma.

22. What are the most common malignant tumors of minor and major salivary glands?

- Mucoepidermoid carcinoma in the parotid gland
- Adenoid cystic carcinoma in the submandibular, sublingual, and minor salivary glands

23. Which are the most common salivary neoplasms in children?

Hemangiomas and lymphangiomas of the salivary glands, followed by pleomorphic adenomas, are the most common benign tumors. Malignant neoplasms are very rare, but the rate of malignancy in children is much higher than in adults. The most common malignant salivary tumor is mucoepidermoid carcinoma, followed by acinic cell carcinoma.

24. Is it possible to accurately determine the actual clinical extent of an adenoid cystic carcinoma? Why?

No. Adenoid cystic carcinoma tends to invade nerves and spread perineurally. Therefore, it can extend well beyond its primary location.

25. Are there central (intraosseous) salivary tumors?

Yes. Although rare, salivary tumors arising in the maxilla and mandible have been reported. These tumors are thought to derive from heterotopic salivary gland inclusions and are mostly mucoepidermoid carcinomas. However, other salivary malignancies, such as acinic cell carcinoma, clear cell carcinoma, and myoepithelial carcinoma in pleomorphic adenoma, have also been reported to occur centrally within the jaws.

26. Is there a role for intraoperative frozen-section evaluation of tumors of the major salivary glands?

Yes. When FNA biopsy is inconclusive and because open biopsy is not indicated, intraoperative frozen sections might provide information that can modify the treatment plan. Frozen section is more accurate in the evaluation of benign tumors, whereas its sensitivity for malignancy is 61.5% and its specificity is 98%.

27. What types of surgical procedures can be used for the management of benign and malignant tumors of the parotid?

- Extracapsular excision or lumpectomy—tumor removal with a safety margin without facial nerve dissection
- Partial superficial parotidectomy—with no need for dissection of the full facial nerve or excision of the entire superficial lobe
- Superficial parotidectomy with preservation of the facial nerve
- Deep lobe parotidectomy with facial nerve preservation

Malignant tumors, based on their TNM stage and histology, can be managed by superficial or total parotidectomy, which can be combined with selective or radical neck dissection. When the facial nerve is involved or in close proximity with the tumor, its sacrifice is inevitable, and repair may follow by immediate or late reconstruction.

28. What is the role of radiation and chemotherapy in the management of malignant salivary gland tumors?

Postoperative radiation therapy should be administered when the tumor is high stage or high grade, the adequacy of resection is in question, or the tumor has ominous pathologic features. Neutron beam therapy shows promise in controlling locoregional disease but requires further study. Currently, chemotherapy is clearly indicated only for palliation in patients with recurrent or unresectable disease.

BIBLIOGRAPHY

1. Carlson ER: The comprehensive management of salivary gland pathology. Oral Maxillofac Clin North Am 1:387–430, 1995.
2. Carvalho MB, Soares JM, Rapoport A, et al: Perioperative frozen section examination in parotid gland tumors. Sao Paolo Med J 117:233–237, 1999.
3. Iizuka K, Ishikawa K: Surgical techniques for benign parotid tumors: Segmental resection vs. extracapsular lumpectomy. Acta Otolaryngol Suppl 537:75–81, 1998.
4. Shintani S, Matsuura H, Hasegawa Y: Fine needle aspiration of salivary gland tumors. Int J Oral Maxillofac Surg 26:284–286, 1997.
5. Spiro RH: Management of malignant tumors of the salivary glands. Oncology 12:671–680, 1998.
6. Spiro RH: Treating tumors of the sublingual glands, including a useful technique for repair of the floor of the mouth after resection. Am J Surg 170:457–460, 1995.
7. Witt RL: Facial nerve function after partial superficial parotidectomy: An 11-year review (1987–1997). Otolaryngol Head Neck Surg 121:210–213, 1999.

35. ORAL AND MAXILLOFACIAL CYSTS AND TUMORS

Chris A. Skouteris, D.M.D., DRDENT (Path)

1. What is the current treatment of solid mandibular ameloblastoma?

Small lesions can be managed effectively by curettage with peripheral ostectomy or marginal resection. Large tumors require block resection. Supraperiosteal resection should be performed in cases of cortical bone perforation.

2. Is there a nonsurgical treatment for aneurysmal bone cysts of the jaws?

Yes. Human calcitonin is administered subcutaneously (100 IU/day) for a period of 6 months. If the cyst shows evidence of osseous regeneration and a decrease in size at the end of this time period, treatment is continued for 12–18 months until complete resolution of the lesion is accomplished.

3. Is there a nonsurgical alternative to the treatment for central giant cell lesions of the jaws?

These lesions have been treated nonsurgically by intralesional injections of a mixture of equal parts of triamcinolone acetonide (10 mg/ml) and a local anesthetic (bupivacaine 0.5% with epinephrine 1:200,000). Antiangiogenic therapy with systemic administration of interferon alpha-2a has been reported to be effective in controlling recurrent lesions. Radiation therapy has been used in rare instances, primarily in elderly patients.

4. How are odontogenic keratocysts treated?

Evidence suggests that these cysts can be managed effectively by a conservative approach. Good results have been achieved with decompression or marsupialization followed by later cystectomy. More aggressive procedures ranging from enucleation with peripheral ostectomy or application of Carnoy's solution to total resection should be reserved for certain cases and recurrent lesions.

5. Is suction drainage required after removal of jaw cysts?

Although vacuum drainage is not common practice in the postsurgical management of cysts of the jaws, it does not seem to adversely affect primary wound healing at the surgical site.

6. What is the incidence of development of cystic lesions around retained, asymptomatic, impacted mandibular third molars?

0.3–37%.

7. Does ultrasonography have a role in the evaluation of intraosseous lesions of the jaws?

Yes. Ultrasound has been found to be a useful complementary imaging technique, particularly for the diagnosis of bone lesions of the jaws that are not surrounded by dense cortex. Ultrasound can correctly identify solid tumors in radiolucent lesions 92.4% of the time, fluid-filled cystic lesions 73.9% of the time, and lesions with both solid and cystic areas 92.8% of the time.

8. Is it possible to assess osseous resection margins during removal of aggressive mandibular tumors?

Yes. Frozen-section analysis of cancellous bone is possible and has been shown to be a good predictor of osseous surgical margins.

9. What is the mechanism of "recurrence" in bone grafts following resection of benign, locally aggressive tumors?

This occurrence can result from positive osseous resection margins and from residual tumor attached to periosteum in cases where, although tumor perforation of cortical bone is present, a subperiosteal resection is performed.

10. What laboratory values should be assessed in patients scheduled for resection of a large central arteriovenous malformation that has been pretreated with embolization?

Complete coagulation profile with special emphasis on platelet count and bleeding time. The incidence of transient thrombocytopenia and precipitous consumption coagulopathy has been reported following preoperative embolization, particularly in lesions that contain significant shunting or dilated venous channels.

11. What are the most common soft tissue cysts and benign tumors in children?

Thyroglossal duct, dermoid, and epidermoid cysts are the most common soft tissue cysts in children. The most common benign soft tissue tumor is hemangioma.

12. What are the most common benign intraosseous tumors in children?

Odontoma is the odontogenic tumor with the highest incidence; ossifying fibroma is the most common nonodontogenic tumor in children.

13. Is it necessary to remove teeth that are in close association with a cyst?

Appropriate imaging techniques should be obtained to ascertain that teeth are indeed involved by the lesion. Usually teeth with displaced but intact roots can be treated endodontically and preserved. Teeth showing root resorption should be extracted. The removal of teeth associated with odontogenic keratocysts is appropriate in order to prevent recurrence.

14. What is the surgical treatment of mandibular giant cell lesions?

In most cases, removal of the lesion with marginal removal of bone provides cure for the patient.

15. What osseous resection margin is considered safe for odontogenic myxoma of the jaws?

The lesion should be resected with a 1-cm margin of normal bone.

16. Is there anything that can be done intraoperatively to prevent a stress fracture from occurring in the remaining mandible at the site of a marginal resection that has been performed for the removal of a benign but locally aggressive tumor?

The remaining mandible can be re-enforced by plates and screws. In addition, a stress fracture is less likely to occur when resection borders are rounded off instead of being perpendicular to the preserved inferior border of the mandible.

17. What should be suspected when a lesion giving the impression of a branchial cyst is noted in the neck of a patient older than 50 years?

The possibility of cystic lymph node metastasis should be ruled out. Carcinoma of the tonsil is known to be associated with cystic metastases in cervical lymph nodes. Therefore, a thorough clinical examination of the patient that might even require a diagnostic tonsillectomy is of utmost importance.

18. Is it possible to preserve the inferior alveolar nerve during surgical ablation of benign cysts and tumors of the mandible?

Yes. Cysts and slowly expanding, well-encapsulated neoplasms usually displace the inferior alveolar nerve without invading it. The relation of the nerve to the lesion can be determined preoperatively by contemporary imaging techniques such as Dentascan. In certain cases where the nerve is encompassed by the tumor, microdissection and exposure of the neurovascular bundle are completed along its course through the neoplasm. The tumor is then resected after the neurovascular bundle has been isolated and protected. Potential disadvantages of this technique are the presence of tumor remnants on the neurovascular sheath and the dissemination of tumor cells in the surrounding tissues.

19. How should fibrous dysplasia be treated?
Recontouring is usually performed in cases where aesthetic and functional improvement is required, but it is more effective when the dysplastic site has undergone maturation. Although complete resection of fibrous dysplasia has been decried in the past, current refined instrumentation and craniofacial surgical techniques allow a more aggressive, nondisabling approach, particularly when vital anatomic structures are affected by the lesion.

20. Can maxillary or mandibular osteotomies be performed in patients with fibrous dysplasia?
Yes. Recent evidence suggests that osteotomy sites can heal without complications. Fixation plates and screws seem to be well tolerated by the dysplastic bone.

21. Is FNA biopsy efficacious in the diagnosis of benign intraosseous lesions?
FNA biopsy can accurately distinguish between benign and malignant tumors, but it is not as accurate in making a definitive diagnosis of benign lesions.

22. What is the method of choice in the treatment of cervicofacial lymphangiomas?
When technically feasible, total removal is the treatment of choice. Aspiration and decompression should be performed only to secure the airway in emergencies.

23. How should the surgeon approach cyst-associated teeth when marsupialization is contemplated for the treatment of dentigerous cysts in preadolescents?
In this setting, cyst-associated teeth should not be removed and should be allowed to erupt with or without orthodontic traction.

24. What is the appropriate treatment for peripheral ameloblastoma?
Conservative surgical removal by local excision.

25. What diagnostic methods can be used for the evaluation of a cystic jaw lesion?

Auscultation for bruits	Dentascan
Panorex and plain films	Aspiration for cytology and culture
Ultrasonography	Open biopsy
CT scan	Fiber-optic endoscopy

26. Does the treatment of cystic ameloblastomas differ from that of solid lesions?
Yes. Evidence suggests that unilocular or multilocular cystic ameloblastomas can be adequately treated initially by marsupialization that is later followed by enucleation with peripheral ostectomy when the lesion has attained a much smaller size.

BIBLIOGRAPHY

1. Assael LA: Benign lesions of the jaws. Oral Maxillofac Clin North Am 7:73–126, 1991.
2. Lauria L, Curi MM, Chammas M, et al: Ultrasonography evaluation of bone lesions of the jaw. Oral Surg Oral Med Oral Pathol 82:351–357, 1996.
3. Marker P, Brondum N, Clausen PP, Bastian HL: Treatment of large odontogenic keratocysts by decompression and later cystectomy: A long-term follow-up and a histologic study of 23 cases. Oral Surg Oral Med Oral Pathol Oral Radiol Endod 82:122–131, 1996.

4. Meara JG, Shah S, Li KK, Cunningham MJ: The odontogenic keratocyst: A 20-year clinicopathologic review. Laryngoscope 108:280–283, 1998.
5. Motamedi MHK: Aneurysmal bone cysts of the jaws: Clinicopathological features, radiographic evaluation, and treatment analysis of 17 cases. J Craniomaxillofac Surg 26:56, 1998.
6. Sampson DE, Pogrel MA: Management of mandibular ameloblastoma: The clinical basis for a treatment algorithm. J Oral Maxillofac Surg 57:1074, 1999.
7. Sato M, Tanaka N, Sato T, Amagasa T: Oral and maxillofacial tumors in children: A review. Br J Oral Maxillofac Surg 35:92–95, 1997.

36. NEOPLASMS OF THE ORAL CAVITY

Chris A. Skouteris, D.M.D., DRDENT(Path)

1. What is the usual clinical presentation of squamous cell carcinoma?

Oral squamous cell carcinoma usually presents as an indurated ulcer with poorly defined borders. The lesion is characteristically painless, unless inflammation from superinfection or chronic mechanical irritation is present. An indolent clinical presentation in the form of a small superficial ulceration, leukoplakia, or erythroplakia is also likely, especially in the early stages of development.

2. What is the current staging system for oral cancer?

The TNM (tumor, node, metastasis) staging system:

Tumor Classification of Cancer of the Oral Cavity

CLASS	TUMOR SIZE
T1	≤ 2 cm at greatest dimension
T2	> 2 cm but ≤ 4 cm at greatest dimension
T3	> 4 cm at greatest dimension
T4	Tumor invades adjacent structures

Node Classification of Cancer of the Oral Cavity

CLASS	DESCRIPTION
NX	Regional lymph nodes cannot be assessed
N0	No regional lymph node metastasis
N1	Metastasis in a single ipsilateral lymph node, ≤ 3 cm at greatest dimension
N2	Metastasis in a single ipsilateral lymph node, more than 3 cm but not more than 6 cm at greatest dimension *or* Multiple ipsilateral lymph nodes, none more than 6 cm at greatest dimension *or* Bilateral or contralateral lymph nodes, none more than 6 cm at greatest dimension
N2a	Metastasis in a single ipsilateral lymph node, > 3 cm but ≤ 6 cm at greatest dimension
N2b	Metastasis in multiple ipsilateral lymph nodes, none > 6 cm at greatest dimension
N2c	Metastasis in bilateral or contralateral lymph nodes, none > 6 cm at greatest dimension
N3	Metastasis > 6 cm at greatest dimension in a lymph node

Metastasis Classification of Cancer of the Oral Cavity

CLASS	DESCRIPTION
MX	Distant metastasis cannot be assessed
M0	No distant metastasis
M1	Distant metastasis

Stage Grouping of Cancer of the Oral Cavity

STAGE	TUMOR CLASS	NODE CLASS	METASTASIS CLASS
Stage 0	Tis*	N0	M0
Stage I	T1	N0	M0
Stage II	T2	N0	M0
Stage III	T3	N0	M0
	T2	N1	M0
	T3	N1	M0
Stage IVA	T4	N0	M0
	T4	N1	M0
	Any T	N2	M0
Stage IVB	Any T	N3	M0
Stage IVC	Any T	Any N	M1

* in-situ

Some inherent inadequacies of this system have prompted the proposal of certain modifications and revisions in an effort to enhance its prognostic significance.

3. Which factors indicate a poor prognosis in oral cancer?
The most important poor prognostic factors include:
Site
Tumor diameter
Tumor thickness and invasion
Degree of histologic differentiation
Lymph node metastasis
Level of lymph node involvement
Number of affected lymph nodes
Extranodal spread
Distant metastasis
Local or locoregional recurrence and nonresponse to radiation and chemotherapy are also factors that adversely influence prognosis of overall patient survival.

4. What is the most common anatomic site for oral cancer?
The tongue and floor of the mouth. Other sites might be more common in different parts of the world through certain predisposing ethnic, cultural, or other factors.

5. What is the most common form of oral cancer?
Squamous cell carcinoma.

6. Explain the main difference between carcinoma in-situ and invasive carcinoma.
Carcinoma in-situ is an epithelial dysplasia that includes all the layers of the epithelium but does not extend beyond the basal layer. Once the malignant cells have penetrated the basal layer into the lamina propria, early invasive squamous cell carcinoma has been established. If tumor invasiveness extends deeper into the tissues, involving fat, muscle, or other structures, then true invasive squamous cell carcinoma has evolved.

7. What features are characteristic of lip carcinoma?
Squamous cell carcinoma usually affects the lower lip and rarely the upper lip. This occurrence has been attributed to greater exposure of the lower lip to sunlight. Lip carcinoma commonly presents as an ulcer. In many cases, a keratin crust covers the ulcer. The rest of the lip vermilion may show actinic changes.

8. Which feature best describes the degree of malignancy of a tumor?

The degree of histologic differentiation. Malignant neoplasms are histologically classified as (1) well differentiated, (2) moderately differentiated, or (3) poorly differentiated
(anaplastic) tumors. From a histologic point of view, poorly differentiated tumors have the
highest degree of malignancy. However, that does not necessarily correlate with the clinical
behavior of a neoplasm or its response to treatment.

9. Name the most common routes of spread of oral carcinoma.

Local spread is achieved by direct invasion and infiltration of adjacent structures.
Perineural invasion and spread is particularly important because it can adversely influence the
actual extent of the tumor. Regional spread to the neck lymph nodes occurs via the lymphatic
route. Usually, the higher echelon nodes that mainly drain the area of the lesion are affected.
Widespread nodal involvement can also occur, as well as direct involvement of a lower level of
nodes, by skipping all other intermediate levels via the so-called fast tracks. Midline lesions
affect nodes on both sides of the neck. Spread to distal organs follows the hematogenous route.

**10. What is the most appropriate management of a small, painful, ulcerative lesion on
the posterolateral aspect of the tongue that has been present for several weeks?**

Remove any suspected source of trauma or irritation. Traumatic ulcers heal within 10–14
days. Ulcers that persist for more than 2 weeks should undergo biopsy, as should deep-seated
large ulcers, particularly those with rolled borders.

**11. Describe the role of the three major treatment modalities (surgery, radiation, and
chemotherapy) in the management of oral cancer.**

1. **Surgery**, with the recent advances in reconstructive techniques, remains the mainstay
of treatment for oral carcinoma. The primary site is resected, and the cervical lymph nodes
are removed through different types of neck dissections.

2. **Radiation therapy** can be the primary treatment modality in certain cases in the form
of external beam radiation or brachytherapy. Radiation therapy also can be combined with
surgery. In such instances radiation therapy can be delivered preoperatively (neoadjuvant), intraoperatively, or postoperatively (adjuvant).

3. **Chemotherapy** is not suitable as the primary treatment modality for oral carcinoma.
However, it can be combined with surgery and radiation in different treatment protocols, particularly for the management of patients with advanced disease. Chemotherapy, in general,
may be administered as induction, primary or neoadjuvant, adjuvant, and palliation therapy.

**12. What are the most common adverse effects of radiation therapy on the oral and
paraoral tissues?**

   Rampant caries
   Radiation mucositis
   Xerostomia
   Difficulty in swallowing
   Varying degrees of trismus
   Radiation dermatitis

Osteoradionecrosis does not develop unless the patient's oral condition is not optimized
prior to radiation therapy and postirradiation dental procedures are performed without proper
precautions.

13. What is the proper management of postmaxillectomy defects?

Some controversy exists over the best way to manage postmaxillectomy defects. One
school of thought holds that immediate reconstruction of such defects is inappropriate because it prevents inspection for possible recurrence. An obturator is used for 1 year, and if recurrence is not detected, a delayed reconstruction is performed.

Other surgeons prefer immediate defect reconstruction following intraoperative frozen-section assessment of resection margins. Defect reconstruction can be performed successfully by nonvascularized grafts, local flaps, regional flaps, and free tissue transfers. The most frequently used methods include the temporalis muscle flap as a simple or composite flap with attached calvarial bone, the buccal fat pad, and free composite flaps that can be combined with osseointegrated implants for oral rehabilitation.

14. Which tests should be included in the metastatic work-up for oral cancer?

Blood and biochemical profiles, chest x-ray, liver ultrasound, and bone scan. In the case of equivocal results, computed tomography (CT) scanning or magnetic resonance imaging (MRI) also may be required to clarify the findings.

15. What is the best way to manage a highly suspicious lesion that is biopsied but determined by the pathologist to be noncancerous?

The lesion should be rebiopsied. Tissue sampling should be obtained from multiple sites of the lesion. If this action does not solve the diagnostic problem, a second opinion from another pathologist might be appropriate before any final treatment decision is reached. However, it can not be overemphasized that all pertinent clinical information and the findings of other diagnostic modalities must be provided to the pathologist at the time of the initial submission of the specimen.

16. Which is the most appropriate imaging study for evaluation of a maxillary sinus neoplasm?

CT.

17. What conditions should be suspected (a) when a patient who has undergone marginal mandibulectomy and postoperative radiation therapy for squamous cell carcinoma presents with a fracture in the area of the marginal mandibulectomy and (b) when a patient who has been treated surgically for carcinoma of the posterior maxilla develops trismus?

a. Osteoradionecrosis and, most importantly, tumor recurrence.

b. Tumor recurrence.

18. Define radical neck dissection, modified radical neck dissection, and selective neck dissection.

1. **Radical neck dissection** (RND) is the *en bloc* removal of the lymph-node–bearing tissues of one side of the neck, from the inferior border of the mandible to the clavicle and from the lateral border of the strap muscles to the anterior border of the trapezius. Included in the resected specimen are the spinal accessory nerve, the internal jugular vein, and the sternocleidomastoid muscle.

2. The **modified radical neck dissection** (MRND) differs from RND in that one, two, or all three of the major anatomic structures that are removed during RND (spinal accessory nerve, internal jugular vein, sternocleidomastoid muscle) are preserved in MRND.

3. The **selective neck dissection** (SND) entails the removal of only those lymph node groups that are at highest risk of containing metastases according to the location of the primary tumor, preserving the spinal accessory nerve, internal jugular vein, and sternocleidomastoid muscle. Currently, the most frequently used SND is the anterolateral neck dissection (supraomohyoid neck dissection and the expanded supraomohyoid neck dissection). In both operations, nodal regions I (submental, submandibular nodes), II (upper jugular, jugulodigastric, and upper posterior cervical nodes), and III (midjugular nodes) are removed *en bloc* together with the lymph nodes found within the fibroadipose tissue located medial to the sternocleidomastoid muscle. The **expanded supraomohyoid neck dissection** also includes the nodes in region IV (lower jugular, scalene, and supraclavicular lymph nodes located deep to the lower one third of the sternocleidomastoid muscle).

19. Which is the best imaging modality to diagnose invasive squamous cell carcinoma?

Soft tissue invasion is best assessed by MRI. Osseous invasion is best assessed by conventional CT or Dentascan imaging.

20. What patient characteristics are suggestive of a malignant neoplasm of the oral cavity?

The following characteristics suggest, but are not conclusive of, advanced disease:

Malnourishment

Halitosis

Drooling

Difficulty in speech and deglutition

BIBLIOGRAPHY

1. Black RJ, Gluckman JL, Shumrick DA: Screening for distant metastases in head and neck cancer patients. Aust N Z J Surg 54:527–530, 1984.
2. Davison SP, Sherris DA, Meland NB: An algorithm for maxillectomy defect reconstruction. Laryngoscope 108:215–219, 1998.
3. Eversole LR: Oral Medicine: A Pocket Guide. Philadelphia, W.B. Saunders, 1996.
4. Howaldt HP, Kainz M, Euler B, Vorast H: Proposal for modification of the TNM staging classification for cancer of the oral cavity. J Craniomaxillofac Surg 27:275–288, 1999.
5. Medina JE, Rigual NR: Neck dissection. In Byron J, Bailey J (eds): Head and Neck Surgery—Otolaryngology. Philadelphia, J.B. Lippincott, 1993, pp 1192–1220.
6. Nakayama B, Matsuura H, Ishihara O, et al: Functional reconstruction of a bilateral maxillectomy defect using a fibula osteocutaneous flap with osseointegrated implants. Plast Reconstr Surg 96:1201–1204, 1995.

37. LASERS IN ORAL AND MAXILLOFACIAL SURGERY

Robert A. Strauss, D.D.S.

1. What does the term laser mean?

The word *laser* is derived from the acronym for *l*ight *a*mplification by *s*timulated *e*mission of *r*adiation.

2. What is the most common laser used in the oral and maxillofacial surgery (OMS) practice?

Carbon dioxide (CO_2) laser.

3. CO_2 laser wavelength is absorbed principally by what tissue component?

At a wavelength of 10,600 nm, the CO_2 laser is almost completely absorbed by water (98%). Its use in OMS is based on the fact that all soft tissues are composed mainly of water and therefore they absorb this wavelength exceedingly well.

4. What are the four basic tissue interactions associated with lasers?

1. Reflection (bouncing off the tissue)
2. Transmission (going through the tissue)
3. Scatter (breaking up inside the tissue)
4. Absorption

Of these, only absorption has any significant beneficial effects on tissue. Therefore, a laser is usually chosen by its percentage of absorption into the intended target tissue.

5. What are the four main reactions seen in tissue after laser energy absorption?

1. Photothermal
2. Photochemical
3. Photoablative
4. Photoacoustic

6. What is a photothermal reaction?

When laser energy is absorbed into a target tissue, one possible result is the generation of heat. This change in energy from light to heat is termed a *photothermal reaction* and results in tissue vaporization. This reaction is used to perform most soft tissue surgeries in OMS.

7. What is a photoablative reaction?

When laser energy is absorbed into a target, another possible result is fragmentation of the chemical bonds of the target, resulting in vaporizing of the tissue. Unique to this reaction is that little or no heat is generated within the target, allowing surgery without lateral thermal damage. For example, this reaction is used in ophthalmology to ablate the cornea for vision correction without damaging the eye.

8. Which basic tissue interaction is used by the CO_2 and Er:YAG lasers?

Both of these lasers are primarily absorbed by tissue water, with a resultant generation of heat. This **photothermal** reaction then causes the intracellular water to vaporize, generating steam that expands and eventually disrupts the cell membrane.

9. What are the two most common lasers used for cosmetic skin resurfacing?

Because of their high affinity for tissue water found in the epidermis and dermis, the CO_2 and Er:YAG lasers are the most common lasers used for skin resurfacing techniques.

10. What is power density (irradiation)?

Power density is a measure of the amount of laser power applied to a given area. Measured in watts per centimeters squared (W/cm^2), it determines how deep the laser's effect will go into the tissue in any given time unit (e.g., 1 second). Therefore, greater power or a smaller spot size causes a deeper laser effect in tissue for each second of use. As the power is diminished or the spot size is increased, the laser's effect becomes more superficial for each second of use.

11. What is energy density (fluence)?

Energy density is a measure of the total amount of laser energy applied to a given unit of tissue during a complete laser pulse. Essentially, this represents the power density over the course of time of the entire laser pulse and is measured as $W/cm^2 \times$ time (in seconds). In other words, the total depth of effect will be greater for a given power density (power and spot size) the longer the laser is applied. As an example, a 2-second pulse will create twice the total effect depth in tissue as a 1-second pulse.

12. What is thermal relaxation time?

Thermal relaxation is the process by which heat diffuses through tissue by thermal conduction. Thermal relaxation time is the time required for a given tissue to dissipate 50% of the heat absorbed from the laser pulse. Any pulse that is longer than the thermal relaxation time for the target tissue would, therefore, lead to some amount of lateral thermal damage.

13. What is coagulation necrosis?

Coagulation necrosis is the area surrounding the intended surgical site that is both reversible and irreversibly damaged by lateral thermal conduction. The longer the laser energy is applied, the greater the zone of lateral thermal damage that occurs through conduction. Conversely, this principle does have the positive effect of contracting blood vessel wall collagen, thereby sealing any blood vessel that is within this zone (300–500 μm diameter). This leads to bloodless surgery in many cases.

14. What is the significance of the thermal relaxation time of approximately 700–1000 μsec for skin?

If a laser can provide a pulse of energy that is shorter in duration than the thermal relaxation time for the target tissue, there will be little or no thermal damage to adjacent and underlying tissue. It is this effect that makes skin resurfacing possible. The time on tissue is maintained below the thermal relaxation time for skin, ensuring that there will be little or no damage to the underlying dermal tissues and allowing rapid re-epithelialization from intact dermal adnexal structures.

15. What three delivery systems for lasers are used currently?

The ideal delivery system is a fiber-optic guide. Unfortunately, many laser wavelengths useful in OMS cannot be transmitted through fiber optics. Articulated arm lasers use a series of connecting hollow metal tubes with prism articulations to transmit the beam, but this is sometimes cumbersome in intraoral use. More recently, hollow wave guide technology using internal mirrored and bendable hollow metal fibers has facilitated the use of lasers in the oral cavity.

16. What is the difference between a focused and a defocused laser beam?

A laser beam can be focused down to a very small spot size or backed away from the target, allowing the spot size to increase. Because spot size is a determinant of power density, the smaller the spot size the greater the power density and the deeper the laser affects tissue during each pulse. A larger spot size will cause a larger but more superficial effect as the power density diminishes. A high-power density and a small spot size are used to make incisions while a large spot size with lower power density is generally used for tissue ablation.

17. What is meant by tissue ablation?

Tissue ablation, or tissue vaporization, is the removal of the surface layers of tissue over a wide area, such as would be used to remove a superficial leukoplakia. This is accomplished by applying the laser at a large spot size, thereby lowering the power density and creating a large but superficial effect in tissue. This technique allows for removal of large surface lesions with little damage to underlying structures but does preclude obtaining an excisional specimen for histologic examination.

18. How is a particular laser chosen?

In general, laser choice is determined by matching the wavelength of the laser with the absorption of that wavelength by the intended target tissue. The greater the absorption, the greater the effect in that tissue.

19. What is the effect of a laser beam on supplemental oxygen being delivered to the patient?

Although oxygen is not flammable, it does support combustion. Hence, in higher concentrations (approximately over 30%), the oxygen would support rapid combustion with disastrous consequences if anything in the surgical field caught fire (e.g., endotracheal tube, hair, gauze). Keeping everything but the target wet, protecting endotracheal tubes, and minimizing exposed oxygen supplementation can help diminish the risk.

20. What is an aiming beam?

Lasers that are not within the visible spectrum of light, such as the CO_2, cannot be seen. Therefore, in order to aim and focus the beam, a secondary laser that is within the visible spectrum (e.g., helium neon [HeNe] or diode) is sent coaxially along with the CO_2 to act as a visible aiming beam.

21. What are YAG lasers?

The crystal of these lasers is made of *y*ttrium, *a*luminum, and *g*arnet and is doped with a rare earth element (e.g., neodymium [Nd], holmium [Ho], or erbium [Er]) as the active lasing medium.

22. What is the typical zone of coagulation necrosis surrounding the CO_2 laser wound?

Using a continuous-wave CO_2 laser, the zone of coagulation necrosis is generally around 500 microns or less. Manipulating the speed of the pulse (e.g., Superpulse or Ultrapulse) can decrease this to less than 100 microns.

23. What is coherent light?

Coherent light is a state in which all light waves are temporally and spatially in phase. In other words, the light is monochromatic (one wavelength), collimated (all the waves are parallel), and uniform of phase (all the peaks and troughs line up on top of one another).

24. What is IPL and what are its main uses?

IPL, the acronym for intense pulsed light, duplicates or improves on some effects of the laser using monochromatic, but not coherent, light. Some generalized and deep vascular and pigmented lesions, for example, can be treated effectively using noncoherent light, which has a greater degree of scatter than most laser light sources.

25. What is a chromophore?

A chromophore is a target tissue for a specific laser wavelength. The primary chromophore for the CO_2 and Er:YAG lasers is water, while the argon laser is absorbed well by hemoglobin and tissue pigments (which are its chromophores) but not by water. It is important to match the intended target with the chromophore for the particular laser being used.

BIBLIOGRAPHY

1. Atkinson T: Fundamentals of the carbon dioxide laser. In Catone G, Alling C (eds): Laser Applications in Oral and Maxillofacial Surgery. Philadelphia, W.B. Saunders, 1997.
2. Strauss RA: Laser management of discrete lesions. In Catone G, Alling C (eds): Laser Applications in Oral and Maxillofacial Surgery. Philadelphia, W.B. Saunders, 1997.

38. MANAGEMENT OF THE PATIENT IRRADIATED FOR HEAD OR NECK CANCER

A. Omar Abubaker, D.M.D., Ph.D.

1. What are the principles of management of irradiated patients?

The overall goals of treatment of patients who have undergone or who are about to receive radiation therapy is the following:
- Better understanding of radiation effects and the pathogenesis of osteoradionecrosis (ORN)
- Better prevention and management of the radiation effects
- Minimize postradiation complications by use of hyperbaric oxygen (HBO) therapy
- Functional bony reconstruction and total oral rehabilitation of radiation patients using dental implants

2. What is the incidence of oral cancer?

According to 1996 statistics, the estimated annual number of new cases of head and neck cancer in the United States is 29,490 cases. This accounts for 3% of all new cancer cases in men and 2% in women. The most common head and neck cancer is squamous cell carcinoma. The most common sites for oral carcinoma are the floor of mouth, retromolar trigone, pharynx, tongue, and lips.

3. What are the methods of treating head and neck cancer?

In early stages of the disease, surgery or radiotherapy is often used as the sole therapy. In more advanced stages of the disease, therapies combining surgery, radiotherapy, and chemotherapy are usually used to minimize recurrence of the disease and to improve the survival rate.

4. What are the types of radiotherapy?

- External radiation sources, which include supervoltage and megavoltage (Cobalt 60 and linear accelerator)
- Low-dose brachytherapy, which includes radium needles and cesium and iridium wires

5. What is the mechanism of action of radiotherapy?

The radiation interacts with the atoms and molecules of the cells and produces free radicals, which diffuse a short distance into the cell to damage critical targets such as DNA. It affects all phases of the cell cycle.

6. How is radiation measured?

The measurement of dose of radiation has changed from rads (100 ergs/gm) to grays (Gy; 1 joule/kg): 1 Gy = 100 rads = 100 cGy.

7. What cell types are most affected by radiation therapy?

Radiation affects all rapidly dividing cells including neoplastic cells, epithelial cells, endothelial cells, and reticuloendothelial cells.

8. Which orofacial tissues are affected by radiation therapy?

Oral mucosa	Cartilage
Skin	Muscles of mastication
Subcutaneous tissue	Temporomandibular joint (TMJ)

Teeth	Thyroid and parathyroid glands
Oral flora	Pituitary gland
Salivary glands	Peripheral and cranial nerves
Nasolacrimal drainage system	Lymphatics
Bone	Paranasal sinuses

9. What are the effects of radiation on teeth and periodontium?

The most common manifestations of radiation therapy on oral tissues are erythema of the oral mucosa and friable and easily injured gingival tissue. The gingival tissue also becomes less cellular and fibrotic. The effects on teeth are mostly in the form of radiation caries.

10. What is radiation caries?

Radiation caries is characterized by circumferential decay of the cervical portion of numerous teeth. It is believed that radiation caries is related, at least in part, to xerostomia. Another possible contributing factor is change in the oral flora. Radiation caries also may be related to pulpal death, dentine dehydration, and enamel loss (similar to dentigerous imperfecta). Radiation caries is most severe within the radiation field.

11. How does radiation affect oral mucosa?

Long-term changes include decreased keratinization, decreased vascularity, easy ulceration, and delayed healing. Short-term effects include short-term taste changes and mucositis.

12. What is irradiation mucositis?

Painful erythema of the oral mucosa, pharynx, and larynx. It usually develops after 1 week of radiation therapy, may become severe after 3 weeks of beginning of treatment, and subsides 2–3 weeks after completion of treatment. Its duration and severity are greatly influenced by daily dose. The most common sites affected are the soft palate, tonsillar pillars, buccal mucosa, lateral border of the tongue, and larynx and pharyngeal walls. Mucositis usually does not develop at the hard palate, alveolar ridges, dorsum of the tongue, or true vocal cords.

13. What are the radiation effects on oral flora?

Radiation causes long-term changes in the microbiological population of oral flora, including increased fungal and anaerobic organisms and high incidence of candidiasis.

14. Does radiation affect the TMJ and muscles of mastication?

Changes in these areas are uncommon with irradiation for oral cancer because the TMJ is often outside the field of radiation. When the TMJ and muscles of mastication are within the field of radiation, trismus and fibrosis of the muscles of mastication are seen along with fibrous ankylosis of the TMJ and myofascial pain.

15. What are the radiation effects on bone?

The decreased vascularity of the bone causes delayed healing after any trauma to the bone. These effects, which are the most serious, are marked after 4 months and progress with time. They are chronic, can occur as late as 30 years after radiation, and occasionally result in ORN.

16. What is the dental management of patients prior to radiation treatment?

- Complete oral/dental examination and treatment plan
- Any necessary extraction and surgery
- Maintenance of teeth and caries control
- Restoration of restorable teeth
- Prosthetic examination to prevent postradiation trauma from ill-fitting dentures

17. What factors should be considered in evaluation of patients prior to radiation of the head and neck?

Condition of the dentition

Level of oral hygiene and patient attitude

Age of the patient

Radiation field and dose

Urgency of radiation treatment

18. What are the methods of caries control and prevention in the preradiation patient?

The goal of preradiation management is prevention of dental and oral diseases, which consists of:

- Prophylactic care before and at the end of therapy
- Oral hygiene instructions
- Daily administration of fluoride
- Weekly follow-up during therapy and every 3–4 weeks afterward

19. Name some guidelines for extraction prior to radiation therapy.

- All carious mandibular teeth in the field of radiation (more than 6000 cGy) should be extracted, except in patients with particularly good oral hygiene and excellent dental condition.
- All questionable teeth should be extracted.
- Full bony impacted teeth can be left in place.
- Optimal time for extraction is 21 days before beginning of radiotherapy (no less than 2 weeks).
- Less optimally, extraction can be done within 4 months after completion of therapy.
- Perform radical alveolectomy with primary soft tissue closure following extraction.

20. How should a patient be managed during radiation therapy?

Management of radiation patient at this phase should be mainly palliative, including only pulpectomy, pulpotomy, incision and drainage, analgesics, and antibiotics. Extractions should not be performed during radiation therapy, and definitive treatment should be delayed until after completion of radiation therapy.

21. Describe the management of a patient who has undergone head and neck radiation.

Patients who have history of radiation therapy should be managed carefully in order to prevent ORN, which may result from any dental or surgical trauma. Obtaining records of radiation fields and dose is essential to determine the best approach to these patients. Once such records are available, the following guidelines should be followed:

- Recall for prophylaxis and home care evaluation every 3 months.
- The patient should continue daily fluoride application for the rest of his or her life.
- Restorative dental procedures may be performed as needed.
- Prosthetic appliances may be constructed as early as 3 months if mucositis has cleared.
- Prosthetic appliances must be adjusted carefully to prevent irritation and trauma to the underlying mucosa.
- Invasive procedures involving the irradiated bone should be avoided, if at all possible.
- Within 4 months of completion of radiation therapy and after resolution of the mucositis, minor surgical procedures such as extraction and minor preprosthetic surgery and vestibuloplasty can be performed.
- If an invasive procedure is necessary within the field of radiation (receiving greater than 6000 cGy) 4 months after radiation or thereafter, the procedure should be performed after HBO therapy.

22. What is the management of a postradiation patient who needs oral and maxillofacial surgery (OMFS)?

Four months after completion of therapy (more than 6000 cGy), all surgical procedures in the field of radiation should be done after prophylactic HBO treatment.

23. How are irradiation mucositis and xerostomia managed?

Treatment of mucositis and xerostomia in patients who received radiation therapy is mostly symptomatic:

- Keep mouth and teeth moist and plaque free.
- Avoid using lip balms that are petrolatum based, commercial mouthwashes, peroxide rinses for longer than 3 days, denture adhesives, and citrus and spicy foods.
- Sugarless candy and gum chewing are encouraged.
- Do not drink excessive alcohol or use tobacco.
- Use a saliva substitute (e.g., Xero-lube, Saliva-lube, Saliva-aide, Moi-stir, Salivart).
- Thin foods with liquid to aid in swallowing.
- Keep dentures out if mucositis is present.
- Filter smoke from room with filtering appliances.
- Use water, beeswax, or vegetable oil–based lubricant or hydrous lanolin to moisten the mouth.
- If toothpaste is irritating, using baking soda.

24. How should pain caused by irradiation mucositis and xerostomia be managed?

- Viscous lidocaine 2%, half an hour before meals
- Benadryl syrup and Kaopectate mixed in equal parts
- Ulcers may be coated with sucralfate suspension
- Analgesics starting with ibuprofen and progressing to narcotics as needed

OSTEORADIONECROSIS

25. What is osteoradionecrosis?

After completion of radiation treatment, an area of exposed, nonviable bone at the field of radiation that fails to show any evidence of spontaneous healing is diagnosed as ORN. The bone, which is exposed because of mucosal or cutaneous ulceration, must be at least 3–5 mm in size and must be present in the field of irradiation for at least 6 months (though some authors require only 3 months for diagnosis).

26. What are the risk factors for ORN?

Risk Factors for Osteoradionecrosis

PATIENT-RELATED FACTORS	TUMOR-RELATED FACTORS	TREATMENT-RELATED FACTORS
Presence of teeth	Anatomic location of the tumor	Field of radiation
Presence of active dental disease	Clinical stage of the tumor	Total dose of radiation
Oral hygiene and preradiation care	Presence of lymph node metastasis	Dose rate/day
Alcohol and tobacco abuse		Mode of radiation delivery
		Tumor surgery

27. What is the incidence of ORN?

Incidence of ORN ranges from 1% to 44.2% with an overall incidence of 11.8% in most studies published before 1968. Recent studies showed incidences of 5–15% with an overall incidence of 5.4%. ORN has a bimodal incidence, peaking at 12 months and again at 24–60 months. However, it can occur as late as 30 years later. It is often related to traumatic injuries such as preirradiation extraction (4.4%), postirradiation extraction (5.8%), and denture trauma (less than 1%). ORN may occur spontaneously (albeit rarely) due to progression of periapical or periodontal disease.

28. What is the difference in incidence between maxilla ORN and mandible ORN?

ORN is more common in the mandible than in the maxilla because of the lower blood supply to the mandible and the compact bone structure of the mandibular bone. Another possible explanation is that the mandible is involved in the field of irradiation more often than the maxilla is in most oral cancers.

29. What is the effect of the anatomic site of the tumor on ORN incidence?

Oral cancers have the highest incidence of ORN, especially those of the tongue, retromolar region, and floor of the mouth. This is likely from the direct involvement of the mandible in the radiation field and the aggressive and radical surgical approach for resection of these tumors.

30. What is the effect of neck lymph node metastasis on the incidence of ORN?

There is no difference in incidence of ORN when the neck is N1, N2m, or N3. However, there is a significantly higher incidence of ORN when the neck is N0. This paradoxical effect is probably because patients with N0 tumors have a better prognosis and live longer than patients with cervical involvement and therefore are at higher risk to develop ORN later in life.

31. How does tumor size affect the incidence of ORN?

No difference in ORN incidence has been reported when the tumor size increases from T1 to T3. However, there is a significant increase in incidence of ORN when the tumor size is T4. This increase is likely caused by bone invasion and the patient being subjected to both surgery and radiation therapy.

32. Does the mode of radiation delivery affect ORN incidence?

There is positive correlation between increased risk of ORN and mode of irradiation. The majority of patients who develop ORN are radiated with an external beam source. This difference may be related to the fact that fewer patients are treated with implants or with external beam source plus an implant source.

33. What is the effect of total radiation dose on the incidence of ORN?

The incidence of ORN is uncommon when the total radiation dose is below 5000 cGy. When the total external radiation dose is between 6000 cGy and 7000 cGy, ORN occurs more frequently. When the total dose is above 7500 cGy, ORN is almost 10 times higher than for doses less than 5000 cGy. Dose of radiation is probably the most important factor affecting incidence of ORN of the jaws.

34. What is the pathophysiology of ORN?

There are two general hypotheses regarding the pathophysiology of ORN: the "older concept" put forward by Watson and Scarborough (1938) and Meyer (1970) and a more recent hypothesis by Marx (1983). For a long time it was believed that ORN developed after a triad of radiation therapy, local trauma, and infection of the irradiated bone. Watson and Scarborough and Meyer speculated the sequence of events leading to ORN to be radiation, trauma, and infection leading to radiation osteomyelitis.

The "new concept" of pathophysiology of ORN is based on findings of several studies that showed that ORN can occur without trauma or suppuration and that microorganisms are found with ORN in only rare instances compared to the usual presence of deep organisms in osteomyelitis. Marx's theory holds that ORN is a radiation-induced, wound-healing defect. According to this hypothesis, the pathophysiologic sequence is (1) irradiation, (2) hypovascular, hypoxic, and hypocellular tissue (the "3 H's"), (3) tissue breakdown, and finally (4) a nonhealing wound in which the tissues' metabolic demand exceeds supply.

35. What is the histopathology of ORN?

The most common histopathologic features of ORN, which includes acute cellular damage, endarteritis, hyalinization, and vascular thrombosis, are evident soon after radiation exposure. Fewer osteocytes are seen along with marrow fibrosis and sequestrum formation. These changes are considered subclinical for 6 months. Hypovascularity and fibrosis are evident 6–12 months after radiotherapy.

36. What are the clinical features of ORN?

Exposed bone, loss of soft tissue and bone   Trismus
Pain and dysesthesia/anesthesia   Pathologic fracture and orocutaneous fistula
Soft tissue necrosis

37. What are the radiographic features of osteoradionecrosis?
- Diffuse radiolucency without sclerotic demarcation is seen.
- Mottled osteoporosis and sclerotic areas can be identified after bone sequestra are formed.
- Computed tomography (CT) and bone scintigraphy can be used to evaluate the extension and behavior of ORN.

38. What are the methods of management of ORN?
Depending on the stage of the disease, the management is based either on a conservative approach or on use of an HBO-surgical approach.

39. What is the conservative management of ORN?
ORN can be managed without the need for HBO or major surgical intervention. This approach consists of:
- Daily local irrigation (saline solution, $NaHCO_3$, or chlorhexidine 0.2%)
- Systemic antibiotics
- Avoidance of irritants (tobacco, alcohol, and denture use)
- Good oral hygiene instructions
- Gentle removal of sequestrum in sequestrating lesions

40. What is the HBO protocol?
Hyperbaric oxygen therapy is an administration of 100% oxygen via head tent, mask, or endotracheal tube within a special chamber at 2.4 atmospheric absolute (ATA) pressure for 90 minutes each session. The treatment should be delivered 5 times ("dives") a week once a day.

41. What is the mechanism of action of HBO therapy?
HBO has been shown to help induce tissue healing by:
Angiogenesis
Inducing fibroplasia and neocellularity
Promoting survival of osteoprogenitor cells
Promoting the formation of functional periosteum

42. What are the indications for HBO therapy in OMFS?
- Prophylaxis to prevent ORN when surgical procedures in the irradiated field are indicated after completion of radiation treatment
- Treatment of ORN
- Before bony and soft tissue reconstruction and before placement of dental implants in irradiated bone
- Treatment of necrotizing fasciitis, gas gangrene, and chronic refractory osteomyelitis

43. What are the general principles of use of HBO therapy and surgery in management of ORN?
HBO therapy alone or in conjunction with surgery (depending on the stage of the disease) is often used to treat ORN of the mandible or maxilla using the following guidelines:

1. HBO and surgery are indicated when the lesion is symptomatic and did not respond to conservative measures alone.

2. HBO with or without surgery is indicated for treatment of ORN. According to the Marx–University of Miami protocol, depending on the extent of the disease, combined surgery and HBO treatment consists of three treatment stages of advanced clinical severity: stages I, II, and III.

3. HBO is indicated when surgery to remove the sequestrum or bony reconstruction is planned.

44. What is staging I treatment of osteoradionecrosis?

All patients who meet the definition of ORN should begin stage I treatment and receive 30 treatments of HBO along with rigorous wound care. After 30 treatments, the wound is reevaluated for definitive improvement, decreased exposed bone, resorption, spontaneous sequestration, and softening of exposed bone. If the wound shows any of these signs, then the patient receives another 10 treatments for a full course of 40 treatments. If no improvement is seen after 30 HBO treatments, the patient is considered a nonresponder to stage I treatment and is advanced to stage II.

45. What is stage II treatment of ORN?

A patient with a chronic, persistent (nonprogressive) form of ORN that persists after 30 treatments of HBO is considered nonrespondent to stage I and should advance to stage II treatment. This stage consists of intraoral surgical debridement (transoral alveolar sequestrectomy) of all necrotic bone to a bleeding bone with primary closure of the wound in a layered fashion. If healing progresses after surgery and the wound remains closed, 10 additional treatments of HBO are given. If no improvement is seen after the surgical debridement and the wound breaks down leaving larger areas of exposed bone, the patient is a nonresponder to stage II treatment and is advanced to stage III treatment protocol.

46. Who is a candidate for stage III treatment of ORN?

A patient with an exposed bone in the field of radiation with one or more of the following features should be considered a candidate for stage III treatment:

1. Nonresponder to stage II therapy

2. Patient who presents initially or after previous treatment of ORN with one of the following:

- Pathologic fracture of the mandible
- Orocutaneous fistula
- Radiographic evidence of osteolysis of the inferior border of the mandible
- Soft tissue dehiscence and continuous bony exposure despite treatment with stage II protocol

47. What is stage III treatment of ORN?

Patients who are candidates for stage III treatment should have had 30 treatments of HBO prior to surgical intervention. This is followed by transoral resection of the mandibular bone to bleeding bone. The remaining segments of the mandible are stabilized with either extraskeletal pin fixation or maxillomandibular fixation. This is followed by 10 additional postresection treatments of HBO. Later, bony reconstruction may be carried out if the patient is a suitable candidate.

48. What are the possible complications of HBO treatment?

Barotrauma	Oxygen toxicity
Ear and sinus trauma	Central nervous system and pulmonary
TMJ rupture	reactions and myopia
Pneumothorax and air embolism	Fire, transient visual problems, claustrophobia

49. What are the contraindications to use of HBO?

Absolute contraindications:	Relative contraindications:
Optic neuritis	Seizure disorder
Untreated pneumothorax	Claustrophobia
Congenital spherocytosis	Pregnancy
Fulminate viral infections	Emphysema

50. What is the HBO protocol for prophylactic use before oral surgical procedures?

This protocol consists of once-daily treatment 5 days per week. The patient should receive twenty consecutive treatments before extraction or before any other oral surgical procedure within the field of radiation. Ten additional treatments should be administered postoperatively.

CONTROVERSIES

51. Should extractions be performed with the use of prophylactic HBO?

Pro. This approach is based primarily on the randomized, prospective study by Marx et al. of 137 patients that compared conservative protocol with that of HBO plus surgery.[10] This study was updated on 1991 to include 300 patients. According to this study, the incidence of ORN in the non-HBO group was 30% compared to 5.4% in the HBO group. Calculation of cost of ORN treatment was found to far exceed the cost of prophylactic HBO. Accordingly, most authors argue that HBO is very cost-effective.

Con. Authors against the use of prophylactic HBO for extractions argue that the incidence of loss of continuity of the mandible after mandibular extractions in irradiated mandible due to ORN is generally low (2.5–4.5%). Considering that HBO is 80% effective in prevention of ORN, the rate of ORN with the use of HBO will be reduced to 0.5–1.0%. Therefore, at best, HBO may preserve 2–3 mandibles while unnecessarily treating 97–98. Accordingly, these authors argue that HBO is not cost-effective.

52. Should prophylactic HBO therapy be instituted before dental implants in the irradiated jawbone?

Pro. Animal and clinical studies showed improved soft tissue wound healing and decreased dehiscence after implants with HBO. These studies also showed improved torque removal forces of implants in irradiated bone with HBO and significantly greater quantity of bone-implant contact in irradiated rabbit tibias treated with HBO compared to implants placed without prior HBO treatment. Furthermore, some authors argue that the previously reported high success rate of dental implants in irradiated bone without prior HBO is explained by the low radiation dose used and the placement of implants outside the field of radiation.

Con. The argument against the placement of dental implants with HBO in irradiated patients is based on the high success rate of integration of implants in humans and improved integration of implants in the animal model without the use of HBO, especially if longer integration time is allowed. Accordingly, the potential benefit of HBO therapy balanced against its cost and potential complications does not justify its use in an irradiated mandible prior to placement of dental implants.

53. What is the protocol for HBO therapy when used prior to implant placement in the irradiated patient?

This protocol is advocated by some authors and consists of:
- Strict oral hygiene regimen before and after implant placement
- Use of the longest and widest implant type and the maximum number of implants possible
- Delay implant surgery until 6 months after irradiation
- Thorough informed consent
- Cessation of smoking

- Preoperative HBO (increase integration time by 3 months)
- Overengineered implant supported prosthesis
- A similar protocol for implants in irradiated maxilla and mandible
- Previously integrated implants should be buried before irradiation and subjected to 20 HBO treatments before uncovering

BIBLIOGRAPHY

1. Curi MM, Laura L: Osteoradionecrosis of the jaws: A retrospective study of the background factors and treatment in 104 cases. J Oral Maxillofac Surg 55:540–544, 1997.
2. Chapman L: Management of dental extractions in irradiated jaws: A protocol without hyperbaric oxygen therapy. J Oral Maxillofac Surg 55:275–281, 1997.
3. Epstein J, Meij VD, McKenzie M, et al: Postradiation osteonecrosis of the mandible. A long-term follow-up study. Oral Surg Oral Med Oral Pathol Oral Radiol Endod 83:657–662, 1997.
4. Johnson R, Marx RE, Buckley SB: Hyperbaric oxygen. In Worthington P, Evans JR (eds): Controversies in Oral and Maxillofacial Surgery. Philadelphia, W.B. Saunders, 1994.
5. Keller EE: Placement of dental implants in the irradiated mandible: A protocol without adjunctive hyperbaric oxygen. J Oral Maxillofac Surg 55:972–980, 1997.
6. Lambert PM, Intrieve N, Eichstaedt R: Management of dental extractions in irradiated jaws: A protocol with hyperbaric oxygen. J Oral Maxillofac Surg 55:268–274, 1997.
7. Larsen PE: Placement of dental implants in the irradiated mandible: A protocol involving adjunctive hyperbaric oxygen. J Oral Maxillofac Surg 55:967, 1997.
8. Marx RE: A new concept in the treatment of osteoradionecrosis. J Oral Maxillofac Surg 41:351, 1990.
9. Marx RE, Johnson RP, Kline SN: Prevention of osteoradionecrosis: A randomized, prospective clinical trial of hyperbaric oxygen versus penicillin. J Am Dental Assoc 111:49, 1985.
10. Parker SL, Tong T, Bolden S, Wingo PA: Cancer statistics, 1996. Ca J Clinician 46:5, 1996.
11. Rosenberg SW, Arm RN: Management of patient receiving antineoplastic and radiation therapy. In Clinician's Guide to Treatment of Common Oral Conditions, 4th ed. Baltimore, American Academy of Oral Medicine, 1997, pp 14–15.
12. Wang JK, Wood RE, McLean M: Conservative management of osteoradionecrosis. Oral Surg Oral Med Oral Pathol Oral Radiol Endod 84:16–21, 1997.

39. ORAL AND MAXILLOFACIAL RECONSTRUCTION

Jeffrey S. Jelic, D.M.D., M.D., and Vincent J. Perciaccante, D.D.S.

1. What is an autograft? An allograft? A xenograft?

An *autograft* is transplanted from one region to another in the same individual. An *allograft* is a transplant from one individual to a genetically non-identical individual of the same species. A *xenograft* is a transplant from one species to another.

2. Define the terms osteoinductive, osteoconductive, and osteogeneic.

Osteoinduction refers to new bone formation from the differentiation of osteoprogenitor cells, derived from primitive mesenchymal cells, into secretory *osteoblasts*. This differentiation is under the influence of bone inductive proteins or bone morphogenic proteins—agents from bone matrix. Osteoinduction implies that the pluripotential precursor cells of the host will be stimulated or induced to differentiate into osteoblasts by transplanted growth factors and cytokines. Such grafts help produce the cells that are necessary to produce new bone.

Osteoconduction is the formation of new bone from host-derived or transplanted osteoprogenitor cells along a biologic or alloplastic framework, such as along the fibrin clot in tooth extraction or along a hydroxyapatite block. Osteoconductive grafts provide only a passive framework or *scaffolding*. These grafts are biochemically inert in their effect upon the host. The grafted material therefore does not have the ability to actually produce bone. This type of graft simply conducts bone-forming cells from the host bed into and around the scaffolding.

Osteogenesis is the formation of new bone from osteoprogenitor cells. *Spontaneous osteogenesis* is the formation of new bone from osteoprogenitor cells in a wound. *Transplanted osteogenesis* is formation of new bone from osteoprogenitor cells placed into the wound from a distant site. Osteogeneic grafts include the advantages of osteinductive and osteoconductive grafts in addition to the advantage of transplanting fully differentiated osteocompetent cells that will immediately produce new bone. Autogenous bone is the only graft that possesses all of these criteria.

3. What is bone morphogenic protein?

Bone morphogenic protein (BMP) is a protein complex responsible for initiating osteoinduction. BMP is part of the cytokine family of growth factors, which occurs in the organic portion of bone called the bone matrix. BMP is osteoinductive: it acts on progenitor cells to induce differentiation into osteoblasts and chondroblasts. The target of BMP is the undifferentiated perivascular mesenchymal cell. BMP may be the main signal regulating skeletal formation and repair; is known to induce bone formation de novo, following the same pathways as edochondral ossification; and is responsible for ectopic bone formation by certain tumor cells, epithelial cells, and demineralized bone.

BMPs appear to be stored within bone matrix and released with resorptive activity. This is why cortical bone, which carries the largest proportion of the total bone matrix, is mixed with cancellous bone to elevate the concentration of BMP in the graft. Recombinant technology has now made purified BMP readily available as a commercial product. As many as 14 BMPs have been identified. Two in particular, rBMP-2 and rBMP-7 (also called osteogenic protein or OP-1), are particularly efficacious and may induce bone formation even without an autogenous bone carrier graft.

4. What other growth factors and cytokines are present in bone matrix?

Transforming growth factor b (TGF-b), insulin-like growth factor (IGF), interleukins (IL-1, IL-6), platelet-derived growth factor (PDGF), colony stimulating factors (CSFs), heparin-binding growth factors (HBGFs), tumor necrosis factor a (TNF-a), prostaglandins (PGs), and leukotrienes.

5. Which contains more BMP: cortical or cancellous bone?

Demineralized cortical bone has been shown to contain more BMP than demineralized cancellous bone.

6. What is platelet-rich plasma?

Platelet-rich plasma is an autologous source of platelet-derived growth factor and transforming growth factor beta$_1$ and beta$_2$. These factors have been shown to increase bone graft maturation rates and bone density. The platelet-poor plasma byproduct produced in the process can be used for fibrin glue, which can be placed in the donor site, such as the ilium, obviating the need for the use of products such as Avitene. Fibrin glue can also be used to help mold the PBCM bone graft at the recipient site.

7. List the steps in bone induction.

The steps during bone induction mimic the steps of endochondral bone formation:
1. Chemotaxis of mesenchymal progenitor cells to the area
2. Synthesis of type III collagen
3. Differentiation of chondroblasts
4. Conversion of connective tissue into cartilage (type II collagen)
5. Invasion by capillaries
6. Calcification
7. Synthesis of type IV collagen
8. Synthesis of type I collagen
9. Ossification.

8. What is creeping substitution?

Creeping substitution describes the process by which a wave of osteoclasts and subsequently a wave of osteoblasts systematically remove nonviable bone, and then replace it with viable bone.

9. Where are osteoprogenitor cells found?

Osteoprogenitor cells are found within bone marrow, endosteum, and the cambium layer of periosteum.

10. What is the prevalence of mesenchymal stem cells in the bone marrow of an adult?

At birth, prevalence is 1 in 10,000 marrow cells. The prevalence diminishes with age, and by teenage years it drops tenfold to 1 in 100,000. At age 35, the prevalence of mesenchymal stem cells is 1 in 250,000 marrow cells. Later in life, it continues to diminish to 1 in 400,000 at age 50 and 1 in 2,000,000 by age 80.

11. What is the piezoelectric effect? How does it affect grafted bone?

It is phenomena that explains Wolff's law, which states that form follows function. In 1957, Fukada and Yasuda discovered that when a bone is deformed by mechanical stress, an electric charge is generated. Bone deposition occurs in areas of **electronegativity**, while bone resorption is associated with **electropositivity**. The separation of charge is attributed to the piezoelectric effect. Clinically, when a bone is flexed, concave surfaces undergo compression and become electronegative, and bone is deposited onto them. In contrast, convex surfaces are placed under tension and become electropositive, and bone is resorbed from these surfaces.

The piezoelectric effect transforms the weak, chaotic architecture of grafted bone into an organized tissue capable of withstanding functional loads.

12. Describe the advantages and disadvantages of *cancellous* bone grafts.

Advantages are mostly based on its rich cellular capability: (1) cancellous bone grafts provide an immediate reserve population of viable bone-forming cells as well as a population of progenitor cells that are capable of differentiating into osteoblasts; (2) the porous microstructure of cancellous grafts allows ingrowth of endothelial buds and provides a large surface area for osteoblastic/osteoclastic activity. The result is an immediate increase in graft density and rapid graft incorporation. These qualities also make the graft more resistant to infection and sequestration if soft tissue coverage is compromised.

Disadvantages arise from the fact that cancellous bone grafts do not possess any macroscopic structural integrity. Thus, the graft cannot be rigidly fixed and will deform, migrate, or resorb if placed under tension or compressive functional forces.

13. Describe the advantages and disadvantages of *cortical* bone grafts.

Advantages of the cortical graft are due to its structural capabilities: (1) its rigid lamellar architecture does not deform with compression or tension, allowing rigid fixation of the graft and its use in load-bearing or structural applications; (2) cortical bone also has a higher concentration of BMP, and cortical chips incorporated into cancellous bone grafts enhance osteoinductive potential of the graft.

Disadvantages are also due to the lamellar architecture: (1) cortical bone does not carry a large population of osteocompetent cells, and the tenuous Haversian system does not allow diffusion of nutrients to maintain the few viable osteoblasts or osteoprogenitor cells that are transplanted; (2) lamellar bone provides little surface area for remodeling activity, so that graft density initially decreases, and the graft weakens as osteoclasts begin a very slow process of incorporation; (3) lamellar bone makes the graft more susceptible to infection and complete graft loss if soft tissue cover is compromised.

14. What do the terms phase I and phase II refer to when describing physiology of bone graft healing?

Axhausen proposed the two-phase theory of osteogenesis. During **phase I**, bone is formed from cells that have been transplanted with the graft. These cells often have survived transplantation, proliferated, and formed new osteoid. This phase is most active within 4 weeks of transplanting the graft and is responsible for immediate increase in graft radiopacity. However, phase I bone is randomly oriented and easily resorbed.

Phase II involves bone production from cells in the recipient bed of the host. Phase II bone is formed by either the osteoblasts existing in host bone or by recipient bed progenitor cells that have been induced to become osteoblasts. This phase also involves resorption and remodeling of the immature bone that was produced in phase I into mature lamellar bone. Phase II bone production begins at about 2 weeks and peaks around 6 weeks, but the remodeling process continues indefinitely.

Phase I determines the *quantity* of bone that the graft will form. During phase II, reorganization of bone from phase I into *quality* lamellar bone occurs. Although phase II bone healing does not contribute to the total volume of bone produced by the graft, if phase II bone is not produced, the phase I bone will resorb.

15. How does a surgeon determine how much bone will be adequate to reconstruct a particular bony defect?

In general, for most oral and maxillofacial defects, 10 cc of noncompacted corticocancellous bone is required for every 1 cm of defect to be reconstructed.

16. What are the different sources of autogenous bone? How much bone can be harvested from each?

- The **anterior iliac crest** can be used to harvest a maximum of 25–50 cc of PBCM or a corticocancellous block of 2 × 6 cm.
- The **posterior iliac crest** can provide for up to 75–100 cc corticocancellous bone or a 5 × 5 cm (2 to 2.5 times the bone harvested from the anterior ilium can be harvested from the posterior ilium on the same individual).
- The **proximal tibial metaphysis** can provide 25 cc of cancellous bone, but such bone is generally of low quality because of the fatty marrow at this site.
- The **rib** can provide for 12–18 cm length bone segment (with up to 1 cm cartilage cap). This bone is generally more useful for condylar reconstruction and for orbital or zygomatic onlay grafting. The rib can also be used as a carrier for corticocancellous bone harvested from other sites.
- The **calvarium** can offer a larger amount (5–6 strips of 3 × 1 cm) of bone from the parietal site, although it is also mostly cortical bone type.
- **Intraoral sites** to obtain bone graft have also been used and include the mandibular symphysis, external oblique ridge, and maxillary tuberosity. The mandibular symphysis offers ease of harvesting, but only 10 cc or less of mostly cortical bone can be obtained. The external oblique ridge also provides mostly cortical bone and of limited amount.

Note that graft volumes and dimensions reported in the literature vary widely with factors such as patient's age, gender, and body habitus, as well as the degree of graft compaction.

17. Should maxillofacial defects be reconstructed immediately, or is delayed reconstruction preferred?

Generally, these defects should be reconstructed *immediately or as soon as possible*, preferably within the first year after resection. Early reconstruction limits scar contracture, facial deformity, and oral dysfunction, and has been demonstrated to promote the fastest and most uneventful return to a normal lifestyle. Most recurrences and second primary tumors begin at the defect site as mucosal lesions, and radiographs are as efficacious as clinical examination at identifying these lesions. For this reason, recurrence is more frequently identified—and earlier—in reconstructed patients. Additionally, salvage surgery and radiation treatments are just as effective in reconstructed as in unreconstructed patients.

Some authors advocate a *3- to 5-year waiting period* before reconstruction because reconstruction would mask recurrence and inhibit tumor surveillance, and the reconstruction would be lost due to the resection. Such masking and inhibition is especially problematic in cases of malignant lesions or tumors that have a high incidence of recurrence. These lesions often can grow substantially within the inherent space in this region before symptoms become apparent and the recurrence is detected. For this reason, standard postoperative waiting periods for tumor control may be prolonged before undertaking maxillary reconstruction to ensure a tumor-free state.

18. What are the criteria for a successful mandibular bone reconstruction?

The ultimate goal for any reconstruction procedure is to achieve restoration of the reconstructed organ and functional rehabilitation of the patient. In regard to reconstruction of the mandible, success is:

- **Restoration of mandibular continuity**, to allow greatest restoration of oral functions, aesthetics, and mechanical advantage, and to provide normal contours/appearance and foundation for future restoration
- **Restoration of alveolar bone height**, to allow for placement of a denture or other prosthetic rehabilitation devices
- **Restoration of osseous bulk**, to allow an adequate volume of tissue to achieve a strong prosthetic base and to prevent fracture and failure under function
- **Maintenance of osseous content for at least 18 months**. Grafts, which are stable after 18 months, usually remain functional. Late graft resorption, which occurs between 6

and 18 months, is directly related to diminished vascularity of recipient soft tissue bed (phase II contribution) or diminished graft cellularity. It is likely to be unrelated to rigid fixation or degree of function
- **Restoration of acceptable facial form**, which is necessary to the patient's self-image and allows a return to normal social activities
- **Acceptability of endosseous implants.** The successful bone graft accommodates placement of a dental implant, and therefore the gamut of restorative dental techniques.
- **Recoverable, nondebilitating donor site surgery.** Even with achieving the other six goals, if the patient sustains permanent donor site morbidity, the reconstruction cannot be considered a completely successful procedure.

19. What are the major considerations in repair of large mandibular defects?
Soft tissue coverage, amount of bone replacement, stabilization of the graft, and future occlusal rehabilitation.

20. What can be used to hold PBCM grafts in place during mandibular reconstruction?
Several materials have been used to contain PBCM grafts at the recipient site. These include alloplasts such as titanium mesh, stainless steel, Teflon, and Dacron-urethane trays. Allogenic bone cribs such as rib, ilium, and mandible have also been used because they are better tolerated by thin or irradiated tissue and are bioresorbable. The recent availability of fibrin glue as a byproduct of plasma-rich platelets has allowed the use of a reconstruction plate as another modality for holding PBCM in place during mandibular reconstruction.

21. True or false: The most difficult defect of the mandible to reconstruct is one that crosses the midline.
True. The reason for this difficulty is due to the need in this area for hard tissue support of the chin's soft tissue as well as suspension of the extrinsic tongue musculature.

22. What is the protocol for preparing the recipient bed for mandibular reconstruction in a previously irradiated site?
Irradiated tissues are hypovascular, hypocellular, and hypoxic. Patients who have received more than 5000 cGy of radiation to the tissue bed prior to mandibular reconstruction often require a **qualitative improvement** to this tissue. If the tissue bed is sufficient quantitatively, consider hyperbaric oxygen (HBO) therapy. The protocol consists of 30 preoperative HBO dives at 2.4 atmospheres for 90 minutes and 10 postoperative HBO dives at 2.4 atmospheres for 90 minutes. If the tissue is lacking in quantity, use a myocutaneous flap or free microvascular flap to provide tissue bulk.

23. Describe the boundaries of the compartment that is harvested in anterior iliac crest bone graft.
The iliac crest has two thick segments, which are suitable for corticocancellous bone harvesting. The anterior and posterior sites are separated by an intervening marrowless segment approximating the sacroiliac joint. The anterior third of the iliac crest contains a marrow compartment, which begins 1 cm behind the anterior superior iliac crest (ASIS). In adults, the anterior ilium at this location averages 1.3 cm in thickness. The tubercle is located approximately 6 cm posterior to the ASIS. The tubercle is the thickest portion of the crest and averages 1.7 cm in the average adult. The posterior boundary of the anterior marrow compartment is actually located 1–2 cm posterior to the tubercle. The marrow space of the anterior ilium only extends 2 cm inferior to the iliac crest. A maximum of 25 cc of compacted corticocancellous bone can be safely harvested from the anterior hip of the average adult.

24. Describe the surgical approach to harvesting bone graft from the anterior iliac crest.
Place a sand bag under the sacral spine to display the landmarks of the iliac crest and allow surgical access. A second sandbag is recommended under the shoulder to prevent

over-rotation of the spine. Palpate and mark the ASIS. Identify and mark the tubercle 5–6 cm posterior to the ASIS. Prior to actually marking the incision line (and at the time of incision), the assistant should press on the skin just above the iliac crest to roll this skin superiorly. In this manner, the postoperative scar will be located below the crest and below the belt line.

Start the skin incision at least 1 cm posterior to the ASIS to prevent damage to the lateral femoral cutaneous nerve, which provides sensation to the lateral thigh. The incision will parallel the iliac crest for approximately 5 cm. It should not extend more than 2 cm beyond the tubercle to limit the possibility of damaging the lateral cutaneous branch of the iliohypogastric nerve.

Incise the periosteum within the white line that represents the approximation of abdominal wall muscles and gluteal muscles. After reflection of the periosteum and overlying musculature from the medial side of the ilium, use an osteotome or a saw to harvest the medial cortex of 3–5 mm of cancellous bone, with the appropriate dimensions desired for reconstruction. It is often possible to harvest additional cancellous bone after removal of the medial cortex. Achieve adequate hemostasis before closure of the wound. Close the wound in layers, and apply pressure dressing with or without suction drain.

25. What is the best storage media to maintain harvested bone cell viability?

The ideal storage medium for a bone graft is tissue culture media (CRML). The solution is balanced and buffered to a pH of 7.42 and contains essential organic and inorganic cell nutrients. In studies comparing bone cell turnover, CRML has shown a significant increase over saline. However, saline is currently the most commonly used storage medium for bone grafting today, because saline is inexpensive and still has graft cell viability of 95% at 4 hours. The disadvantage of saline is that it causes washing of the harvest bone and, therefore, loss of growth factor after several hours of immersion. This loss may lead to a decrease in overall graft ossicle size.

Note that antibiotics and blood are cytotoxic, and sterile water is hypotonic and has the potential to lyse cells.

26. List the advantages of the posterior ilium approach over the anterior ilium for autogenous bone harvest in major jaw reconstruction.

The **advantages** of the posterior ilium approach include: ability to harvest more bone; fewer complications, including less postoperative pain; and less disturbance in ambulating, with possible reduction in postoperative hospitalization. These differences from the anterior ilium approach are mostly related to differences in soft tissue and osseous anatomy.

Disadvantages of the posterior approach include increased operating time and increased hazards in moving the patient during anesthesia.

27. What are the possible complications to the donor site associated with harvest of anterior iliac crest bone graft?

Possible complications can be acute or chronic, and major or minor. **Acute complications** include superior gluteal artery or sciatic nerve injury, pain, infection, ileus, herniation at the donor site, seroma, hematoma, pelvic fracture, and perforation of the peritoneum. **Chronic complications** include long-term, disabling pain; paresthesia and anesthesia of the skin of the lateral thigh and/or lateral hip and buttocks; gait disturbances; hernia; hip click; and scar at the incision site.

28. What are the possible complications associated with harvest of posterior iliac crest bone graft?

Nerve injury is possible, including dysthesias and paresthesias of the buttocks due to injury to the superior and middle clunial nerves, which are cutaneous sensory nerves. The superior nerve passes over the superior portion of the crest and travels inferiorly to supply sensation over the posterior buttocks. The middle nerve emerges medially through foramina in the sacrum and travels laterally to supply sensation to the medial buttocks.

Hemorrhage may occur due to transsection of the superior gluteal artery and may require a laparotomy to prevent exsanguinations.

Dislodging of the endotracheal tube can occur during repositioning from prone to supine position, but can be prevented with careful repositioning.

Loss of lower extremity motor functions, though rare, may occur due to injury to the motor enervation to the lower extremity by the sciatic nerve. The sciatic notch and sciatic nerve are 6–8 cm inferior to the posterior iliac crest.

Fractures of the pelvis also are rare complications, when proper technique is followed.

29. Which nerves are most commonly injured in the anterior ilium bone harvest approach?

The incision can affect two peripheral sensory nerves: the **lateral cutaneous of the subcostal nerve** (T12) and the **lateral cutaneous branch of the iliohypogastric nerve** (L1). Both nerves cross the anterior iliac crest from medial to lateral between the tubercle and the anterior iliac spine. Both nerves provide sensory innervation to the skin overlying the gluteus medius and gluteus minimus muscles. Transection or retraction injury to these nerves may result in anesthesia or paresthesia in this area.

The lateral femoral cutaneous nerve of the thigh (L2 and L3) runs approximately 1 cm below the anterior iliac spine and courses on the medial aspect of the ilium and iliacus and almost always below the inguinal ligament—thus, it is protected from surgical injury. However, perforation of the muscle may injure this nerve, causing similar symptoms to the skin over the upper and middle thigh below the level of the acetabulum.

30. What is the average incidence of neurosensory deficit following anterior ilium harvest?

In a study by Marx and Morales, 19 of 50 patients had an average neurosensory deficit of 45 cm^2.

31. What is the incidence of neurosensory deficit following posterior ilium harvest?

Marx and Morales found that 10 of 50 patients had an average neurosensory deficit of 16 cm^2. The superior cluneal nerves (L1, L2, L3) and the middle cluneal nerves (S1, S2, S3) are involved. An oblique incision parallel to the course of the superior cluneal nerves may affect them less frequently or to a lesser degree.

32. List the seven anatomic structures that attach to the anterior iliac crest.

The fasciae latae, inguinal ligament, tensor fasciae latae, sartorius, iliacus, and the internal and external abdominal oblique muscles attach to the anterior iliac crest.

33. What are the surgical options for total temporomandibular joint (TMJ) replacement?

- Alloplastic fossa and condyle (custom design and stock design)
- Free vascularized (fibula, ileum, second metatarsophalangeal joint, and scapula)
- Autogenous (costochondral, clavicle, ileum)
- Allogeneic cadaveric/ banked bone

34. What are the *indications* for alloplastic reconstruction of the TMJ?

- Ankylosis or re-ankylosis with severe anatomic abnormalities
- Failed autogenous graft
- Failed previous alloplastic reconstruction
- Resorption of autograft by foreign body reaction (e.g., Proplast-Teflon)
- Severe inflammatory joint disease
- Patient with multiple previous operations and compromised vascular bed.

35. What are the *contraindications* for TMJ reconstruction with an alloplastic prosthesis?

- Young age, because of the limited longevity of the prosthesis and the potential need for a second surgery, and because of skeletal immaturity and lack of growth potential

- Compromised immune system, because such nonvascularized grafts may increase the risk for infection
- Presence of an active infection (acute or chronic)
- Allergy to the materials used for manufacturing of the prosthesis.

36. List the advantages of alloplastic TMJ reconstruction.
1. There is no need for maxillary-mandibular fixation or mandibular immobilization.
2. Physical therapy can begin immediately.
3. There is no donor site morbidity.
4. Surgery time is decreased.
5. An alloplastic prothesis can be easily designed to accommodate irregular anatomy (e.g., destructive lesions or growth asymmetries).
6. It offers more reliable/predictable control of occlusion and occlusal correction.
7. It is more resistant to autoimmune destruction.

37. List the disadvantages of alloplastic TMJ reconstruction.
1. Cost.
2. There is less mechanical longevity—intrinsic implant failure due to material fatigue.
3. Biological longevity is less—failure due to break down of tissue-implant interface (e.g., loose screws or cements) or possible tissue reactions.
4. The implant has no growth potential.

38. What length of cartilage should be harvested with a costochondral graft used for TMJ reconstruction?
To decrease the lever arm and risk for separation at the bone-cartilage interface, the length of the cartilage harvested should be minimized: 3–5 mm of cartilage is sufficient for TMJ reconstruction. Leaving a periosteal perichondral sleeve helps reinforce this junction.

39. Which donor rib is the most preferable for costochondral graft reconstruction?
Because the sixth rib harvest lends itself to a cosmetic incision at the inframammary crease, and the dissection in this area can be carried out between the terminal extent of the pectoralis major and rectus abdominus muscles, the **right sixth rib** is the best rib for harvest. Harvesting from other ribs on the right side, although acceptable, may cause a more unaesthetic scar, and the dissection may increase the chances of hemorrhage, pain, and pneumothorax.

Note that when rib harvest is performed on the left side, it is important to differentiate postoperative pain from cardiogenic pain.

40. What are the possible donor site complications in rib harvest?
Complications associated with rib and costochondral graft harvest include pain, scar, paresthesia or anesthesia of the lateral chest wall, tear of the pleura leading to a pneumothorax, and atelectasis. The incidence of pneumothorax is higher when harvesting a costochondral graft than with rib harvest because of the relatively greater difficulty in reflecting the perichondrium off the cartilage compared to reflecting the periostium off the bone when harvesting rib without cartilage. Most of the complications associated with rib and costochondral graft harvest are, however, transient and resolve within a few days to weeks. Also, in most instances of pleural perforation, it can be managed without the need for insertion of a chest tube.

41. Describe the different flap classification methods.
There are many methods for classifying tissue used for reconstruction, but the most common are:

Tissue composition—cutaneous, muscle, fasciocutaneous, myocutaneous, osseocutaneous, and innervated (sensate) cutaneous

Source of blood supply—in *axial flaps* (also called direct), the blood supply is provided by a known vessel that runs within the base of the flap. The artery usually runs along the longitudinal axis of the flap, and perforators extend directly between the skin and this artery. In *random flaps* (also called indirect), a distributing artery gives rise to multiple unnamed perforating arteries. These multiple unnamed perforating arteries then enter the base of the flap in a random pattern. These unnamed perforators not only supply the tissue comprising the base of the flap, but also contribute multiple, random, cutaneous perforators to the dermal plexus. Thus, the blood supply to the skin takes an indirect route through a hierarchy of arterioles.

Method of transfer to donor site—*local* occurs via advancement, rotation, and interpolation. *Distant* transfer occurs via direct, tube, free (i.e., split-thickness skin graft, ICBG, cartilage), and free vascularized.

42. What are the most commonly used regional flaps for maxillofacial reconstruction?

Flaps that have proved to be predictable, single-stage soft tissue transfers, with known axial and random vascular patterns, are the **sternocleidomastoid flap, temporalis muscle, pectoralis major, trapezius, latissimus dorsi, and platysma flaps**. These have elevated maxillofacial soft tissue reconstruction to new level. Other known but less commonly used flaps include masseter muscle, deltopectoral, and forehead flaps. These can be used as isolated muscle flap or in combinations with other tissues such as the skin, fascia, or bone.

43. What are the major sources of blood supply to these flaps?

FLAP	DOMINANT BLOOD SUPPLY
Pectoralis major myocutaneous	Thoracoacromial artery Superior and lateral thoracic arteries contribute
Deltopectoral skin	Perforators from internal mammary artery
Temporalis muscle	Anterior and posterior deep temporal arteries
Platysma myocutaneous	Submental branch of facial artery
Trapezius myocutaneous	Transverse cervical artery
Latissimus dorsi myocutaneous	Thoracodorsal artery
Sternocleidomastoid myocutaneous	Branches of occipital and superior thyroid arteries

44. Which factors most affect aesthetics and function following reconstruction with local flaps?

Using the physical characteristics of tissue can lead to better functional and aesthetic results after reconstruction with local flaps. Such characteristics include integration of relaxed skin tension lines, taking into consideration the cosmetic units of the face, and better use of the physical properties of the skin.

45. Differentiate free flap failure and pedicle flap failure.

Failing pedicle flaps tend to show distal necrosis. This occurs when the design of the flap prevents the random cutaneous vascular supply from adequately perfusing the peripheral tissue, or because of external cause of vascular occlusion such as hematoma or compression. *Free flaps failure* is classically described as an all-or-none survival pattern (although segments of distal necrosis are possible), mostly caused by intrinsic intraluminal vascular occlusion at the level of the anastomosis.

46. How can a flap be monitored postoperatively?

Although not always reliable, clinical observation of skin color, skin temperature, capillary refill, and dermal puncture bleeding are the most useful methods to monitor a flap in the postoperative period. Cool and pale tissue suggests arterial (inflow) problems. Venous (outflow) problems are characterized by a congested, bluish appearance, with brisk capillary refill and puncture bleeding. More advanced monitoring methods include intravenous injection of fluorescein dye, conventional or LASER Doppler flowmetry, surface temperature probe, transcutaneous tissue oxygen tension, tissue pH, and radioactive tracer clearance.

47. Are there any measures that can prevent microvascular flaps from failing?

Emergent exploration of the anastomosis may be necessary to salvage free flaps (note that, overall, free flap survival is 95% or better). Unfortunately, close observation is often the only means of treatment available because venous congestion is the most common intrinsic reason for failure of technically correct flaps (pedicle or free). Some surgical techniques and postoperative maneuvers, however, increase the chances for flap survival:

- Use noncrushing instruments when handling the flap, as well as noncompressive tissue manipulation and noncompressive dressings.
- Obtain absolute surgical hemostasis, and use drains to avoid hematomas and seromas.
- Prevent graft mobility by adequate suture anchorage and by immobilizing the donor site.
- Sutures should be tension free and parallel to blood vessels. Promptly remove compromising sutures when necessary.
- Control the initial swelling phase with cooling compresses and liberal use of steroids.
- Use appropriate antibiotics.
- Avoid vasoactive drugs such as caffeine and nicotine.
- In appropriate circumstances, hyperbaric oxygen therapy, topical nitroglycerine, lidocaine, papavarine, aspirin, dextrans, and surgical leaching are often used for salvage of free flaps.

48. What is the difference between a random pattern flap and an axial pattern flap?

Random pattern flaps consist of skin, subcutaneous tissues, and possibly muscle. The blood supply is from the dermal and subdermal plexuses. Axial pattern flaps derive their blood supply from dominant vessels within the flap that can be identified during the dissection.

49. What size of lip defect can be closed primarily?

Defects of approximately one-third of the lower and one-quarter of the upper lip can be closed primarily without resulting in a significant microstomia.

50. What are some flaps that can be used for lip reconstruction?

Some of the local flaps used for closure of lip defects include the Abbe flap, the Abbe-Estlander flap and the Karapandzic flap.

51. Which skin donor site for nasal defect grafting provides the best type and quality match of nasal skin?

The best donor site for grafting of small defects of the nose is the nose itself. When bilobe advancement flaps cannot be used, the next best site for color and texture match is the preauricular skin between the tragus and hair-bearing sideburns. The next most commonly desired site is the supraclavicular skin, followed by the posterior upper arm.

Denuded nasal cartilage may be perforated to increase blood supply to the skin graft of the nose. Larger lateral nose and alar defects are best matched with nasolabial flaps. Forehead flaps will supply enough skin to cover all nine nasal cosmetic units.

52. What are the boundaries for the largest possible buccal mucosa grafts?

Buccal mucosa grafts can be harvested from the pterygomandibular raphae to the commissure and then closed primarily without functional deficits. Grafts wider than 2 cm in a vertical dimension, however, may cause trismus.

53. What is the difference between full-thickness and split-thickness skin grafts?

Split-thickness skin grafts (STSGs) are 0.30 to 0.45 mm thick. The skin is sectioned below the papillary dermis so it will only contain the epidermis and a portion of the upper reticular dermis. Since the skin adenexa (hair follicles and associated sebaceous glands, eccrine and apocrine sweat glands) originate in the mid-reticular dermis or in the subcutaneous fat layer (hypodermis or panniculus adiposis), they are generally not included in STSGs.

In **full-thickness skin grafts** (FTSG), the dermis is not split. The plane of cleavage is designed to separate the subcutaneous fat from the dermis. The actual thickness of an FTSG is extremely variable and depends upon the location on the donor site and the sex, age, and health of the patient.

The eyelid, supraclavicular, and postauricular skin are the thinnest on the body, whereas the palms, soles, and trunk are the thickest. Women have thinner skin. The dermis is very thin in children, increases until age 50, and then atrophies. Conditions such as malnutrition, chronic steroid therapy, and insulin-dependent diabetes mellitus also affect dermal thickness. Be aware of these variables when planning graft harvesting.

54. Differentiate primary and secondary contraction.

Primary contraction refers to the immediate shrinkage of a harvested graft as it is cut free. This form of contraction is due to elastic fibers within the dermis. More dermis means more elastic fibers, so FTSGs have more primary contraction than STSGs. *Secondary* contraction, or wound contraction, is the more significant concern clinically. This type of contraction is caused by the myofibroblasts located in the donor site and is characteristic to the healing of all open wounds. Secondary contraction predominates during the first 2 weeks of healing, but peaks at 8 days.

55. What percent contraction can be expected from STSGs and FTSGs?

Generally, the exact percent of contraction of skin graft cannot be predicted simply on the basis of whether the skin graft is an FTSG or STSG. In relation to *primary contraction*, the proportion of the skin graft harvested, compared to the skin's total thickness, is important in determining the amount of primary wound contracture. If STSGs of identical thickness are harvested from various regions of the body, the grafts harvested from thick skin will contract more than those from thinner areas. Thus, **the thickness of the graft relative to donor skin thickness** is the most important factor in determining primary wound contraction.

In *secondary contraction*, the thickness of a graft is not as important as **the percentage of the dermis being transplanted**. The larger the percentage of dermis that is grafted, the less secondary contraction. A wound covered with a $\frac{3}{4}$ STSG of 0.25 mm may contract less than a wound covered with a 0.5 mm $\frac{1}{4}$ STSG. A $\frac{1}{2}$-thickness STSG, if taken from an area with thin skin, may perform clinically more like an FTSG.

56. What are the advantages and disadvantages of STSGs?

Advantages: STSGs tolerate less vascularity than FTSGs and may survive in less than ideal conditions. Because blood vessels arborize as they ascend into the dermis, STSGs have a higher number of blood vessels on the undersurface of the graft. This higher potential for vascularity gives STSGs a large capacity to absorb nourishment from the underlying bed. In addition, nutrient fluids have shorter distances to diffuse, and thinner grafts have fewer cellular elements requiring nourishment. STSGs can therefore be applied to any vascular surface or any surface where healthy granulation tissue exists.

STSG donor sites heal spontaneously. Epithelial cells migrate from adenexal structures to re-epithelialize the harvested site. In addition, if necessary, the same donor can be used to re-harvest skin in the future. Also, meshing STSGs greatly increases the surface area that can be re-epithelialized, and therefore a larger defect can be covered with a smaller graft.

Disadvantages: significant amount of contracture; inability of the graft site to accommodate growth well in children; abnormal pigmentation at both harvest and donor site; and poor mechanical strength.

57. What are the advantages and disadvantages of FTSGs?

Advantages: FTSGs are the ideal choice for epithelial coverage. They are much more resistant to contracture than STSGs, grow in children, have a texture and pigmentation that is more similar to normal skin, and are functionally more durable.

Disadvantages: Because of thickness and limited exposure of the microvasculature, it is difficult for simple diffusion to maintain cell viability throughout the graft. Therefore, FTSGs can only be placed in very clean, highly vascular donor sites. For this reason harvesting is limited to sites such as palpebral, postauricular, supraclavicular, and dorsal pedal skin. Since the donor site can only be harvested once and the graft cannot be meshed and expanded, FTSGs provide much more limited coverage.

58. Describe STSG healing.

During the ischemic phase 0-48 hours postoperatively, the graft appears pale. During this phase, nutrition and excretion are by exudation and diffusion. During the period 24–72 hours postoperatively, the graft gains a pinkish tint as reanastomosis between tissue surface vessels of the graft and those of the host bed are established. At 3–6 days postoperatively, the graft becomes cherry red, with demonstrable capillary refill if neovascularization occurs. Endothelial buds grow into the graft from the host bed and reestablish the microcirculation.

Note that these phases may be longer in thicker grafts and/or only occur in the deeper regions of thicker grafts, with the superficial layers sloughing off.

59. What are the most common causes of STSG failure?

- Inadequate recipient site (poor vascularity)
- Hematoma under the graft
- Graft mobility
- Infection
- Technical errors (e.g., placement over epithelium or necrotic tissue, placed upside down, cut too thick or too thin)
- Poor storage of graft

60. Describe the changes that occur in FTSGs placed into the oral cavity.

In general, no surface tissue changes occur after placement of FTSGs in the oral cavity. Mucosalization of a skin graft does not occur. There may be a thinning of the keratin layer, but transplanted skin maintains most of its original characteristics.

61. What are the disadvantages associated with intraoral STSGs and with mucosal and palatal tissue grafts?

Problems associated with skin grafts include possible hair growth, disagreeable color and odor, and a tendency to excessive keratinization when placed under a denture base. Oral mucosa is certainly the preferred tissue for intraoral grafting, but it does present some difficulties. Disadvantages of buccal mucosa grafts are poor load-bearing qualities, technical difficulties obtaining and handling thin grafts, and limited surface available for harvest.

Disadvantages of palatal mucosa are technical difficulty procuring split-thickness grafts of any size, limited availability, and rugated surface texture. Full-thickness palatal grafts are technically easier to obtain, but they have protracted, painful, and often unsatisfactory healing at the donor site.

62. Describe the important aspects of lateral canthus reconstruction.

The goal of lateral canthus reconstruction is mobilization of the lateral canthal soft-tissue complex, which includes mobilization of the ligament periosteum and orbicularis muscle. This soft-tissue complex can be approached by a variety of incisions, including hemicoronal, lateral canathotomy, and brow, or via existing lacerations and/or incisions. The lateral canthusrea is undermined subperiosteally until the complex can be elevated without resistance.

The confluence of tissue then can be reattached to the lateral orbital rim by either plate or screw fixation through a hole secured with suture or wire, or to the periorbital tissue when the correction is for only a minor deformity. The canthopexy should be positioned superiorly approximately 3–4 mm above the medial canthal ligament. An inferior tilt of the lateral canthus usually is unaesthetic. This type of canthal deformity is called antimongolian and is often seen in certain craniofacial abnormalities, such as Treacher Collins syndrome, or in traumatic cases associated with residual, inferior, displaced zygomatic fractures.

Soft-tissue revisions of the canthal region should be the final phase of post-traumatic orbital reconstruction. To optimize aesthetic results after reconstruction, it is important to develop revisions so that the bulk of the scar falls within the relaxed skin tension lines. This can be achieved by using fusiform excision, Z-plasty, W-plasty, and geometric excisions.

63. What is the pathophysiology of enophthalmos? How it is corrected?

Loss of bone and ligament support allows posterior displacement of the globe by gravity and scar contracture, leading to enophthalmos. Enophthalmos may also result from fat necrosis, tethering of orbital contents, and neurogenic conditions. Clinically, enophthalmos is not evident until at least a 4-mm change occurs in the position of the globe when measured in an anteroposterior plane from the lateral orbital rim to the zenith of the cornea.

Enophthalmic corrections involve accurate restoration of the shape and size of the bony orbit.

64. What are the different approaches to surgical access of the orbit?

For extensive reconstructive procedures involving the nasoethmoidal region, the **hemicoronal or coronal approach** has been used successfully. Incisions placed through scars from **previous incisions or lacerations** can also be used, although they may require some lengthening. Circumvestibular, subciliary, lower lid crease, transconjunctival, and inferior orbital rim incisions are used to approach the inferior orbital rim and orbital floor. However, the **inferior orbital rim approach** generally is avoided because it may leave some unfavorable scarring. The **circumvestibular incision** may be used with a facial degloving procedure, although with some difficulty. The **subciliary and inferior lid crease incisions** provide excellent access and favorable healing characteristics. The **transconjunctival incision** provides excellent cosmesis and superior lateral orbital rim exposure, especially when the lateral canthotomy incision is added. There is an increased risk of lid deformity (especially entropion) if the wound is not reapproximated properly. The lateral orbital rim is best approached through hemicoronal, brow, or **lateral canthotomy** approaches. Scarring from the **brow approach** can be minimized by keeping the incision beveled parallel to the hair follicles or making the incision above or below the brow instead of within the brow, thereby avoiding the possibility of alopecia.

BIBLIOGRAPHY

1. Banwart JC, Asher MA, Hassanein RS: Iliac crest bone graft harvest donor site morbidity Spine 20:1055–1060, 1995.
2. Bardach J: Local flaps and free skin grafts in head and neck reconstruction. St. Louis, Mosby, 1992, pp 42–49.
3. Bloomquist DS, Turvey TA: Bone grafting in dentofacial deformities. In Bell (ed): Modern Practice in Orthognathic and Reconstructive Surgery. Philadelphia, W.B. Saunders, 1992, pp 831–853.
4. Burget CG, Menick FJ: Aesthetic Reconstruction of the Nose. St. Louis, Mosby, 1994.
5. Carlson ER: Regional flaps in oral and maxillofacial reconstruction. Oral Maxillofac Surg Clin North Am 5:667–685, 1993.
6. Carlson ER: Mandibular bone grafts: Techniques, placement, and evaluation. OMFS Knowl Update: 1:35, 1994.
7. Cutting CB, McCarthy JG, Knize DM: Repair and grafting of bone. In McCarthy JG (ed): Plastic Surgery. Philadelphia, W.B. Saunders, 1990, pp 583–629.

8. Feinberg SE, Fonseca JF: Biologic aspects of transplantation of grafts. In Fonseca RJ, Davis WH (eds): Reconstructive Preprosthetic Oral Maxillofacial Surgery. Philadelphia, W.B. Saunders, 1986, pp 19–39.

9. Ferraro N, August M: Reconstruction following resection for maxillofacial tumors. Oral Maxillofac Clin North Am 5:355–383, 1993.

10. Gerard DA, Hudson JW: The Christensen Temporomandibular Prosthesis System: An overview. Oral Maxillofac Clin North Am 11:61–72, 2000.

11. Habal MB, Reddi AR: Introduction to bone grafting. In Habal MB, Reddi AR (eds): Bone Grafts and Bone Substitutes. Philadelphia, W.B. Saunders, 1992, pp 3–5.

12. Hall MB, Vallerand WP, Thompson D, Hartley G: Comparative anatomic study of anterior and posterior iliac crest as donor sites. J Oral Maxillofac Surg 49:560–569, 1991.

13. Haug RH, Buchbinder D: Incisions for access to craniomaxillofacial fractures. Oral Maxillofac Surg Clinic North Am 1:1–29, 1993.

14. Marx RE, Morales MJ: Morbidity from bone harvest in major jaw reconstruction: A randomized trial comparing the lateral anterior and the posterior approaches to the ileum. J Oral Maxillofac Surg 48:196–203; 1988.

15. Marx RE, Saunders TR: Reconstruction and rehabilitation of cancer patients. In Fonseca RJ, Davis WH (eds): Reconstructive Preprosthetic Oral Maxillofacial Surgery. Philadelphia, W.B. Saunders, 1986, pp 347–428.

16. Marx RE: Physiology and particulars of autogenous bone grafting. Oral Maxillofac Surg Clin North Am 5:599–613, 1993.

17. Manson PN, Clifford CM, Su CT, et al: Mechanisms of global support and posttraumatic enophthalmos: I. The anatomy of the ligament sling and its relation to intramuscular cone orbital fat. Plast Reconstr Surg 77:203–214, 1986.

18. Mercuri LG: The TMJ concepts patient-fitted total temporomandibular joint reconstruction prosthesis. Oral Maxillofac Surg Clin North Am 1:73–91, 2000.

19. Hoffman DC, Pappas MJ: Hoffman-Pappas Prosthesis. Oral and Maxillofacial Total Temporomandibular Joint Reconstruction. Philadelphia, W.B. Saunders, 2000, pp 105–132.

20. Rudolph R, Ballantyne DL: Skin grafts. In McCarthy JG (ed): Plastic Surgery. Philadelphia, W.B. Saunders, 1990, pp 221–274.

21. Skouteris CA, Sotereanos GC: Donor site morbidity following harvesting of autogenous rib graft. J Oral Maxillofac Surg 47:808–812, 1989.

40. FACIAL AESTHETIC SURGERY

Vincent B. Ziccardi, M.D., D.D.S.

1. What considerations should soft tissue envelope assessment take into account in the planning of facial aesthetic surgery?

First and foremost is the overall health of the skin and the degree of actinic damage. Healing capacity will be adversely affected by highly damaged skin, and this must be discussed with the patient preoperatively. Any lesions that are present should be evaluated, documented, and possibly biopsied before surgery. Other factors for evaluation include the general elasticity and recoil quality of the skin. This is especially important when considering lower eyelid blepharoplasty and submental liposuction. The amount of subcutaneous tissue affects the overall aesthetic result of surgical rejuvenative procedures. Some patients may require soft tissue augmentation in the lips, cheeks, or natural folds. Finally, the facial animation of a patient during speech and laughter and while at rest should be assessed. In some cases overactive mimetic muscles of facial expression may create wrinkles and folds that the patient finds objectionable. These may be managed with botulinum toxin type A injections.

2. What are the objectives of rhytidectomy?

Rhytidectomy ("face-lift") removes the lax and redundant skin of the face and neck, including the prominent nasolabial folds, jowls, and submental redundancy, that add to the aged-appearance of the face. During the aging process, the elastic fibers of the dermis and the superficial musculoaponeurotic system (SMAS) layer begin to undergo degeneration and are replaced by fibrous connective tissue. The SMAS should be addressed during the face-lift operation to assist in the maintenance of the surgical procedure. Factors that contribute to the aging process include genetics, ultraviolet (UV) light damage, gravity, and tobacco smoking. As gravity causes the skin to sag, the lines of fascial attachment between the skin and mimetic muscles becomes accentuated. Most face-lift operations involve a skin-flap technique with some manipulation of the SMAS.

3. Describe some potential complications of the rhytidectomy procedure.

Anticipated sequelae include swelling and ecchymosis. The significant complications involve sloughing of the flap due to a compromised blood supply. Active smokers should not undergo face-lift operations. Hematoma formation can also result in loss of the skin flap. This is managed by pressure dressing, drain placement, surgical hemostasis, and evacuation of hematomas when clinically evident. Injury to the facial nerve is a significant complication. Understanding the anatomy and not violating the SMAS plane will prevent facial nerve injury. Infection is another potentially significant complication that rarely occurs following use of prophylactic antibiotic coverage. Other potential complications including unfavorable scarring, earlobe deformity, and telangiectasia, which can be covered with make-up or possibly removed with laser treatment.

4. What characteristics make the ideal surgical candidate for submental liposuction?

The ideal candidate for submental liposuction is a patient with distinct supraplatysmal fat deposition and skin with good recoil that allows for postoperative draping of the soft tissue envelope. Traditionally, patients older than 40 years have been excluded; however, it is better to make the assessment on an individual basis. Because the procedure is carried out through one or more small skin incisions, there is no excision of excess skin. Therefore, a patient with excessively redundant skin or very poor recoil would have an unpredictable outcome. The skin would not redrape uniformly with the pressure support dressings, and the outcome would be affected. Ideally, the fat that is blindly removed by the tumescent cannula technique is located above the platysma muscle. Any fat located below the platysma muscle is best approached by an open approach under direct vision. The platysma muscle could be plicated if indicated at that point as well.

5. At what anatomic plane is submental liposuction safely performed?

Submental liposuction is performed at the supraplatysmal plane, a distinct layer of subcutaneous fatty tissue located below the dermis at which the procedure is safely performed in an almost bloodless field. The area safely treated from the submental incision is bounded by the anterior border of the sternocleidomastoid muscle, inferior border of the mandible, and superior border of the thyroid.

6. What is the tumescent technique? What purpose does the tumescent fluid serve in liposuction?

The tumescent technique is a local anesthetic technique that allows submental liposuction to be performed easily and safely. The tumescent fluid is essentially a tenfold diluted local anesthetic. This provides for profound anesthesia and wound hemostasis. Using either a spinal needle or multiport injector, the tumescent fluid is injected into the appropriate surgical plane. One hundred cubic centimeters or more of tumescent fluid can be used in the submental region. After injection of the fluid, adequate time is allowed for the onset of anesthesia and analgesia. The region may often even take on a blanched appearance. The liposuction cannulas are then inserted into this already established plane, which essentially has been hydrodissected by the tumescent fluid.

7. By what mechanisms does submental liposuction achieve its results?

Submental liposuction achieves its results on several levels. First, there is the physical removal of fat from the supraplatysmal plane. The amount of fat removed varies depending on the patient and operator but ranges between 5 and 25 cc on average. The creation of multiple tunnels radiating from the entry port creates a potential dead space that is then compressed with the postoperative pressure dressing. Additionally, scar contracture of the fatty tissue is violated by the suction cannulas. Most important, however, is the compression and redraping of the soft tissue envelope afforded by the pressure dressing. Patients must understand the importance of the pressure dressing. It is an absolute contraindication to perform the surgery if a patient will not be compliant with the postoperative management. The author's protocol includes 72 hours of continuous pressure dressing (except while bathing), followed by 4 weeks of wearing the dressing for 12 hours/day. Pressure garments are commercially available for this purpose, although 3-inch wide Ace bandages may also be used.

8. What are some of the surgical options available to improve the submental region aesthetics?

A relatively significant improvement in the draping of tissues can be achieved with chin augmentation using either alloplastic implants or osteoplastic osteotomy techniques. This will improve the neck-chin angle and more aesthetically drape the tissues in the submental region. Additional methods to improve the submental region aesthetics include skin excision, platysma muscle plication, and formal neck-lifting procedures. Many of these techniques can be incorporated to a create comprehensive treatment plan. The disadvantage to most of the adjunctive techniques is that they require additional surgery and external skin incisions.

9. Name several complications associated with submental liposuction. How are they best prevented and treated?

Submental liposuction is a relatively safe procedure; however, proper informed consent that outlines all potential complications must be obtained before surgery. Expected postoperative sequelae including bruising, swelling, pain, and numbness in the skin overlying the surgical site are to be expected at least temporarily. Patients must be informed of additional complications including contour abnormality or inadequate fat removal that might require treatment by repeat surgery. Infection can occur in any surgical wound but is minimized with sterile technique and at least prophylactic antibiotic coverage. Bleeding resulting in a hematoma can occur in any potential dead space. This risk is minimized by the postoperative pressure dressing that should be worn up to 1 month after surgery at least 12 hours per day. In addition, the use of a pressure dressing enhances the recontouring of the submental region during the healing process. Facial nerve injury may occur to the marginal mandibular branch if the operator is overzealous in the region above the inferior border of the mandible when approached from the submental portal. This may be prevented by strict adherence to the appropriate plane of dissection and keeping the cannulas below the inferior border of the mandible. Finally, all patients must have realistic expectations of the procedure and an understanding that it is not a substitute for neck-lifting or rhytidectomy procedures.

10. In which circumstances is lipoinjection or fat transfer a useful adjunctive aesthetic procedure?

Lipoinjection or fat transfer is a useful adjunctive technique for soft tissue augmentation of the face. It is widely used in the augmentation of the lips, nasolabial fold, and contracted scar augmentation. Microinjections have been described for the use in acne scar rejuvenation. The fat is autologous and well tolerated by the patient; however, it has a somewhat unpredictable resorption pattern that must be overcontoured intraoperatively to offset the resorption. Patients may require repeat fat injections in the future. Alternative materials include collagen injections into the dermis or the use of alloplastic materials.

11. What are the advantages and disadvantages of the open rhinoplasty technique?

The major disadvantage of an open rhinoplasty technique is the transcolumnellar incision, which could be potentially problematic if unfavorable scarring occurs. In addition, prolonged edema of the nasal tip could take months to resolve. Paresthesia of the nasal tip also persists for a variable period of time. The surgical procedure is more time consuming and there is the potential for skin loss or slough. The advantages of an open technique, however, are numerous and include direct visualization of the structures to be modified, precise surgical manipulation of exposed elements, and an excellent teaching modality to clearly demonstrate the effects of surgical techniques.

12. What aesthetic change results from performing a cephalic excision from the lower lateral cartilage?

The cephalic or upper edge excision of the lower lateral cartilage in rhinoplasty is a common surgical manipulation. The purpose of this procedure is to reduce the bulk of the nasal tip width along with some cephalic elevation of the nasal tip. One must be sure to preserve at least 5–7 mm of residual lower lateral cartilage after excision to prevent elimination of some support for the nasal tip. Over resection will give the appearance of a pinched and elevated tip that is not aesthetically pleasing.

13. Why are intradomal sutures used in nasal surgery?

The intradomal region is located at the nasal tip where the lateral crura curve to form the medial crura. This defines the nasal tip, which is seen externally on the nasal skin as two light reflexes approximately 5 mm apart. An individual with thick skin may not have a well-defined tip and a unilateral broad light reflex may be seen. In narrowing and redefining the nasal tip region, some surgeons will use an intradomal suture to narrow and cephalically elevate the nasal tip. This is generally done in conjunction with other surgical manipulations such as cephalic trimming of the lower lateral cartilage and placement of a nasal tip shield graft.

14. Why is dorsal nasal reduction usually accompanied by lateral osteotomies?

Reduction of the nasal dorsum usually results in the creation of an open roof deformity. This is essentially thought of as the roof being taken off the nasal dorsum with two lateral bony struts and a central septal strut. If this open roof deformity is not collapsed upon itself with the lateral osteotomies, a broad and irregular deformity will result from the adaptation of the soft tissues into the broad dorsum creating the open roof deformity.

15. What is one of the most important considerations for evaluation before performing lower eyelid blepharoplasty? Why?

The assessment of lower lid laxity should be undertaken by all surgeons. In general, the lower lid is pulled away from the eye and the time for recoil to occur is documented. A young person will have a "snap" as the lid quickly recoils in place, whereas an elderly person may demonstrate an ectropion, which slowly returns to normal position. The patient with moderate to severe lid laxity will be at risk for postoperative ectropion or eversion of the lower eyelid. These patients must have detailed informed consent about the possible ramifications of lower eyelid surgery and the possible need for additional procedures such as lateral lid shortening.

16. What is the most common technique used for lower eyelid blepharoplasty?

The most commonly used approach for lower eyelid blepharoplasty is the skin-orbicularis muscle flap technique. The excess skin and herniated orbital fat along with any hypertrophic orbicularis muscle can be excised by this technique. This is a relatively easy approach in an avascular plane above the orbital plane. In this surgical technique, the incision is created approximately 1.5 mm below the lash line and extended about 1 cm laterally in the lateral canthal region following the crow's feet lines. The incision is started with a scalpel, and the area of the lateral canthal region is undermined below the orbicularis muscle above the orbital retinaculum and then extended along this plane at the level of the subciliary incision. Blunt dissection may be assisted with the use of cotton swabs. Once the dissection is complete, the orbital fat pads are identified and the septum is incised over the designated region while applying some gentle pressure on the globe to allow for the extrusion of orbital fat. The fat is clamped, cut, and cauterized before releasing to prevent retrobulbar hemorrhage. The skin-muscle flap is rolled laterally and superiorly while the patient looks upward and the excess tissue is excised with scissors. Additional orbicularis muscle may be excised if the patient tends to have a hypertrophic orbicularis bulge.

17. How many fat pads are generally encountered in the upper and lower eyelid blepharoplasty procedures?

The upper eyelid has two fat pads including the nasal and middle pad. The nasal pad is the smaller of the two. Remember that the lacrimal gland is located laterally and should not be mistakenly excised during upper lid blepharoplasty. The lower eyelid has three fat pads: nasal, middle, and temporal. The nasal fat pad is the smallest, and the fat generally has a white color appearance. The middle fat pad is the largest of the three and is separated from the nasal pad by the inferior oblique muscle. The temporal pad is of variable size and may have more than one compartment. Any blood vessels that traverse the fat pads must be thoroughly cauterized to prevent postoperative retrobulbar hemorrhage.

18. What other facial anatomic structures should be assessed before performing upper eyelid blepharoplasty?

In conjunction with the evaluation of the upper eyelids prior to blepharoplasty should be the assessment of the brow. In many cases, the brow will be ptotic and worsen the appearance of the upper eyelids. If the upper lid blepharoplasty was performed without correction of the brow, the result would be less than desirable and possibly more eyelid skin would be removed than necessary. Generally, male patients have a straight and relatively flat brow whereas females should have a laterally elevated brow. The distance from the pupil center to the brow is usually at least 20 mm. When assessing these patients, the brow should be elevated with the examiner's hand to determine the effect of concomitant brow lifting.

19. What is the Mustardé technique of otoplasty?

The Mustardé otoplasty technique is primarily designed to produce a cartilaginous fold in the antihelical area through the use of horizontal mattress sutures. The site of the proposed antihelical fold is marked with methylene blue after an elliptical strip of skin is removed from the posterior aspect of the ear. This is determined simply by bending the ear toward the head and observing where the fold develops. Three to five horizontal mattress sutures are introduced equidistant from the designated fold and tightened to establish the desired depth of fold. Abrasion or scoring of the cartilage can be used to weaken the cartilage in a patient with a very thick cartilaginous ear structure.

20. What are some of the advantages and disadvantages of alloplastic implants for facial augmentation?

Alloplastic implants are frequently used in facial rejuvenation surgery. The desirable features of these implants include their ease of placement through intraoral incisions, their availability, and the large number of anatomic sizes and shapes commercially available. Most implants can be secured with a screw for immediate stabilization. Most importantly, the alloplastic implants obviate the need for a donor surgical site with its concomitant morbidity. The downside to the use of alloplastic materials is that they are foreign bodies that are usually encapsulated with fibrous tissue capsules. They are susceptible to infection since there is no true tissue ingrowth and vascularization, and they may migrate causing local morbidity. Silicone chin implants have been shown to cause underlying bone resorption after many years. The most critical component to the successful use of alloplastic facial implants is maintaining adequate soft tissue coverage. This translates into placing the implants only where they can be situated under well-vascularized tissues. If an implant becomes infected, the prognosis for maintaining the implant is very poor. There is some local morbidity associated with the removal of implants including scar contracture and associated soft tissue deformities.

21. Which techniques are used for the revision of facial scars?

The simplest procedure is the fusiform or elliptical excision, which is used for scars that fall within the resting skin tension lines of the face. Scar repositioning techniques are used to move scars located near facial landmarks or better align the scar with the resting skin tension lines. Included within the category are the Z-plasty, W-plasty, and geometric revision procedures. The Z-plasty is most commonly used near the commissure of the mouth, lateral alar region of the nose, and periorbital region. The W-plasty is used in most other areas of the face or when the scar diverges from the resting skin tension lines by more than 35°. Dermabrasion is a useful adjunct for scar camouflage allowing for the blending of scar margins with the surrounding skin. It may be performed as the initial procedure for scar revision or as a secondary procedure on a scar that has previously undergone excision or revision surgery.

22. What is dermabrasion best suited for today?

The crater type of acne scar is suitable for dermabrasion because of the gradual blending of the edges into the surrounding tissue leaving less of a shadow cast by the crater ridge. The remodeling of the region results in a smoothing of the depressed defects of the skin and a less noticeable scar. Removal of tattoos and the blending of scars are other important uses of the dermabrasion procedure. A number of other dermatologic conditions traditionally have been treated with dermabrasion, such as the removal of fine rhytids, but these are better managed with laser resurfacing. The dermabrasion may be carried out to the level of the reticular (deep) or papillary (superficial) dermis depending on the desired result. The author's preference for dermabrasion is for facial scars that may have undergone excision or revision procedures but require dermabrasion for final camouflage. This is performed with diamond fraises or wire brushes using local anesthesia with or without conscious sedation. Wire brushes tend to gouge the skin if not properly used; therefore, diamond fraises may be better. The surgery may be completed using either spray refrigeration or skin tension. Pinpoint bleeding indicates the level of the papillary dermis. Wounds are covered with antibiotic ointment, sterile petrolatum, or nonadherent dressings. Patients must observe strict adherence to sun avoidance for up to 6 months after surgery to prevent pigmentary changes.

BIBLIOGRAPHY

1. Aiach G, Levignac J: Aesthetic Rhinoplasty. Edinburgh, Churchill Livingstone, 1991.
2. Epker BN: Aesthetic Maxillofacial Surgery. Philadelphia, Lea & Febiger, 1994.
3. Johnson CM, Toriumi DM: Open Structure Rhinoplasty. Philadelphia, W.B. Saunders, 1990.
4. Putterman AM, Warren LA: Cosmetic Oculoplastic Surgery, 3rd ed. Philadelphia, W.B. Saunders, 1999.
5. Thomas JR, Holt GR: Facial Scars: Incision, Revision, and Camouflage. St. Louis, Mosby, 1989.

41. DENTAL IMPLANTS

Frank Iuorno, Jr., D.D.S., and A. Omar Abubaker, D.M.D., Ph.D.

1. What are the different dental implant categories?

Dental implants are divided into three categories based on their relationship to the oral tissues: (1) subperiosteal, (2) endosteal, and (3) transosseous. Endosteal implants are subdivided into root-form implants and plate-form or blade implants. Root-form implants can be smooth, threaded, perforated, and solid or hollow, vented, coated, or textured. Currently, the most commonly used implants are root-form implants. Only endosseous and transosseous implants are considered true osseointegrated implants.

2. Define osseointegration.

Several definitions have been proposed over the years to describe a successful dental implant in the human jaw. However, the most inclusive definition to date describes osseointegration as "a process whereby clinically asymptomatic rigid fixation of alloplastic materials is achieved and maintained in bone during functional loading."[2]

3. What criteria were used to determine the success of an implant prior to 1986?

Before 1986, the criteria for a successful implant were different from those used today. According to the 1978 Harvard–National Institutes of Health (NIH) consensus conference on implantology, an implant was considered successful despite the presence of one or more of the following clinical features:
- Mobility of less than 1 mm in any direction
- Bone loss of no greater than one-third of the vertical height of the implant
- Gingival inflammation amenable to treatment
- Absence of symptoms such as infection, numbness, pain, or maxillary sinus or nasal symptoms
- Implant functional for 5 years in 75% of cases

4. What became the criteria for successful implants after 1986?

In 1986, with the introduction of osseointegration, the criteria for successful implants were revised:
- Implant is clinically immobile
- No radiographic evidence of any peri-implant radiolucency
- Vertical bone loss of less that 0.2 mm following the first year of function
- Absence of any symptoms such as pain, infection, numbness, or maxillary sinus or nasal symptoms
- Success rate of 85% after 5 years and 80% after 10 years

5. When are dental implants indicated?

Dental implants are used to achieve rehabilitation of the oral and facial tissue after tooth loss with and without bone loss, after jaw bone loss due to tumor resection, after tooth loss from trauma, and for partially or completely congenitally missing teeth. More specifically, implants are used to achieve one of the following purposes:
- Fixed restoration of single or multiple teeth in partially edentulous jaw
- Retention of removable prosthesis in partially edentulous jaw
- Retention of a prosthesis in a completely edentulous jaw
- Retention of fixed prosthesis in completely edentulous maxilla or mandible

- Retention of maxillofacial prosthesis following loss of jawbone from trauma or following tumor resection
- As a fixture for orthodontic tooth movement when conventional anchorage is not feasible or is cumbersome

6. List Branemark's surgical principles for ensuring osseous integration of implants.

Branemark established a set of surgical principles based on animal and human research that, if followed during implant placement, ensure osseointegration of the dental implants:

- The implant should be placed in direct contact with the bone.
- Implants should be inserted in bone in a surgically prepared site, using a graded series of drills followed by a tap rotating at 15 rpm.
- Absolute temperature control at the surgical site should not exceed 47° to minimize thermal necrosis of bone adjacent to implant.
- The mucosa should remain sutured over the newly inserted implant and the implant should remain functionless for 3–6 months.
- At a second stage (3–6 months later), the implant is exposed, and an abutment and the implant are connected to the prosthesis. Consequently, loading of the implant is done only after the implant is osseointegrated.

7. How much space is needed between implants for successful integration?

Imagine that a square box is drawn around the implant. In the buccal-lingual dimension, a minimum of 0.5 mm of bone is required around the implant. Therefore, for a standard 3.75-mm implant, the operator would need approximately 5 mm of bone in this dimension. Mesiodistally, for implant survival, the same 0.5 mm is required for implant survival. Prosthodontically, at least 3 mm is necessary on both sides of the implant to create the proper emergence profile of a restoration. Consequently, the recommendation for distance between implants for single tooth restoration is 7 mm from the center of one implant to the other.

8. How much space is observed between implant and bone in an osseointegrated titanium implant?

The chemical properties and the interface chemistry are determined by the oxide layer and not by the metal of the implant. Therefore, the dense oxide film of a titanium implant, for example, is about 100 angstroms (Å) thick.

9. Can an implant be placed in an extraction site? What is the prognosis for such a procedure?

Limitations to placing immediate implants include lack of bone to gain initial stability and inability to cover the site with soft tissue when using a two-stage system. Provided no acute infection is present and adequate bone for initial stability (usually found in the apical one-third to two-thirds) is available, the soft tissue defect may be overcome using a "bio-col" technique. This is a technique whereby a membrane is used to prevent soft tissue ingrowth at the implant-bone interface in conjunction with a collagen plug to ensure watertight closure.

10. Can an implant be placed into grafted bone?

Implants can be placed into grafted bone immediately if native bone is adequate for initial stability of the implant or if the graft was done 3–6 months earlier. Successful placement of implants into bone graft using either alloplastic or autogenous material has been reported.

11. How much is the surface area of an implant increased by increasing the diameter of an implant compared to increasing its length?

For each 0.25-mm increase in implant diameter, there is a 10% increase in surface area. Therefore, a 1-mm increase in diameter increases surface area by 40%. Studies have shown that for implants larger than 15–18 mm, there is no further significant biomechanical advantage regardless of implant diameter.

Some authors have shown that increasing the length of an implant to more than 18 mm provides no additional mechanical advantage and possibly increases the incidence of failure rate because of the difficulty of adequately irrigating during the preparation of the site.

12. What major anatomic structures in the maxilla and mandible can affect implant placement? How can these problems be overcome?

In the posterior maxilla, a pneumatization of the maxillary sinus can result in a decrease in the available bone in this region. This deficiency can be overcome by bone grafting of this region. If the interarch space is adequate for restoration (implant-to-crown ratio), a sinus lift bone graft procedure is indicated. However, if there is an excessive interarch space, onlay bone graft with or without sinus lift procedure is a better choice. Distraction osteogenesis both to increase the bone height and to close the interarch space is another option when there is an increased interarch space.

In the anterior maxilla, bony defects are occasionally observed on the buccal surface caused either by traumatic extraction or by buccal concavity around the apical one-third of the root. These defects must be treated prior to or during implant placement. Angulation of the implant to engage existing bone often will result in an implant that is unable to receive a direct axial load and will be more prone to failure after a restoration is placed.

In the posterior mandible, the inferior alveolar nerve is one of the most common impediments to implant placement. Frequently, there is insufficient bone height to place even an 11.5-mm implant in the posterior mandible without the risk of nerve injury. Remedies for this problem depend mostly on restoration length and available interarch space. As in the maxilla, if there is sufficient interarch space, the nerve must be surgically repositioned (lateralized) to gain adequate bone length to achieve a proper crown-to-root ratio and anchorage for the implant. If there is excessive interarch space, onlay bone grafting or distraction osteogenesis should be considered to gain vertical bone height and decrease the interarch space prior to implant placement.

The lingual concavity of the mandible in the posterior and anterior regions is another anatomic area to be considered during placement of mandibular implant. Computed tomography (CT) or plain tomography should be considered if there is any question as to whether or not an implant can be placed without perforating the concavity and risking implant failure or damage to the lingual nerve.

13. What is the ideal fixture depth in relation to the adjacent tooth?

In order to gain proper emergence profile, a single tooth restoration should be placed 3–4 mm apical to the cementoenamel junction of the adjacent tooth. This will allow for tissue covering of any metal margins and provide more natural emergence of the implant from the soft tissue. At the same time, the dental papilla will be able to grow between the natural tooth and restoration, and the patient will find it easier to maintain the implant.

14. Is it necessary to have attached gingiva when placing implants?

Ideally, implants are more easily maintained if an adequate cuff (1–2 mm) of attached tissue is left around the restoration. This does not mean, however, that attached tissue is necessary at the time of placement. In the edentulous mandible, there is often a paucity of attached tissue at the time of placement, and most patients have high mentalis muscle attachments that extend to the crest of the remaining alveolus. At the time of placement or at a later time but prior to uncovering the implant in a two-stage implant system, measures can be taken to lower these muscle attachments (lipswitch or other vestibuloplasty procedures) to gain immobile tissue.

15. How do you test for osseointegration at the time of implant uncovering?

Torque testing can be done to test for osseointegration at the time of implant uncovering. Ideally, one should be able to place a force of 10–20 N/cm without unscrewing an implant if it is successfully osseointegrated. Other clinical subjective signs of integration are percussion and immobility when placing a fixture mount or impression coping on the implant. When a lateral force of 5 pounds is applied, no movement should be seen. Horizontal mobility of greater than 1 mm or movement < 500 gm of force indicates a failed implant.

16. What methods are used to uncover implants? Can a laser or electrocautery be used?

Conventional uncovering is done with a blade. If there is a minimal band of keratinized tissue, an incision is made to split this band and the tissue is sutured to either side of the healing abutment. If there is adequate attached immobile tissue, a punch biopsy can be used after localization of the implant with a needle. Lasers can also be used, but care must be taken to avoid reflecting energy off the implant to the adjacent bone, which will cause irreversible thermal damage. Electrocautery can also be used carefully without touching the fixture to avoid transmitting heat throughout the socket.

17. Can bone be grafted to a failing implant?

If an implant is mobile, it must be removed as soon as possible to prevent further bone resorption. If the implant is integrated and has a bony fenestration or dehiscence, then guided tissue regeneration or bone grafting procedures may be performed. However, a dehiscence or fenestration must be significant and growing prior to considering grafting.

18. What are the radiographic signs of implant failure?

The most useful radiographic sign of implant failure is loss of crestal bone. Early crestal bone loss is a sign of stress at the perimucosal site. At least 40% of the trabecular bone must be lost to be detected radiographically. Rapid progressive bone loss indicates failure. This will usually be accompanied by pain on percussion or function.

19. What preoperative radiographs are necessary for adequate work-up prior to implant placement?

Panoramic and periapical radiographs are helpful and necessary although they offer no information regarding the internal anatomy of the alveolar process or residual ridge. In addition, they do not permit accurate three-dimensional superimposition of a clinically verified radiopaque template, which can be used as a surgical guide. Multiplanar reformatted CT can be used to obtain this information if it cannot be obtained easily by a combination of conventional radiographic techniques and clinical examination.

20. How many implants are adequate for support of mandibular removable prosthetic replacement in an edentulous mandible?

In general, a minimum of two implants are necessary for support of an implant-retained, tissue-supported prosthesis. It is best to place these as far apart on the ridge as possible while avoiding the mental nerve. For an implant-supported and retained prosthesis, at least three implants should be used with the length of the cantilever being 1.5 times the distance between the most anterior and posterior implants as measured in the horizontal plane.

21. Are MRI or CT scans contraindicated in a patient with dental implants?

MRI and CT scans are not contraindicated in patients with pure titanium implants. Most CT scanners can subtract titanium and other metals from the image and eliminate the scatter images.

22. Are there any absolute contraindications to implant placement?

No. However, because smoking affects the healing of bone and overlying tissue, it should be considered a relative contraindication to implant placement. Similarly, in patients with uncontrolled systemic diseases such as diabetes, immunocompromised patients, and patients with bleeding disorders, implant placement should be considered with extreme caution.

23. What are the most common reasons for endosseous dental implant removal?
Lack of integration
Lack of bone support
Loss of bone
Surgical malposition
Psychiatric reasons

24. What are the possible complications of endosseous dental implants?
The most commonly reported reasons for dental implant failure are:
• Infection
• Loss of implant
• Bone resorption around implant
• Nerve injury and numbness
• Perforation of the maxillary sinus and nasal cavity
• Cost and long-term treatment period
• Fracture of the mandible

25. What is the long-term success rate of endosseous implants?
According to Kent et al., the 5-year combined success rate of maxillary and mandibular dental implants is 94.6%. Albrektsson et al. reported maxillary implants with a success rate of 84.9% for 5–7 years. For irradiated maxilla, the success rate of implants is 80%; in grafted maxilla, the success rate is 85%.

In large, long-term studies of mandibular and maxillary endosseous implants, the success rate ranges from 84% to 97%. Specifically, the maxillary implant success rate after 1 year is 88% and is 84% after 5–12 years. In the mandible, the 1–2-year success rate is 94-97%, 5–12 years is 93%, and the 15-year success rate is 91%. The success rate in the mandible posterior region is 91.5% and in the maxillary posterior region is 82.9%, while the success rates are higher in the anterior mandible in the 94–97% range.

26. What is the success rate of endosseous implants placed into an autogenous bone graft site?
In a study by Keller et al., 248 commercially pure titanium endosseous implants were placed in 54 consecutive patients who required bone grafting. Types of grafts included cortical, corticocancellous, and particulate bone. All 74 antral sites received a block graft. Endosseous implant success over the 12-year period was 878 and bone graft success reached 100%. A higher loss of implants occurred in the Le Fort I fracture groups compared with other grafting approaches.

27. Can endosseous implants be successfully placed in an irradiated bone?
Many studies indicate successful integration of endosseous implants in irradiated fields even without the use of hyperbaric oxygen (HBO) therapy. A study by Anderson et al. demonstrates a success rate of 97.8% for endosseous implants placed into an irradiated field. This study evaluated 90 implants placed in 15 patients for treatment of malignancies in the maxillofacial region with radiation doses ranging from 44 cGy to 68 cGy. Other studies show similar rates of success without the use of HBO.

28. When is a transmandibular implant indicated?
A transmandibular implant (TMI) can be placed in a totally edentulous mandible of any bone height. However, TMI works particularly well in the prosthetic restoration of a severely atrophic mandible (less that 12 mm of bone vertically).

29. What is the success rate of a transmandibular implant?
According to a multicenter study published in 1989, the success rate of TMI after a follow-up of between 3 months and 12 years was 96.8%. One long-term study (13-year

follow-up) by Bosker et al. provided data on 1356 patients treated with TMI placement; this study reported an overall success rate of 96.8%. The incidence of complications was found to be closely related to the experience of the individual placing the TMI.

30. What are the possible complications of TMI?
- Numbness of the lip due to inferior alveolar nerve injury
- Fracture of the mandible
- Infection
- Fracture of the post
- Pain and psychological problems

BIBLIOGRAPHY

1. Adell R, Lekhholm U, Rockller B, Branemark P-I: A 15-year study of osseointegrated implants in treatment of the edentulous jaw. Int J Oral Surg 18:387–416, 1981.
2. Albrektsson CJ, Sennerby L: What is osseointegration? In Worthington P, Evans JR (eds): Controversies in Oral and Maxillofacial Surgery. Philadelphia, W.B. Saunders, 1997, pp 436–446.
3. Albrektsson T, Branemark P-I, Hansson HA, Lindstrom J: Osseointegrated titanium implants. Requirements for ensuring a long-lasting, direct bone-to-implant anchorage in man. Acta Orthop Scand 52:155–170, 1981.
4. Albrektsson T, Dahl E, Enbom L, et al: Osseointegrated oral implants. A Swedish multicenter study of 8139 consecutively inserted Nobelpharma implants. J Periodontal 59:287–296, 1988.
5. Anderson G, Andreasson L, Bjelkengren G: Oral implant rehabilitation in irradiated patients without adjunctive hyperbaric oxygen. Int J Oral Maxillofac Implants 13:647–654, 1998.
6. Becker W, Becker BE, Alsuwyed H, Al-Mubarak S: Long-term evaluation of 282 implants in maxillary and mandibular molar positions. A prospective study. J Periodontol 70:896–901, 1999.
7. Bosker H, Jordon R, Sindet-Pedersen S, Koole R: The transmandibular implant: A 13-year survey of its use. J Oral Maxillofac Surg 49:482–492, 1991.
8. Branemark P-I: Precision, Predictability. Gothenburg, Sweden, Institute for Applied Biotechnology, 1990.
9. Branemark P-I: Introduction to osseointegration. In Branemark P-I, Zarb G, Albrektsson T (eds): Tissue Integrated Prostheses. Chicago, Quintessence, 1985, pp 11–76.
10. Keller EE, Eckert SE, Tolman DE: Maxillary antral and nasal one-stage inlay composite bone graft: Preliminary report on 30 recipient sites. J Oral Maxillofac Surg 52:438–448, 1994.
11. Noack N, Willer J, Hoffmann J: Long-term results after placement of dental implants: Longitudinal study of 1,964 implants over 16 years. Int J Oral Maxillofac Implants 14:748–755, 1999.
12. Schliephake H, Schmelzeisen R, Husstedt H, Schmidt-Wondera LU: Comparison of the late results of mandibular reconstruction using nonvascularized or vascularized grafts and implants. J Oral Maxillofac Surg 57:944–950, 1999.
13. Steinemann SG, Eulenberger J, Maeusli PA, Schroeder A: Adhesion of bone to titanium. Adv Biomater 6:409, 1986.
14. Zarb G, Albrektsson T: Osseointegration: A requiem for the periodontal ligament? [editorial]. Int J Periodontal Rest Dent 11:88, 1991.

42. PREPROSTHETIC SURGERY

Vincent J. Perciaccante, D.D.S.

1. How does the blood supply of the edentulous mandible differ from that of the dentate mandible?

As edentulous bone loss (EBL) progresses, there is a change in the blood supply to the mandible. The inferior alveolar vessels become smaller. The primary blood supply to the dentate mandible moves **centrifugally** from the inferior alveolar artery. The primary blood supply to the edentulous mandible flows **centripetally** from the periosteum. Elevation of the periosteum on mandibles that have had severe bone loss could compromise blood supply. Therefore, during surgical procedures, elevation of the periosteum should be done judiciously in the edentulous atrophic mandible.

2. Does alveolar bone resorb more quickly in the mandible or in the maxilla?

EBL in the maxilla is usually more rapid and severe. This may be due to the lack of muscle attachments to the maxilla and therefore lack of functional stimulus after tooth loss.

3. What skeletal relationship results from EBL?

The skeletal relationship that results from EBL is **pseudo class III**. Most EBL in the maxilla takes place on the lateral and inferior aspects of the ridge; therefore, the crest moves posteriorly and superiorly. As the height and width of the mandibular ridge deteriorate the crest moves further anteriorly. As vertical dimension collapses, the mandible autorotates forward as well.

4. How are edentulous alveolar ridges classified?

Kent Classification of Edentulous Ridges (1986)

CLASS	DEFINITION
I	Alveolar ridge is of adequate height but inadequate width, with lateral deficiencies or undercut areas
II	Alveolar ridge deficient in both height and width, with a knife-edge appearance
III	Alveolar ridge has been resorbed to the level of basilar bone, producing a concave form in the posterior areas of the mandible and sharp ridge form with bulbous, mobile soft tissues in the maxilla
IV	Resorption of the basilar bone, producing a pencil-thin, flat mandible or maxilla

Caywood Classification of Edentulous Ridges (1988)

CLASS	DEFINITION
I	Dentate
II	Immediately postextraction
III	Well-rounded ridge form, adequate in height and width
IV	Knife-edge ridge form, adequate in height but inadequate in width
V	Flat ridge form; inadequate in height and width
VI	Depressed ridge form, with some basilar loss evident

5. What is combination syndrome?

Combination syndrome is excessive resorption of the edentulous alveolar ridge of the anterior maxilla, caused by the forces generated by opposition of natural mandibular anterior teeth.

6. When and how are torus mandibularis and torus palatinus treated?

Mandibular tori usually need to be removed when a mandibular denture is being planned. The denture flange typically will impinge on these exostoses of bone. Palatal tori often do not need to be removed. Dentures often can be constructed over them. However, if a palatal torus is extremely large and fills the vault, extends beyond the dam area, has traumatized mucosal coverage, has deep undercuts, interferes with speech, or poses a psychological problem for the patient, it should be removed.

The tissue over mandibular tori is extremely thin and friable. Great care should be taken elevating it. This tissue can be "ballooned" out by injecting some local anesthesia directly under it. The incision should be crestal or lingual circumdental. No releasing incisions should be made. After careful elevation of tissues, a groove can be cut along the intended line of removal with a fissure bur. Mallet and osteotome may be used to cleave the torus in this plane. After the bone has been smoothed and the area thoroughly irrigated, the wound can be closed. Gauze should be placed under the tongue to minimize the chance of hematoma.

Prior to removing a palatal torus, a stent should be fabricated. This should be done on a study cast that has had the exostosis removed. A double-Y incision should be made over the midline of the torus. After careful elevation of the flaps, the torus should be scored multiple times in the anterior, posterior, and transverse dimensions. An osteotome can be used to remove each of these small portions. This decreases the risk of fracturing into the floor of the nose. A large bur or bone file is used to smooth the area. After thorough irrigation, the wound is closed with horizontal mattress sutures, and the stent is placed.

7. How can an abnormal frenum be excised?

Z-plasty
V-Y advancement
Diamond excision

8. What is epulis fissurata and how is it treated?

Epulis fissurata is submucosal fibrosis secondary to chronic denture irritation. The denture must first be relieved in the area to treat inflammation and irritation. The denture can then be lined with tissue conditioner and left out as much as possible. After maximum resolution has occurred, surgical excision or cryosurgery removes the epulis fissurata.

9. What is papillary hyperplasia and how is it treated?

Papillary hyperplasia of the palate is of unknown etiology and is seen in patients with ill-fitting dentures. It presents as numerous papillary projections that cover the hard palate. Initially the ill-fitting denture should be removed or relined with tissue conditioner. The tissue can be removed using a large curette, electrocautery, mucoabrasion, acrylic bur, or cryosurgery.

10. In denture reconstruction, how much space is needed between the crest of the tuberosity and the retromolar pad?

At the correct vertical dimension, the distance from the crest of the tuberosity to the retromolar pad should equal at least 1 cm.

11. What can be done if there is inadequate intermaxillary distance at the tuberosity?

A tuberosity reduction can be performed to remove excess tuberosity. An elliptical incision is made over the tuberosity and carried down to bone. This wedge is resected. The buccal and palatal tissues are undermined subperiosteally. Submucous wedges are removed from each flap and the wound is closed. This decreases the vertical and horizontal dimensions of the tuberosity.

12. What can be done for super-erupted but healthy maxillary posterior teeth that interfere with a restorative plan?

Over time after loss of mandibular posterior teeth, maxillary teeth may super-erupt into the edentulous mandibular space. This impinges on the room needed for mandibular restoration as well as freeway space. Often, these teeth are healthy and periodontally sound. They may be planned as abutments for a maxillary prosthesis. In these cases, extraction may not be the best choice and the amount of super-eruption may be too great for crown preparation and full coverage. The maxillary posterior segmental osteotomy can be used to reposition these segments superiorly.

13. What is the average size of the maxillary sinus?

The average size of the maxillary sinus is 14.75 cc, with a range of 9.5–20 cc. On average the width is 2.5 cm; height, 3.75 cm; and depth, 3 cm.

14. How should tears of the sinus membrane be managed during sinus lift?

Tears over corticocancellous grafts will heal. Particulate grafts may be lost if they migrate through perforations. Small tears may not pose a problem because the membrane folds over itself as it is lifted. Larger tears should be patched with a material such as Surgicel or Collatape.

15. How much native bone is required for immediate placement of implants with sinus lift?

A minimum of 4–5 mm of alveolar bone.

16. What is the proper size of the window for a sinus lift?

The window for a maxillary sinus lift begins at the anterior aspect of the sinus and continues inferiorly to several millimeters above the sinus floor. The window extends posteriorly approximately 20 mm. The superior osteotomy is approximately 10–15 mm above the inferior osteotomy.

17. What is guided tissue regeneration (GTR)?

Different cell types migrate into a wound at different rates during repair. Membranes can be used to hinder the migration of undesirable cell types (fibrous connective tissue). This will allow repopulation of the wound with the desirable cell type (bone).

18. What is the goal of anterior maxillary osteoplasty?

In situations where implants are desired in a maxilla with adequate height but inadequate width, an anterior maxillary osteoplasty may provide the solution. It is used to widen the crest of the ridge. An incision is made labial to the vestibule, and a submucosal dissection is carried down to the crest of the ridge. At the crest of the ridge, the periosteum is incised, and the dissection continues palatally in the subperiosteal plane. A vertical bone cut is made obliquely from the crest of the ridge to the floor of the nose. The labial segment is mobilized, and an interpositional bone graft is placed.

19. What is a visor osteotomy?

The visor osteotomy is a procedure to increase the vertical height of the mandible by vertically splitting the anterior portion of the mandible (anterior to the mental foramen) and repositioning the lingual segment superiorly in relation to the buccal segment.

20. What is the sandwich osteotomy?

The sandwich osteotomy horizontally splits the mandible, the cranial fragment is repositioned superiorly, and an interpositional bone graft is placed. There is also a modification called the sandwich-visor osteotomy, which is a combination of these two techniques.

21. What is the desired thickness of a split-thickness skin graft (STSG)?

STSGs can be of varying thickness. An STSG is composed of the epidermis layer and part of the dermis layer. The STSG can be classified as thin, intermediate, or thick, based on the amount of dermis included. STSGs are between 0.010 and 0.025 inches.

22. Which types of skin grafts contract the most? The least?

The thinner a skin graft, the more the contraction. A thin STSG contracts more than an intermediate STSG, which contracts more than a thick STSG. Full-thickness skin grafts hardly contract at all.

Primary contraction is caused by elastic fibers in the skin graft as soon as it has been cut. This can be overcome when a graft is sutured in place. Secondary contraction begins about postoperative day 10 and continues for up to 6 months.

23. What is plasmic imbibition?

Plasmic imbibition is the process by which a skin graft absorbs a plasma-like fluid from its underlying recipient bed. It is absorbed into the capillary network by capillary action. This process is the initial means of survival for a skin graft and continues for approximately 48 hours.

24. Does grafted skin most resemble the donor site or the recipient site?

Grafted skin maintains most of its original characteristics, except that sensation and sweating more closely resemble the recipient site.

25. Name the goals of vestibuloplasty.

Vestibuloplasty, skin grafting, and floor of the mouth lowering increase the depth of the sulcus, which helps control lateral displacement of a denture. The skin graft also provides attached tissue, which will not be elevated by movement of the lip, cheeks, and tongue, providing a stable denture seating area. Skin grafts provide more comfortable load-bearing tissue than mucosa. The mandibular resorption rate beneath skin is probably slower.

26. List the possible graft donor sites for vestibuloplasty.

Skin

Palatal mucosa

Buccal mucosa

27. What are the advantages of using a stent to secure a graft in place for a vestibuloplasty?

A stent can be used to adapt the skin with accuracy to any contour in the labiobuccal area and undercuts in the lingual area. A stent also provides additional graft stabilization and protects the graft from food in the oral cavity.

28. What are the advantages of suturing a graft in place for a vestibuloplasty?

Patients are more comfortable without the stent. Stent construction and adaptation materials are not necessary.

29. Describe the lip-switch procedure.

The lip-switch procedure is a transpositional flap vestibuloplasty. An incision is made in the labial mucosa. A thin mucosal flap is elevated, continuing into a supraperiosteal dissection on the anterior aspect of the mandible to the crest of the ridge. The mucosal flap is sutured to the depth of the vestibule covering the anterior aspect of the mandible, and the denuded tissue on the inner surface of the lip heals by secondary intention. A modification transposes the lingually based mucosal flap with an inferiorly based facial periosteal flap.

30. What is a submucous vestibuloplasty?

Submucous vestibuloplasty can be used for improvement of the maxillary vestibule in situations where the alveolar ridge resorption is not severe but mucosal and muscular attachments exist near the crest of the ridge. Through a midline incision, submucosal and subperiosteal dissections are performed. The tissue between these two tunnels is cut and allowed to retract. A splint is relined and secured in place for 7–10 days.

31. How is floor of the mouth lowering performed?

An incision is made on the lingual aspect of the alveolus. A supraperiosteal dissection is carried inferiorly, and the mylohyoid and genioglossus muscles are sharply dissected from their insertions. No more than half of the superior aspect of the genioglossus muscle should be released. The mucosal margins are then sutured to the new depth, either with sutures passed externally or in a circum-mandibular fashion.

32. What is the minimum distance from the inferior border that the mentalis must remain attached, during vestibuloplasty, to prevent a sagging chin?

A minimum of 10 mm of muscular tissue must remain attached to the vestibular periosteum in order to avoid a sagging chin.

33. What is a tuberoplasty?

Tuberoplasty is hamular notch deepening. The hamular notch occurs where the posterior border of the maxillary denture rests. The posterior palatal seal is placed in the deepest portion of the notch. Patients with decreased vertical height of the tuberosity may have an inadequate notch. In tuberoplasty, a curved osteotome is used to fracture the pterygoid plates free from the tuberosity and displace them in a posterior direction. The tissue is then sutured to the depth of the area creating a new notch. This procedure has limited predictability of success.

34. What procedures can be done to augment a severely atrophic maxilla with a good palatal vault?

In the severely resorbed maxilla that still retains an adequate palatal vault, the Le Fort I osteotomy with anterior-inferior repositioning and interpositional bone graft can be used.

35. What procedures can be done to augment a severely atrophic maxilla with a poor palatal vault?

In a severely resorbed maxilla with a poor palatal vault, onlay grafting may be useful. This can be accomplished with onlay grafting of rib or horseshoe-shaped corticocancellous ilium. Implants may or may not be placed at this time, depending on the residual maxillary bone. Soft tissue procedures are often needed secondarily.

BIBLIOGRAPHY

1. Davis WH, Sailer HF: Preprosthetic surgery. Oral Maxillofac Surg Clin North Am 6:4, 1994.
2. Fonseca RJ, Davis WH: Reconstructive Preprosthetic Oral and Maxillofacial Surgery, 2nd ed. Philadelphia, W.B. Saunders, 1995.
3. MacIntosh RB: Autogenous grafting in oral and maxillofacial surgery. Oral Maxillofac Surg Clin North Am 5:4, 1993.
4. Marx RE, Carlson ER, Eichstaedt RM, et al: Platelet-rich plasma: Growth factor enhancement for bone grafts. Oral Surg Oral Med Oral Pathol Oral Radiol Endod 85:638–646, 1998.
5. Marx RE, Morales MJ: Morbidity from bone harvest in major jaw reconstruction: A randomized trial comparing the lateral anterior and posterior approaches to the ilium. J Oral Maxillofac Surg 48:196–203, 1988.
6. Peterson LJ, Indresano AT, Marciani RD, Roser SM: Principles of Oral and Maxillofacial Surgery. Philadelphia, J.B. Lippincott, 1992.

43. SLEEP APNEA AND SNORING

Kenneth J. Benson, D.D.S.

1. Define snoring.
Snoring is a partial airway and pharyngeal flow obstruction that does not awaken the individual. Movement of air through an obstructed airway creates the snoring sound.

2. Does snoring always indicate the presence of obstructive sleep apnea syndrome (OSAS)?
No. Although patients who have OSAS are typically loud snorers, and snoring usually indicates some degree of obstructed breathing, not all people who snore have OSAS. In fact, about 25% of adult males snore, and this number increases with age, reaching about 60% at age 60 years. Most snoring, however, is not pathologic and may be reduced or prevented by lifestyle changes.

3. Can a snoring patient with excessive daytime somnolence but without other classic symptoms have OSAS?
Yes. The lack of other classic symptoms of OSAS does not mean the diagnosis of OSAS can be ruled out. Because snoring is an indication of partial airway obstruction, understanding the potential of the process to worsen over time is important.

4. How is snoring treated?
Laser-assisted uvulopalatoplasty (LAUP) and Bovie-assisted uvulopalatoplasty (BAUP) are the most commonly used procedures for treatment of snoring. Both procedures involve amputation of the uvula and creation of a 1-cm trench in the soft palate on either side of the uvula. After healing, the soft palate stiffens, reducing its ability to vibrate, and thus reduces snoring. Occasionally the procedure is repeated to resect more tissue without causing velopharyngeal insufficiency. The procedure is usually done under local anesthesia in the office. The advantage of LAUP over the BAUP is the prevention of deeper tissue damage and possibility of less postoperative pain, but both procedures are equally effective.

5. What is obstructive sleep apnea (OSA)?
OSA is repetitive, discrete episodes of decreased airflow (hypopnea) or frank cessation of airflow (apnea) for at least 10 seconds' duration in association with greater than 2% decrease in oxygen hemoglobin saturation.

6. Is there a difference between OSA and OSAS?
Yes. These are not the same processes. OSA is an objective laboratory finding. OSAS involves sleep apnea with signs and symptoms of disease.

7. What are the differences between apnea and hypopnea?
Apnea is the cessation of airflow lasting for greater than 10 seconds. Hypopnea refers to a greater than two-thirds decrease in tidal volume. Both show a decrease in oxygen saturation of at least 2%.

8. How many sleep stages are there in normal sleep patterns?
There are five sleep stages: one rapid eye movement (REM) stage and four non-REM stages.

9. During which sleep stages do most obstructive events occur?
Stages III and IV and the REM stage, which are the deeper stages of sleep. Pharyngeal wall collapse is more common during these stages because the muscles are most relaxed.

10. What factors may contribute to OSA events?
Anything that effectively causes patient drowsiness may contribute to OSA. Alcohol, sedatives, and narcotics are good examples. Weight gain can also potentiate OSA events as can allergies and upper respiratory infections.

11. What is the primary symptom of OSAS?
Excessive daytime sleepiness.

12. What other symptoms of OSAS may be present?
Morning headache
Restless sleep and frequent arousal at night
Impotence
Hypertension

13. What are the important elements of the physical examination of a patient suspected of having OSA?
A thorough head and neck examination should be performed in any patient who presents with possible OSA. Examination should include the nose for signs of obstruction or septal deviation, hypertrophic turbinates, and allergic rhinitis. The oral cavity should be examined for large tonsils, redundant soft palate and uvula, redundant lateral pharyngeal walls, macroglossia, and retrognathia. The neck examination should evaluate for thick neck and laryngeal obstruction. The patient should also be examined for signs of cor pulmonale and hypertension.

14. What is the main objective test for diagnosing OSAS?
Polysomnography is the most commonly performed evaluation for diagnosis of OSAS. It comprises the following tests:
Electroencephalography (EEG)
Electrooculography (EOG)
Chin and leg electromyography (EMG)
Electrocardiography (EKG)
Nasal and oral airflow
Thoracic and abdominal efforts
Pulse oximetry
The less formal home sleep study and multiple sleep latency tests (MSLT) may also be included.

15. What is the respiratory disturbance index (RDI)?
RDI represents the number of obstructive respiratory events per hour of sleep. The RDI along with oximetry is the primary clinical indicator in the diagnosis of OSAS.

16. How is RDI calculated?
RDI = apnea + hypopnea/total sleep time × 60
An RDI of 5 is the upper limit of normal.

17. What is the modified Mueller technique?
While undergoing a fiber optic nasopharyngoscopy, the patient performs an inspiratory effort against a closed mouth and nose. The examiner observes any oropharyngeal or hypopharyngeal obstruction.

18. How are lateral cephalograms used in evaluation of patients for OSAS?

Cephalometric analysis helps confirm physical examination and fiber optic nasopharyngoscopy examination results. The following are normal measurements of the cephalogram.

Sella nasion A point (SNA): 82
Sella nasion B point (SNB): 80
Posterior airway space (PAS): 11 mm
Posterior nasal spine–palate (PNS-P): 35 mm
Mandibular plane–hyoid (MP-H): 15 mm

19. What is Fujita's classification of upper airway obstruction?

Type I Fujita—upper pharyngeal obstruction including palate, uvula, and tonsils; normal base of tongue

Type II Fujita—type I obstruction plus base of tongue obstruction

Type III Fujita—obstruction at tongue base, supraglottis, and hypopharynx; normal palate

20. What are the classes of sleep apnea?

Obstructive, central, and mixed.

21. Differentiate between central and obstructive sleep apnea.

With OSA, there is a normal inspiration effort, but upper airway obstruction causes intermittent cessation of airflow. Central sleep apnea is marked by a lack of inspiratory effort secondary to failure of respiratory centers in the central nervous system to provide the phrenic nerve with appropriate afferent information to activate the diaphragm.

22. Who usually treats central apnea?

Neurologists and sleep specialists.

23. How is OSA classified?

The combination of RDI and oxyhemoglobin desaturation (SaO_2) is a good parameter for scoring OSA severity.

	RDI	SaO_2
Mild OSA	10–30	> 90%
Moderate OSA	30–50	< 85%
Severe OSA	> 50	< 60%

24. List some systemic complications associated with OSAS.

Cor pulmonale	Stroke
Death	Hypoxia
Polycythemia vera	Depression
Hypertension	Daytime somnolence

25. What are the criteria for cure for OSAS?

The surgical cure would have respiratory and sleep results equal to the second night of continuous positive airway pressure (CPAP) titration.

For patients on CPAP, a nonsurgical treatment, cure is determined as:

- A postoperative RDI reduction of at least 50% with a maximum of 20 (i.e., an RDI of 26 should be reduced to 13, and an RDI of 80 should be reduced to 20)
- Postoperative SaO_2 that is normal or with only a few brief falls below 90%
- Normalization of sleep architecture

26. Describe the nonsurgical methods of treatment for OSAS.

Nasal CPAP is the most effective nonsurgical treatment for OSAS. It consists of an air-tight mask held over the nose by a strap wrapped around the patient's head. CPAP is maintained by a machine that is similar to a ventilator. Although nasal CPAP is nearly 100% effective in relieving OSAS, it is very poorly tolerated. Even when it is initially successful, many patients (30% or more) eventually stop using it because of the discomfort.

Tongue-retaining devices and mandibular positioning devices are other nonsurgical methods of treating OSAS. These devices open the airway by holding the tongue or mandible forward during sleep. As with CPAP, discomfort and poor compliance are major problems.

Behavioral modifications, such as weight loss and avoidance of alcohol and sedatives, may also reduce OSAS. Again, patient compliance is a major stumbling block.

27. What are the potential complications of CPAP?

Mask related:	Pressure/airflow related:
Skin rash	Rhinorrhea
Conjunctivitis from air leak	Nasal dryness/congestion
	Chest discomfort
	Sinus discomfort
	Tympanic membrane rupture (rare)
	Massive epistaxis (rare)
	Pneumothorax (rare)

28. What are the surgical options for management of OSAS?

Tracheotomy
Uvulopalatopharyngoplasty (UPPP)
LAUP
LA-UPPP
Mandibular osteotomy with genioglossus advancement
Hyoid suspension
Tongue reduction
Maxillary and mandibular advancement

29. What is a "U-triple-P"?

UPPP is a surgical procedure performed to enlarge the oropharyngeal airway in an anterior-superior and lateral direction. The tonsils are removed (if they have not been removed previously), along with the posterior edge of the soft palate, including the uvula. The tonsillar pillars are then sewn together, and the mucosa on the nasal side and oral side of the cut edge of the soft palate are sewn together. This is the most common surgical procedure performed for treatment of OSAS.

30. What are the results of UPPP in treatment of OSAS?

UPPP offers promising results to many patients suffering from OSAS, but success rates vary:
• Elimination of snoring in 80–100% of cases
• Subjective decrease and improvement in excessive daytime somnolence of 80–100%
• Measured RDI decrease by approximately 50% in 50% of patients

Despite having an approximate 50% reduction in RDI, a patient may still have significant OSA; therefore, UPPP may not improve an OSA patient enough to decrease mortality. CPAP and tracheostomy are still the gold standards to decrease OSA mortality rates.

31. What are the potential complications of UPPP?

Bleeding is the most common postoperative complication. Velopharyngeal insufficiency occurs in 5–10% of patients but is rarely permanent. Nasopharyngeal stenosis is rare but can be a complication. Other minor complaints include dry mouth, tightness in the throat, and an increased gag reflex.

32. What is the role of LAUP in OSAS?

LAUP is highly effective in the treatment of snoring, with successful results in 85–90% of patients. However, the effectiveness of LAUP in the treatment of OSAS has not been well established. Snoring and OSAS probably represent a continuum of a similar pathology, but it is still difficult to determine where LAUP is effective and where it is not. Therefore, the current recommendation is that all patients should undergo a sleep study prior to surgery for snoring or OSAS. Additional research is still needed to support the use of LAUP in the treatment of OSAS.

33. What is an appropriate phase I surgical treatment plan for an OSAS patient with an oropharyngeal site of obstruction?

UPPP is excellent for snoring but has only a 40% success rate with OSAS at this obstruction site.

34. What phase I treatment would be appropriate for OSAS in the presence of oropharyngeal and hypopharyngeal obstruction?

UPPP and genioglossus advancement. A modified hyoid myotomy may also be used in phase I surgical treatment.

35. What is the next step after phase I treatment?

CPAP treatment is continued for 6 months, at which time the patient is reevaluated with polysomnogram. If phase I treatment is unsuccessful, then phase II surgery would be appropriate. Phase II surgery involves orthognathic surgery, which consists of combined maxillary and mandibular advancement.

36. What is the most effective surgical management of OSAS?

Tracheostomy.

37. What is the success rate of maxillomandibular advancement (MMA) in the treatment of OSAS?

Many consider MMA the most promising surgical alternative to tracheostomy. Although there are currently no long-term studies, recent evidence suggests 100% effectiveness of MMA based on the polysomnographic data. MMA is very effective because it increases upon airway space.

BIBLIOGRAPHY

1. Davila DG: Medical considerations in surgery for sleep apnea. Oral Maxillofac Surg Clin North Am 7:205–217, 1995.
2. Hausfeld JN: Snoring and sleep apnea syndrome. In American Academy of Otolaryngology–Head and Neck Surgery Foundation: Common Problems of the Head and Neck. Philadelphia, W.B. Saunders, 1992, pp 85–96.
3. Munoz A: Sleep apnea and snoring. In Jafek BW, Stark AK (eds): ENT Secrets. Philadelphia, Hanley & Belfus, 1996, pp 144–149.
4. Nelson PB, Riley RW: A surgical protocol for sleep disorders breathing. Oral Maxillofac Clin North Am 7:345, 1995.
5. Nimkam Y, Miles P, Waite P: Maxillomandibular advancement surgery in obstructive sleep apnea syndrome patients: Long-term stability. J Oral Maxillofac Surg 53:1414–1418, 1995.
6. Prinsell J: Maxillomandibular advancement surgery: A site specific treatment approach for obstructive sleep apnea in 50 consecutive patients. Chest 116:1519–1520, 1999.
7. Riley RW, Powell NB, Guilleminault C: Maxillofacial surgery and obstructive sleep apnea: A review of 80 patients. Otolaryngol Head Neck Surg 101:353, 1989.
8. Riley R, Troeh R, Powell N: Obstructive sleep apnea syndrome: Current surgical concepts. Oral Maxillofac Surg Knowledge Update 2:79–97, 1998.
9. Sher AE: Obstructive sleep apnea syndrome: A complex disorder of the upper airway. Otolaryngol Clin North Am 23:593–605, 1990.
10. Tina B, Waite P: Surgical and non-surgical management of obstructive sleep apnea. Principles Oral Maxillofac Surg 3:1531–1547, 1992.

44. FACIAL ALLOPLASTIC IMPLANTS: BIOMATERIALS AND SURGICAL IMPLEMENTATION

Steven G. Gollehon, D.D.S., M.D., and John N. Kent, D.D.S.

1. Define the term *alloplast*. What advantages do these materials offer today's surgeon?

The term *alloplastic* is synonymous with *synthetic*. This indicates that the material is produced from inorganic sources and contains no animal or human components. Alloplastic materials offer a prepackaged solution to common reconstructive surgical problems without the need for autogenous grafting and donor site morbidity. Moreover, they may greatly decrease operative time and complexity of surgical procedures.

2. How does biocompatibility factor into the choice of alloplastic augmentation materials?

The success of any alloplastic material depends on its biocompatibility with surrounding host tissues. Material biocompatibility is influenced by the chemical and physical characteristics of the implant material itself, the surgical technique involved, tissue site of implantation, and host reaction to the implant. These complex interactions between the human body and implant explain why so few safe and effective biomaterials exist despite the tremendous advances that have been made in biomaterial development and engineering over the past half century.

3. In the final healing stages after placement of an alloplastic implantable material, what "barrier protection" is essential for long-term implant success?

The final stage of healing after placement of an alloplastic material requires the formation of an encapsulating fibroconnective tissue scar. The formation of this end-stage tissue is initiated by the surgical placement of the alloplast, which produces an initial acute inflammatory response of the adjacent tissues. The response becomes chronic, and the tissue begins to granulate to form an encapsulating foreign body reaction that evolves into the enveloping fibrotic scar. This resulting barrier protects the "foreign" alloplastic material from "self" tissues. In some form, all alloplastic implants will develop fibrous encapsulation. Several features, especially the implant's surface characteristics, have been shown to influence the degree and composition of this capsule.

4. What tissue characteristics are essential for successful placement of an alloplastic material?

The composition of the alloplastic material implanted clearly has an impact on biocompatibility, but the anatomic location and the surgical technique used for alloplast placement exhibit an equal and often greater impact on long-term clinical success. Ensuring that the biomaterial is appropriately matched to the tissue plane within which it will be implanted is ultimately the responsibility of the treating surgeon.

The tissue quality of the area in which the implant is to be placed must be carefully scrutinized for vascularity and soft tissue coverage. Patients with previous irradiation of the area in question may not be candidates for implant placement because the resulting decrease in vascularity impedes the ability of the body to mount an adequate inflammatory response to microbial invasion should the implant become inoculated or secondarily infected.

Tissue overlying an implant should be as thick as possible. Implanting material under thin tissue significantly increases the chances of wound dehiscence, implant exposure, and extrusion in the postoperative period. Implants placed immediately under the dermis or under a thin, subcutaneous tissue layer may eventually cause further thinning, especially if the implant lacks sufficient flexibility or if it is placed in an area of significant tissue mobility. In all cases, the overlying dermis of the skin thins from the pressure of the underlying avascular implant.

5. Describe the sequelae of placing alloplastic materials in inflamed or chronically infected tissue.

Placement of alloplasts in or through a contaminated or infected tissue bed greatly increases the chances of implant infection and subsequent failure. Because most implants are unable to tolerate host tissue vascular ingrowth, the lack of vascular supply added to the surface affinity of many alloplasts for bacterial adhesion creates an intolerable environment for alloplast materials. Nothing less than optimum aseptic technique and clean tissue planes are required for alloplast placement.

6. Describe the characteristics of an ideal alloplastic implant material.

Kent et al. defined the requirements for an ideal facial implant material:

1. The material is readily available in block and precarved forms and can be carved easily.

2. It can be steam-autoclaved repeatedly.

3. It can be bent or molded to improve bone interface and overlying facial contour.

4. It should be low modulus, permitting deformation to clinical requirement, but not have "memory" characteristics that may lead to mobility, extrusion, or resorption.

5. It should have surface porosity for rapid tissue ingrowth and immediate stabilization on bone and surrounding soft tissue.

6. Deformation or resorption of bone beneath implants from soft tissue and muscle tension should not be clinically significant.

7. Redistribution of soft tissue overlying the face of implant materials should be minimal so that the clinician can determine implant size predictably.

8. The healed tissue implant matrix should have gross physical characteristics approaching bone with supple overlying soft tissue and skin.

9. The material should be osteoconductive or osteophilic to satisfy the clinical requirement of calcified tissue ingrowth and stabilization.

10. The material should have no objectionable color characteristics when used in areas with less than ideal skin coverage.

11. The material should be excised easily if the surgical result is not satisfactory.

12. The material should permit additional augmentation when necessary.

13. The material should be highly biocompatible, exerting no local or distant cytotoxic effects.

Although no single implant material satisfies all the requirements for craniofacial augmentation, several polymers and ceramics satisfy many clinical requirements (see Table, next page).

7. What special techniques should be used when handling alloplastic materials in the operating theater?

Patients undergoing alloplastic biomaterial placement should receive an intravenous antibiotic infusion during placement and an oral course of antibiotics after surgery. Coverage for staphylococcus or streptococcus infection (depending on the path of insertion), 1 gm of a first-generation cephalosporin or 600–900 mg of clindamycin, should be given. No other specific antibiotic amount or duration of administration has been shown to be of superior clinical advantage. Because of the hydrophilic nature of some implants, additional antibiotic coverage can be achieved by washing or soaking the implant before intraoperative insertion. Finally, the implant should be kept in its sterile packing until ready for placement. Clean instruments should be used to handle the implant; handling the implant with the gloved hand should be kept to a minimum. Some authors even advocate donning fresh sterile gloves if the implant is to be handled.

Commonly Used Facial Alloplasts: Clinical Considerations

	SOLID SILICONE RUBBER	PMMA	POROUS PMMA	HA PTFE	EXPANDED PTFE	MESHED POLYMER	POROUS POLY-ETHYLENE	DENSE HA	POROUS HA
Surface porosity	–	–	+	+	–	+	+	–	+
Modules of elasticity	–	–	–	+	–	+	–	–	–
Memory	–	±	±	+	–	+	±	±	±
Adaptability	+	+	+	+	+	+	–	–	–
Color	+	+	+	+	+	+	+	+	+
Ease of removal	+	+	–	–	+	–	–	+	–
Osteophilic	–	–	–	–	–	–	–	+	+
Displacement	–	–	+	+	–	+	+	+	+
Bone resorption	–	–	–	–	±	±	±	+	+
Soft tissue reaction	+	–	–	+	+	–	+	+	+
Degradation	+	+	+	+	+	–	+	+	+

+ = advantages; – = disadvantages; PMMA = polymethylmethacrylate; HA = hydroxyapatite; PTFE = polytetrafluoroethylene

Contact with the surrounding skin, soft tissues, and oral cavity should be kept to a minimum to prevent bacterial inoculation onto the implant's surface. Currently, no studies confirm that this treatment has a significant effect on preventing postoperative infections. However, these precautions will limit contamination and therefore improve implant success and survival.

8. Name the advantages of dimethylsiloxane (silicone) implant materials.

A combination of bulk and preformed silicone rubber implants with or without polymer fabric has been used to augment frontal, zygomatic, nasal, chin, parasymphyseal, paranasal, orbital, maxillary, malar, nasal dorsum, columella, ear, and mandible deficiencies. Their history of clinical acceptance is the longest of all facial implant materials. Despite recent criticism stemming from the breast implant controversy, silicone implants have been used since the 1950s. Preformed silicone is available commercially for many facial applications, and room temperature, vulcanizing silicone may be used to customize implant shapes for specific deformities. Because implant migration and extrusion remain a major problem, other advantages are the ease of intraoperative modification with scalpel or scissors and the stability with screw or suture fixation. The material's "memory" demands adaptation to bone contour in the relaxed state because bending may lead to extrusion or bone resorption. Silicone implants are easily sterilized by steam autoclave or irradiation without damage to the implant composition. In addition, silicone is widely used throughout the medical and surgical community because of the lack of adverse tissue reactivity; only a thin to moderate fibrous tissue capsule forms without ingrowth, and tissue reactions are acceptable if there is adequate soft tissue coverage and bony stabilization. Porous silicone implants and silicone bonded to Dacron with Silastic Medical Grade Adhesive Type A (Wright Dow Corning) have been used to enhance stability. Porous silicone can be used successfully only where functional load and tissue movement will not induce implant tearing and fracture.

9. Discuss the evolution of the use of polytetrafluoroethylene (PTFE).

PTFE was originally marketed as Proplast in the 1980s. The Food and Drug Administration (FDA) withdrew Proplast from the market because of material fragmentation and subsequent foreign body reactions due to mechanical loading as a glenoid fossa replacement in temporomandibular joint (TMJ) reconstruction. It has reappeared as Gore-Tex, an expanded microporous polymer of PTFE that is useful in the subcutaneous augmentation of bony and soft tissue contour defects associated with craniofacial deformities.

Gore-Tex is available in 1-, 2-, and 4-mm sheets that can be trimmed easily and placed subcutaneously by a variety of open and closed techniques. Gore-Tex, as demonstrated in several animal model studies, produces minimal foreign body reaction and elicits a delicate fibrous encapsulation. The microporous nature of this material allows minimal soft tissue ingrowth, which stabilizes the alloplast but allows easy removal if indicated. It was approved by the FDA as an implant material for facial applications in 1994 and has been used for subdermal implantation in the lip, nasolabial folds, glabella, nasal dorsum, and other subcutaneous facial defects. In addition, it has gained in popularity for bony augmentation of the midface, malar, and mandibular areas. The fibrillar composition results in noninterconnected surface openings with pore sizes between 10 and 30 µm. This allows for microvascular ingrowth and minimal fibroconnective tissue encapsulation.

10. Why has the use of polyethylene increased recently?

Polyethylene (Medpor) is a nonresorbable, porous (pore size: 125–250 µm) material that possesses high tensile strength. This biocompatible alloplast can be carved, contoured, and adapted three-dimensionally in the reconstruction of facial deformities. Animal studies demonstrate minimal foreign body response to the thin, fibrous capsule that forms around the polyethylene implant. In addition, this encapsulation is not associated with significant contraction. The porosity of Medpor allows rapid tissue and vascular ingrowth, but it is hard, difficult to sculpt, and not truly osteoconductive (although, some limited bony ingrowth may occur). This material currently is being used in applications such as temporal contour reconstruction and midfacial and mandibular augmentation.

11. What are the disadvantages of polymethylmethacrylate (PMMA) as an implant material?

Acrylic biomaterials are derived from polymerized esters of either acrylic or methylacrylic acids. With a long history of use in orthopaedic surgery as a bone cement for joint prostheses, PMMA resin is fabricated intraoperatively by mixing a liquid monomer with a powdered polymer to create a rigid, nearly translucent plastic. Unfortunately, PMMA has some downsides:

- PMMA has an offensive odor when mixed.
- Its fumes are teratogenic, so female personnel who are pregnant or who are planning to become pregnant must leave the operating theater.
- The exothermic reaction created as the two polymers cure (8–10 minutes) can reach as high as 80°C. Cool irrigation is necessary to prevent adjacent tissue damage secondary to this high curing temperature.
- Bacteria have a high affinity for adherence to the surface of the material. Therefore, it cannot be placed in areas where indigent opportunistic microbes reside, such as the oral cavity or the paranasal sinuses.

12. How can PMMA's disadvantages be bypassed?

1. Preoperative wax-up models can be fabricated and subsequent impressions can be reproduced in stone. From this model, an accurate acrylic implant can be fabricated, gas sterilized, and brought to the operating theater for placement, ensuring accurate fit, decreased operative time, and the absence of tissue damage from the heat of polymerization.

2. Antibiotics can be combined with the acrylic mixture to further reduce the incidence of microbial inoculation and implant failure.

3. Although PMMA is rigid, the adjunctive use of metal mesh reinforcement decreases the risk of fracture on impact and more closely approximates the strength of cranial bone.

13. What are the most common uses of PMMA today?

PMMA is used most often in forehead contouring and cranioplasty procedures for full-thickness skull defects.

14. What is HTR-PMI?

Hard tissue replacement (HTR) is a composite of PMMA and polyhydroxyethyl-methacrylate that has significant strength, interconnected porosity, marked hydrophilicity, and a calcium hydroxide coating that imparts a negative surface charge. Although it has a long clinical history of use in dentistry and jaw implantation as a granular bone replacement material, it is also available as a preformed craniofacial implant that is custom manufactured to the patient's defect from a computed tomography (CT) scan (HTR-PMI; Walter Lorenz Sugical, Jacksonville, FL). It is useful as a replacement for large, full-thickness defects involving the cranial, frontal, and orbital regions where sufficient autologous material may not be available or where there is significant morbidity with the size of the donor defect.

15. What are the major advantages and disadvantages of calcium phosphate ceramic implantable materials?

Hydroxyapatite and related calcium materials interact with and may ultimately become an integral part of living bone tissue. All current calcium phosphate biomaterials can be classified as **polycrystalline** ceramics. Either porous or dense ceramic forms can serve as a permanent bone implant, because they show no tendency to bioresorb. Limitations of calcium phosphate implant materials subtend their mechanical properties. These materials are brittle, with low-impact resistance and relatively low strength. Biocompatibility of calcium phosphate ceramics is excellent, and body response is characteristic whether solid or porous. They appear to become directly bonded to bone by natural bone-cementing mechanisms; bone is deposited without intervening fibrous tissue. A great advantage of these alloplasts is their ability to osteoconduct with actual tissue ingrowth and incorporate into the surrounding tissue.

Unfortunately, these alloplasts offer no osteoinductive potential. Hydroxyapatite granules became available in the early 1980s for maxillofacial reconstruction, particularly alveolar ridge augmentation. Block forms (Interpore, Ceramed) of these alloplasts have been successful as interpositional grafts in facial osteotomies; however, because of their potential for fracture or fragmentation, they should not be used in load-bearing areas. Nonceramic hydroxyapatite is available in powder and liquid forms. Either form may be mixed intraoperatively and used to fill bony defects. Within 10–15 minutes after placement, the substance undergoes direct crystallization to form pure hydroxyapatite. Currently, two forms of calcium carbonate cement are available, Bone Source and CRC. The current thinking is that these cements will develop significant bony ingrowth and the alloplast will eventually need to be replaced. Prospective studies will need to be done to see if this is true.

16. Compare and contrast intraoral versus extraoral access in the placement of alloplastic facial implants.

Adequate native or transplanted covering without excessive tension is necessary to ensure the acceptance of any graft or facial implant. The extraoral approach for facial augmentation offers the advantages of accurate placement and ease of access. The intraoral approach has the advantage of no visible scar but carries a higher rate of infection.

17. What perioperative and intraoperative techniques help ensure consistent success of facial alloplasts?

Implants should lie in healthy tissue away from regions of excessive scarring or areas of irradiation. The implant should be buried as deeply as possible in a supraperiosteal pocket or placed directly on bone if the implant is porous or osteophilic. Preoperatively determined landmarks, measurements, facial moulage, or three-dimensional imaging should be used to ensure accurate placement. Frequent scalpel blade changes are required when carving the implant to feather edges that would otherwise be palpable. A broad, firm contact of the implant with underlying closures is preferred, particularly with intraoral techniques. Compression of implant pores should be avoided. Appropriate antibiotic protocol should be followed before and after surgery, and a porous implant should be soaked in antibiotic or vacuum impregnated upon implantation. The implant should be sutured, wired, or screwed into position firmly and further supported with a compressive dressing to minimize dead space and hematoma formation.

18. What information should patients understand about alloplastic augmentation materials and surgery in order to give true informed consent?

The success of implants is dependent on physical characteristics, biologic response, proper preparation and handling, clinical experience, surgical technique, and postoperative patient management. Patient compliance, ensured through proper selection and thorough explanation, is extremely important. Potential complications include:

Infection
Untoward reaction to medication, anesthesia, or surgical procedures
Poor wound healing
Hematoma
Seroma
Motor or sensory nerve damage or irritation
Neuralgia
Loss of sensation
Intolerance to any foreign implant
Unremitting previously established symptoms
Changes in surrounding tissue
Implant migration
Extrusion or structural failure
Additional surgical intervention

19. Which intraoral or extraoral approaches should be used for the placement of alloplastic materials in the mandibular symphysis, ramus, or inferior border?

These deficiencies are either vertical or lateral and may be corrected by either an intraoral or extraoral approach. Preformed and carved alloplasts can be constructed to exact specification using facial three-dimensional CT or moulage. Autogenous bone or hydroxyapatite grafts can be fashioned to correct these contour defects as well. The **intraoral approach** requires a standard genioplasty incision and dissection of the mandibular symphysis; a vertical vestibular incision similar to that used for ramus osteotomy through periosteum and a subperiosteal dissection is completed along the lateral surface of the angle and ascending ramus. Curved elevators facilitate release of the soft tissue attachments along the inferior border and posterior ramus. An appropriately contoured ramus angle implant is inserted into the subperiosteal pocket, and bone screws are used to secure the implant to the lateral cortex of the mandible.

The **extraoral technique** for angle and inferior border augmentation involves the standard submandibular approach. A modified Risdon incision is made, preferably in an existing rhytid through subcutaneous fat down to the platysma muscle. The platysma is then divided segmentally with blunt hemostats. A nerve tester set at 2 mA is used to test selectively for the cervical and marginal mandibular branches of the facial nerve as they dip below the inferior border of the mandible. Once divided, the platysma is retracted superiorly and inferiorly in the surgical field, exposing the superficial layer of the deep cervical fascia. Great care must be taken because the facial nerve lies in this layer. Once encountered, the nerve is selectively freed and retracted superiorly. In addition, anteriorly, the facial artery and vein are usually encountered near the submandibular lymph node. These vessels must be ligated if they become an obstacle in the proper placement of the implant. Should they become breached during the surgical procedure, the likelihood of a postoperative hematoma is extremely great and will adversely affect the successful integration of the implant without infection or need for repeat surgery. After the nerve and vessels have been addressed, careful dissection of a pocket along the posterolateral border of the mandibular angle under the pterygomasseteric sling is done and atraumatic placement of the implant and subsequent fixation can be done with ease. The site is irrigated with copious amounts of antibiotic-impregnated saline, and a careful layered closure is achieved with resorbable suture. Placement of a Jobst jaw bra with 4" × 4" dressings over the mandibular angles for 48 hours achieves good postoperative stability and minimizes swelling. Most patients tolerate this postoperative regimen extremely well because they can resume their normal activities within 1–2 days.

20. How are asymmetric mandibular excesses corrected?

Vertical inferior border excesses and outward bowing of the mandible in patients with condylar hyperplasia may require reduction by either an inferior border resection or a horizontal wedge osteotomy procedure, usually through an intraoral vestibular approach. Inferior border leveling by this technique also provides autogenous bone, which may be required for augmentation of the contralateral angle ramus or inferior border. A horizontal wedge osteotomy procedure relocates the inferior border and its soft tissue attachments superiorly but requires difficult repositioning of the inferior alveolar nerve.

21. What implant considerations must be made prior to augmentation of the chin in a vertical versus horizontal dimension?

The versatility of the sliding horizontal osteotomy of the mandibular symphysis is well documented and is used to correct asymmetries of the chin by reducing or increasing the vertical height of the chin or its anterior and posterior projection. Hydroxyapatite blocks and autogenous grafts are most suitable for lengthening; whereas, silicone rubber and other polymer implants have been used successfully in the correction of parasymphyseal contour deficiencies (either lateral or anterior), occasionally in conjunction with a horizontal osteotomy.

22. Which access is best for augmentation of the mandibular symphysis? What methods of fixation of osteotomies or implants are indicated?

The osteotomy or alloplast implant placement is accomplished most easily by an intraoral approach through a mucosal incision anterior to the depth of the mucobuccal fold through the underlying mentalis muscle. The symphysis and inferior border soft tissue are degloved for placement of the implant in order to advance soft tissue; the soft tissue remains attached to the symphysis when a horizontal osteotomy is performed. Implants are stabilized with screws or sutures, and the osteotomized symphysis is stabilized with screws or bone plates.

23. Compare and contrast the use of zygomatic complex osteotomies versus the placement of zygomatic implants to correct malar deficiencies.

Residual depression or flattening of the malar eminence is noted before or, more clearly, after conventional osteotomies to correct the maxillary and mandibular deformities. Occasionally, the correction of malar deficiency is significant enough to warrant zygomatic complex osteotomies. The use of autogenous tissues for onlay grafting sometimes is unpredictable secondary to variable resorption. Alloplasts are used to correct these problems.

24. What implant materials could be considered for placement of malar implants?

Particulate hydroxyapatite may be used, but preventing migration of hydroxyapatite from the desired augmentation site during placement is a technically demanding procedure. Block forms of hydroxyapatite have been used successfully for infraorbital augmentation; however, their brittle nature makes lateral malar augmentation difficult. The use of polyethylene (Medpor) makes augmentation of this aspect of the facial skeleton much more simple and predictable.

25. What surgical approach is indicated for the placement of malar implants? How are they stabilized?

For the intraoral approach to zygomatic augmentation:

1. A standard horizontal vestibular incision is made above the maxillary canine and premolar teeth through the small facial muscles overlying the anterior maxilla and zygomatic bone.

2. A subperiosteal dissection extending from the medial infraorbital rim across the body of the zygoma is completed.

3. The infraorbital nerve is identified and isolated, thus preventing inadvertent injury.

4. The implant is carved to fit into the preformed soft tissue pocket, over the zygomatic arch, and stabilized with screws, sutures, or wires.

26. Describe the use of alloplastic materials in the correction of saddle nose deformities in the nasal dorsum.

In a saddle nose deformity, the nasal dorsum lacks adequate ventral projection. The condition is occasionally congenital but more often results from trauma, infection, or excessive resection of the septum. The saddle formation may affect the bone or the cartilaginous nasal dorsum in isolation or include both structures. The guideline for correction includes the outer deformity in addition to a thorough analysis of the function of the internal nasal airway. The collapse of the nasal dorsum is always associated with impairment of nasal airflow, which becomes greater as the saddle formation extends further caudally. Alloplastic implants are readily available, preformed, and easy to use for these purposes. They do not deform and are negligibly resorbable. Conversely, there remains the lifelong risk of extrusion or infection because of their anatomic location.

27. Discuss the role of alloplastic implants in the correction of craniofacial defects.

Alloplasts have done very well in recent years in improving the long-term results of craniofacial defect reconstruction. These defects usually are approached through a coronal incision, exposing the defect in a subperiosteal plane. The temporal branches of the facial nerve are avoided through careful dissection lateral and superior to the supraorbital ridges beneath the deep layer of the superficial temporal fascia. Once the defect is exposed, the underlying dura is thoroughly neurosurgically evaluated with repair, if necessary, using pericranium or lyophilized dura. Various alloplastic augmentation materials may be used including PMMA and the newer calcium carbonate cements. Once fixed or set, the contours of these materials may be adjusted with burrs to achieve an acceptable aesthetic result. Reinforcement with titanium mesh to achieve optimum postoperative strength and stability can be done easily and offers extra protection and comfort to the patient.

BIBLIOGRAPHY

1. Artz JS, Dinner MI: The use of expanded polytetrafluoroethylene as a permanent filler and enhancer: An early report of experience. Ann Plast Surg 32:457–462, 1994.
2. Bessette RW, Casey DM, Shatkin SS, Schaaf NG: Customized silicone rubber maxillofacial implants. Ann Plast Surg 7:453–457, 1981.
3. Chisholm BB, Lew D, Sadasivan K: The use of tobramycin-impregnated polymethylmethacrylate beads in the treatment of osteomyelitis of the mandible: Report of three cases. J Oral Maxillofac Surg 51:444–449, 1993.
4. Eppley BL: Alloplastic implantation. Plast Reconstr Surg 104:1761–1783, 1999.
5. Eppley BL, Prevel CD, Sadove AM: Resorbable bone fixation: Its potential role in craniomaxillofacial trauma. J Craniomaxillofac Trauma 2:56–61, 1996.
6. Kent JN, Craig MA: Secondary autogenous and alloplastic reshaping procedures. Atlas Oral Maxillofac Surg Clin North Am 4:83–105, 1996.
7. Kent JN, Misiek DJ: Biomaterials for cranial, facial, mandibular and temporomandibular joint reconstruction. In Fonseca R, Walker R (eds): Oral and Maxillofacial Trauma. Vol. 2. Philadelphia, W.B. Saunders, 1991, pp 781–1026.
8. Kent JN, Misiek DJ, Kinnebrew MC: Alloplastic materials for augmentation in cosmetic surgery. In Peterson L (ed): Principles of Maxillofacial Surgery. Vol. 3. Philadelphia, J.B. Lippincott, 1992, pp 1769–1813.
9. Lacey M, Antonyshyn O: Use of porous high-density polyethylene implants in temporal contour reconstruction. J Craniofac Surg 4:74–78, 1993.
10. Lin PH, Hirko MK, von Fraunhofer JA, Greisler HP: Wound healing and inflammatory response to biomaterials. In Chu CC, von Fraunhofer JA, Greisler HP (eds): Wound Closure Biomaterials and Devices. New York, CRC Press, 1997, pp 7–24.

11. Maas CS, Gnepp DR: Expanded polytetrafluoroethylene (Gore-Tex soft tissue patch) in facial augmentation. Arch Otolaryngol Head Neck Surg 119:1008–1017, 1993.
12. Park JB, Lakes RS: Polymeric implant materials. In Park JB, Lakes RS (eds): Biomaterials: An Introduction. New York, Plenum, 1992, pp 141–167.
13. Ripamonti U, Petit JC, Moehl T, et al: Immediate reconstruction of massive cranio-orbito-facial defects with allogeneic and alloplastic matrices in baboons. J Craniomaxillofac Surg 21:302–308, 1993.
14. Rubin JP, Yaremchuk MJ: Complications and toxicities of implantable biomaterials used in facial reconstructive and aesthetic surgery: A comprehensive review of the literature. Plast Reconstr Surg 100:1336–1356, 1997.
15. Schoenrock LD, Reppucci AD: Correction of subcutaneous facial defects using Gore-Tex. Facial Plast Surg Clin North Am 2:373–389, 1994.
16. Silver FH, Maas CS: Biology of facial implant materials. Facial Plast Surg Clin North Am 2:241–254, 1994.
17. Szabo G, Suba Z, Barabas J: Use of Bioplant HTR synthetic bone to eliminate major jawbone defects: Long-term human histologic examinations. J Craniomaxillofac Surg 25:63–68, 1997.
18. Yukna RA: Clinical evaluation of HTR polymer bone replacement grafts in human mandibular class II molar furcations. J Periodontol 65:342–349, 1994.

INDEX

Page numbers in **boldface type** indicate complete chapters.

Mucoepidermoid carcinoma, 260
Mucormycosis, 228
Mucosa, oral, effect of radiation on, 276
Mucosal skin grafts, 295
Mucositis, radiation-related, 276, 278
Mucus escape, as lesion cause, 260
Mueller technique, modified, 316
Multiple endocrine neoplasia syndromes (MENS), 141
Muscle cramps, hypocalcemia-related, 62
Muscle relaxants, use in liver disease patients, 131
Muscles
    of mastication
        embryologic development of, 249
        origin and insertion points of, 167
        effect of radiation on, 276
    orofacial, involvement in cleft lip and palate, 250
Mustardé technique, of otoplasty, 302
Mycobacterium avium complex infection, in AIDS patients, 157
Mylohyoid muscles, in suprahyoid myotomy, 248
Myocardial infarction, 101–104
    acute, diagnostic laboratory tests for, 24–25
    conditions which mimic, 84–85
    ECG signs of, 12
    perioperative, 71, 102, 103–104
        in congestive heart failure patients, 117
        prior, as perioperative myocardial infarction risk factor, 103–104
Myocardial injury, ECG signs of, 12
Myocardial ischemia, 101–104
    as chest pain cause, 76
    ECG signs of, 12
    silent, 102
Myocardium, oxygen supply and demand of, 101
    during myocardial infarction, 102
Myofascial pain, temporomandibular disorders–related, 238
Myoglobinuria, malignant hyperthermia–related, 97
Myotomy, suprahyoid, 248
Myotonia, malignant hyperthermia associated with, 96
Myxoma, odontogenic, osseous resection margin of, 263

Naloxone, 51
    administration via endotracheal tube, 85
Narcotics, adverse effects of, 70, 316
Nasal bones, 168
    fractures of, 203
    traumatic injury to, radiographic evaluation of, 31
Nasal cavity, anatomic relationship with nasolacrimal duct, 171
Nasalis muscle, paralysis of, 182–183
Nasal process, medial, merger with intermaxillary segment, 249
Nasal septa, hematoma of, 199, 202
Nasal skin grafts, 293

Nasoduodenal intubation, for enteral nutrition administration, 76, 77
Nasogastric intubation
    contraindication in midfacial fractures, 201
    for enteral nutrition administration, 76, 77
Nasojejunal intubation, for enteral nutrition administration, 76
Nasolabial angle, 247
Nasolacrimal duct, anatomic relationships of, 171
Nasopharyngeal carcinoma, 228
Nausea, postoperative, 70
Neck
    anatomic zones of, 204
    dissection of, 269
    lymph node metastases of, 260, 263, 279
    necrotizing fasciitis of, 225–226
    parotidomasteric fascia extension in, 178
    penetrating trauma to, 204
    radiographic evaluation of, 31
    soft-tissue infections of, diagnostic imaging of, 34
    superficial musculoaponeurotic system extension in, 178
Necrosis
    coagulation, 272
    of pulp, 188
    tubular, 134, 140
Nephropathy, diabetic, 134, 148
Nephrotic syndrome, antithrombin III in, 18
Nerve grafts, 194, 195
Nerve impulse transmission, effect of local anesthetics on, 39–40
Nerve injury
    anterior ilium bone graft harvesting-related, 290
    closed, 194
    delayed repair of, 194, 195
    open, 194
    posterior iliac crest bone grafting–related, 289
    repair of, 194
Neurapraxia, 191
Neurologic disorders, hypertension-related, 115
Neuromuscular blockade agents, as malignant hyperthermia trigger, 96
Neurons, nociceptive, 240
Neuropathy, diabetic, 148
Neurosensory deficits, ilium bone graft harvest-related, 290
Neurotmesis, 191
Nitrite, urine content of, 22
Nitroglycerin, perioperative administration of, 104
Nitrous oxide
    use in chronic obstructive pulmonary disease patients, 54
    contraindication in conditions involving closed gas spaces, 53
    as diffusion hypoxia cause, 57
    minimal alveolar concentration of, 55
    partition coefficient of, 57
Nitrous oxide cylinders, 53